RHEUMATISM AND MUSCULOSKELETAL DISORDERS

PERIOPERATIVE PRACTICE IN TRAUMA AND ORTHOPAEDIC SURGERY

RHEUMATISM AND MUSCULOSKELETAL DISORDERS

Additional books in this series can be found on Nova's website under the Series tab.

Additional e-books in this series can be found on Nova's website under the e-book tab.

RHEUMATISM AND MUSCULOSKELETAL DISORDERS

PERIOPERATIVE PRACTICE IN TRAUMA AND ORTHOPAEDIC SURGERY

WASIM S. KHAN
EDITOR

NOVA BIOMEDICAL

New York

Library of Congress Cataloging-in-Publication Data

ISBN: 978-1-63483-325-7
Library of Congress Control Number: 2015944481

Published by Nova Science Publishers, Inc. † New York

CONTENTS

PREFACE

There has been a shift in the delivery of trauma and orthopaedic services from the specialised to the sub-specialised, while being coupled with a greater multidisciplinary involvement. There are many healthcare professionals involved in the care of trauma and orthopaedic patients, ranging from surgeons, other medical specialities, ward and nursing staff, as well as podiatrists, orthotists, physiotherapists, occupational therapists and social workers. As a result, there is no other up-to-date book available that adequately covers the generality of trauma and orthopaedics, and at the same time appreciates the multidisciplinary approach. This book provides a platform allowing all disciplines to learn about the multifaceted care of these patients with an aim to enhance understanding, promote collaboration and allow the optimisation of care for trauma and orthopaedic patients. The book is aimed at doctors, nursing staff, physiotherapists, occupational therapists and all other staff involved in the care of trauma and orthopaedic patients.

Chapter 1 – Joseph Lister is often seen as a hero of surgery, but his famous method of antisepsis was not solely his work. The commonly told account of the development of antisepsis displays several characteristics of whig history. This investigation will highlight these whiggish features, showing that Lister's original antiseptic technique was not without its failures and that there were other important figures who contributed to its development.

Chapter 2 – Methicillin Resistant *Staphylococcus aureus* (MRSA) is defined as any strain of *Staphylococcus aureus* resistant to beta-lactam antibiotics including the penicillin's and cephalosporins. Over the past ten years the UK has seen a dramatic increase in MRSA prevalence in healthcare facilities and the community with an estimated 30-50% of healthy adults thought to be colonised with MRSA. Surgical patients are among those at highest risk. With potential sequelae including septicaemia, septic shock, septic arthritis, osteomyelitis, meningitis, pneumonia or endocarditis, it is vital that all care facilities have up to date evidence-based guidelines to tackle this problem. The purpose of this chapter is to highlight the current evidence supporting some of the key perioperative measures which may be implemented in preventing MRSA.

Chapter 3 – With the ever increasing number of diabetic patients undergoing surgical procedures, the effective perioperative management of diabetes mellitus has become progressively more important. This article will discuss a number of approaches to improving the perioperative management of patient with this condition, and explore the fine balance of blood glucose management that should prevent hypo and hyperglycaemia. Also discussed will be the complications of diabetes mellitus, particularly where these directly compromise patient health and interventional outcomes.

Chapter 4 – Cardiac pathologies are common and need to be managed well in the perioperative period to reduce complications. In this chapter the authors discuss the management of common cardiac pathologies including coronary artery disease, hypertension, arrhythmias and cardiac failure. The authors also discuss the management of anticoagulation.

Chapter 5 – Respiratory disease contributes significantly to the perioperative challenges of surgery. Pre-existing pulmonary comorbidities and respiratory complications can have profound effects on patient outcomes. Knowledge of these conditions and the potentially deleterious effects of anaesthesia and surgery can enable clinicians to optimize lung function, reduce complications and improve results.

Chapter 6 – With the increasing use of oral anticoagulation therapy the appropriate management of perioperative anticoagulation is of surgical importance. There is a delicate balance between the risk of a perioperative thromboembolic event and the risk of operative bleeding from anticoagulation. Whilst there are a range of options available to the clinician, there appears to be no precise agreement as to how to best manage this problem.

Chapter 7 – Children are not just 'small adults.' They have specific physical, psychological and social requirements that must be identified and addressed to optimise their well-being in the perioperative period. The health care practitioner should be trained to understand the needs of the paediatric patient in hospital, such as the potential triggers for anxiety and distress, in addition to the ever-increasing need to take into account cultural differences.

Hospital policy should include a preoperative preparation programme, specially aimed at the paediatric population, where parental involvement is encouraged throughout, with a structured care plan continuing into the post-operative period. Factors involved the success of these preoperative programmes include their early commencement, orientation tours and role-play over potentially distressing points of care, along with appropriate resources to inform the child and parents. While day-case surgery is associated with improved outcomes and decreased anxiety, care must be taken to ensure parents are adequately placed to manage their children's needs after discharge.

Chapter 8 – Diathermy has revolutionised modern surgery and is an important tool for efficient and safe surgical practice. It has evolved to become the modern day scalpel, cutting and coagulating tissues. This article aims to elicit the functioning and safe usage of diathermy in the perioperative setting. The various precautionary checks before surgery, which are prerequisite for safe usage, are highlighted along with the necessary safety drills taken during and after operation. A specific note is included about the usage of electrical equipment when used in specialised surgeries like cardiac and laparoscopic surgery. A quick insight to issues regarding the maintenance and repair and finally, the anticipation for a future with precise and safer cutting and coagulation devices is addressed.

Chapter 9 – Patient positioning in theatre pertains to how a patient is transferred and positioned for a specific procedure. Patient safety is a central focus of care within the NHS and every healthcare practitioner must ensure that patients are protected from harm where possible. Mal-positioning of the patient has important implications in terms of associated problems of pressure sores, nerve compressions, deep vein thromboses and compartment syndrome, and should be avoided.

Chapter 10 – Ionising radiation is used extensively in trauma and orthopaedic perioperative practice for operative planning and intraoperative decision making. Radiation poses risks to patients and theatre staff, and it is important to always justify, optimise and limit the exposure. This is facilitated by a thorough understanding and awareness of radiation, as well as a sound knowledge of the precautions required for using this technology to minimise the risks of radiation.

Chapter 11 – Plain cervical spine radiographs are the first line investigation in trauma patients to exclude cervical spine fractures and dislocations. Adequate views are essential to reduce the risk of missing diagnoses. Injuries may however not be visible on plain cervical spine radiographs despite adequate views. Additional imaging such as computer tomography scanning is indicated in the event of a normal plain radiograph if there is any clinical suspicion of injury.

Chapter 12 – The chest radiograph is used as a screening test to exclude significant thoracic injuries in cases of major trauma. A systematic approach to reviewing chest radiographs is necessary for accurate interpretation. Radiographic findings should be considered in conjunction with clinical assessment.

Chapter 13 – Pelvic fractures are often high energy injuries and are associated with a high morbidity and mortality. The plain antero-posterior pelvis radiograph is part of the Advanced Trauma Life Support radiographic trauma series and is used as a screening test. As the main limitation of plain antero-posterior pelvic radiographs is the difficulty in identification of some fractures, in particular posterior fractures, radiographic findings should be considered in conjunction with clinical assessment.

Chapter 14 – Bone cement has been increasingly used in orthopaedic surgery over the last 50 years. Since Sir John Charnley pioneered the use of polymethylmethacrylate cement in total hip replacements, there have been developments in cementing techniques and an expansion in the number of orthopaedic procedures that use cement. This chapter covers the perioperative issues surrounding bone cement including storage, cementing techniques and complications. It also discusses specific orthopaedic applications of bone cement and future developments.

Chapter 15 – Fractures are common injuries, and their management has evolved over the last 30 years with a greater propensity to treat fractures surgically. There have also been accompanying advances with a better understanding of the principles of bone healing and their implications on implant choice. The purpose of this chapter is to highlight the various surgical fixation devices available for the management of fractures and their underlying principles.

Chapter 16 – The wrist and hand are important in helping perform activities of daily living. Fractures of the wrist and hand are common injuries and, if inappropriately managed, can result in significant functional deficit. In this chapter some common fractures are discussed including Colles' fractures, Smith's fractures, Bennett's and Rolondo's fractures, scaphoid fractures, peri-lunate fracture dislocations, metacarpal fractures and phalangeal fractures.

Chapter 17 – The ankle and foot are functionally important and complex joints. Bony fractures and ligamentous injuries are common. In this chapter the authors will discuss the functional anatomy, imaging, classification and the management of common ankle and foot injuries including ankle fractures, achilles tendon ruptures, Lisfranc joint injuries, calcaneo fractures and fractures of the metatarsals and phalanges.

Chapter 18 – Acute compartment syndrome is a life and limb threatening condition.

Clinical assessment is the diagnostic cornerstone of compartment syndrome but pressure monitoring also has a role in equivocal cases, in unconscious or uncooperative patients, and patients with nerve blocks and other forms of regional and epidural anesthesia. A high degree of suspicion and early decompression of all compartments at risk are important for a satisfactory outcome.

Chapter 19 – Fractured necks of femur are becoming increasingly common with an ageing population. These fractures could be divided into intra-capsular and extra-capsular fractures. The management of these fractures varies significantly depending on the patient and fracture configuration including location and displacement. In this chapter the authors discuss the surgical management of these fractures.

Chapter 20 – Hip fracture is a major cause of morbidity, mortality and loss of independence for the elderly. Surgical fixation of the fractured hip remains the standard of care to allow for early mobilisation and a return to independence. Operative management in this population carries its own set of problems. The altered physiological state of the older person, often coupled with significant co-morbidity, can present challenges for the anaesthetist, the surgeon and the rest of the perioperative team. This chapter provides an evidence-based review of these important perioperative factors associated with hip fractures in the older person and their management.

Chapter 21 – Bone metastasis is a common problem affecting a significant proportion of patients with metastatic cancer. Bone metastasis can present in a number of ways and the patients may need surgical stabilisation of their lesions. There are many important considerations in the care of these patients that need to be borne in mind including their increased anesthetic risks and potential risk of complications. There are continuous developments in the prevention, diagnosis and treatment with advances in imaging, orthopaedic technique and medication, particularly radiopharmaceuticals and cytotoxic, endocrine treatments with newer treatments based around the tumour cell-osteoclast interaction. Having a better understanding of these considerations and developments is important in allowing the optimisation of the care of the patient with bone metastasis.

Chapter 22 – Knee arthroscopy is a minimally-invasive technique that allows intra-articular assessment and treatment of knee joint pathology. It has proven benefits of reduced patient morbidity, earlier recovery and mobilisation, and it is cost-effective. In this chapter the authors review the anatomy of the knee joint, indications and contra-indications to knee arthroscopic use, and consider the main techniques of knee arthroscopy including types of anaesthetic, prophylactic antibiotics, theatre setup and arthroscopic portals, and post-operative care.

Chapter 23 – Ever since Themistocles Gluck described the use of an ivory cup as a tibial hemiarthroplasty in 1894, knee arthoplasty has continued to evolve. Both human ingenuity and intensive clinical research has led to an improved understanding of biomaterials and knee kinematics, resulting in the modern total knee replacement which has enjoyed such a clinical and commercial success. As it increases in popularity, attempts to improve knee arthroplasty have been driven by demands for improved function and implant survival, particularly in younger, more demanding patients. Research continues to see if advances in implant instrumentation, materials and design will translate into improved clinical outcomes and longevity.

Chapter 24 – Since the introduction of modern implants in the 1970's, Total Knee Replacement surgery has been a great clinical and commercial success. Implants and techniques have continued to evolve, driven by the desire for improved function and longevity. However, inaccurate insertion of these implants may cause them to loosen and fail. Computer navigation has been introduced as a modification to existing surgical techniques to improve the accuracy with which the bones are cut prior to inserting the knee replacement implants. Research continues to see if this potentially costly and time consuming technique can contribute to improved longevity of knee replacements.

Chapter 25 – Total hip replacement is a commonly performed procedure with good results. The implants could be cemented or cementless, and there has been a resurgence of resurfacing procedures. It is important that special consideration is given to the choice of the material used at the bearing surfaces. There have been many developments in recent years that influence the authors' choice of implant and have shaped their practice including minimal invasive surgery and computer-assisted surgery. This chapter aims to provide an overview of these developments.

Chapter 26 – Non-steroidal anti-inflammatory drugs are powerful and effective anti-inflammatory, analgesic and anti-pyretic drugs. They are routinely used in orthopaedic conditions and in the perioperative setting. They are however associated with potentially life-threatening side-effects and it is important to appreciate these before these drugs are given. There is evidence suggesting that these drugs adversely affect bone formation, and this has implications on their use in patients with fractures and other pathologics that involve bone remodelling.

Chapter 27 – There has been an increasing interest in stem cell applications and tissue engineering approaches in surgical practice to deal with damaged or lost tissue. Although there have been developments in almost all surgical disciplines, the greatest advances are being made in orthopaedics, especially in bone repair. Significant hurdles however remain to be overcome before tissue engineering becomes more routinely used in surgical practice.

In: Perioperative Practice in Trauma and Orthopaedic Surgery ISBN: 978-1-63483-325-7
Editor: Wasim S. Khan

Chapter 1

THE HISTORY OF ANTISEPSIS

Alexander Smart and Wasim Khan*
[1]University College London Medical School, Gower Street, London, UK
[2]University College London Institute of Orthopaedic and Musculoskeletal Sciences, Royal National Orthopaedic Hospital, Stanmore, Middlesex, UK

ABSTRACT

Joseph Lister is often seen as a hero of surgery, but his famous method of antisepsis was not solely his work. The commonly told account of the development of antisepsis displays several characteristics of whig history. This investigation will highlight these whiggish features, showing that Lister's original antiseptic technique was not without its failures and that there were other important figures who contributed to its development.

Keywords: Lister, antisepsis, whig history, surgery

INTRODUCTION

In this chapter we discuss the history of antisepsis and the role of Lister (Smart and Khan 2012). Although Joseph Lister had a huge impact in the field of surgery with his method of antisepsis, the commonly told account of its development, where Lister is portrayed as the only important character in the story as he virtually 'single-handedly revolutionised modern surgery' (Granshaw 1992), may be an example of whig history. In this essay, the commonly told story of antisepsis will be analysed in order to identify whether it possesses any of the characteristics of whig history.

The term 'whig history' was first coined by Herbert Butterfield in his book *'The Whig Interpretation of History'* in 1931.

* Corresponding author: Mr W. Khan, Clinical Lecturer, University College London Institute of Orthopaedic and Musculoskeletal Research, Royal National Orthopaedic Hospital, Stanmore, Middlesex, HA7 4LP, UK. Telephone number: +44 (0) 7791 025554, fax number: +44 (0) 1707 655059, e-mail: wasimkhan@doctors.org.uk.

He defines it as "the tendency in many historians to write on the side of Protestants and Whigs, to praise revolutions provided they have been successful, to emphasise certain principles of progress in the past and to produce a story which is the ratification if not the glorification of the present" (Butterfield 1931). This definition provides several characteristics of whig history which will be useful in identifying the extent to which the common story of antisepsis is whiggish. The first of these characteristics is the emphasis of certain principles of progress. This often leads to the omission of certain events in the story, tailoring the story to meet the intentions of the historian. It allows the historian to create an easy path from the past to the present (Butterfield 1931), showing only the elements of progress and omitting any complexities in the story, making this type of history usually very inaccurate. The second trait of whig history which will be looked for is whether there seems to be a ratification or glorification of the present. As Butterfield says, "it is part and parcel of the whig interpretation of history that it studies the past with reference to the present" (Butterfield 1931). Instead of attempting to view the past through the eyes of those who were living then, the whig historian tries to find similarities between the past and present. He is then able to construct a story depicting continuous progress over time to "produce a scheme of general history which is bound to converge beautifully upon the present" (Butterfield 1931). Finally, this interpretation of history produces a division between the people involved in the story into those on the side of progress, and those who tried to hinder progress (Butterfield 1931), which can result in the creation of heroes and villains within history. The creation of a hero figure who is striving for progress distorts the truth by introducing bias on the side of the hero, and ignoring the role that others played in history.

Such a division, with Lister portrayed as the hero, will therefore be searched for within the commonly told story.

Next, the commonly told history of the development of antisepsis must also be described, so that it can be established whether it possesses any characteristics of whig history. Lister's biographies, such as those written by Richard B. Fisher and Douglas Guthrie, books on the history of surgery, and surgical lectures all tell the history of antisepsis in a similar fashion. They portray Lister as the sole hero of a surgical 'revolution', fighting against adversity to make his ideas and theories heard. They detail how Lister first came up with the idea of antisepsis, through the use of the then novel germ theory, proposed by Louis Pasteur, and consequently made surgery 'scientific' (Worboys 2000). The story then identifies how Lister made antisepsis applicable to surgery, with the application of carbolic acid to wounds, initially as a dressing in 1867 (Guthrie 1949) and then by spraying it onto the wound in 1871 (Fisher 1977). It continues with details of how the effect of Lister's new techniques were opposed by those who claimed that the lower mortality rates following surgery were as a result of improved cleanliness in hospitals, but then tell of how Lister finally won over his opponents. The main focus of the commonly told story of antisepsis appears very much to be Joseph Lister, although this may be expected in Lister's biographies. However it seems that the story neglects many of the other individuals involved and the compromises made by Lister, concentrating mainly on the scientific progress which was being made. Having now described the commonly told story of how antisepsis was introduced into surgery, it seems that there are definitely some aspects of this story which could be considered whiggish.

The first aspect which can be considered to be whiggish is the portrayal of Lister as the only character to play a key role in the incorporation of antisepsis into surgical procedures. The commonly told story of antisepsis disregards the work of several important individuals, without whom it may have been impossible for Lister to make his breakthroughs. One such individual is George Callender, a surgeon at St. Bartholemew's Hospital, who claimed that he used an "alternative, superior method" (Granshaw 1992) to antisepsis, which was termed 'cleanliness.' He advocated 'scrupulous cleanliness' (Granshaw 1992) to the wounds, as well as the patients and their surroundings, to ensure they were dirt-free, as opposed to the purely chemical actions of antiseptics, which had the aim of removing and preventing germs from the wound. His method of cleanliness had more success than Lister's in its application to surgery, largely due to its lower post-operative mortality rates (Granshaw 1992).

Lister consequently amended his method of antisepsis, incorporating practices from the method of cleanliness, such as placing surgical instruments in carbolic lotion to clean them thoroughly (Granshaw 1992). This was the start of a compromise between antisepsis and cleanliness, which eventually led to the recognition of much of Lister's work, yet rendered Callender's work largely forgotten. Although Joseph Lister produced some brilliant work, the commonly told story 'whiggishly' elevates him to the heights of a hero whilst forgetting the work of others, such as George Callender, Ignaz Semmelweis, who worked on the first antiseptics during the 1840s (*Blood and Guts: A History of Surgery* 2008), and Thomas Spencer Wells, who in 1864 was one of the first to comment on the possibility that germs may be the cause of sepsis (Worboys 2000).

The next whiggish characteristic to be looked for is the depiction of continuous progress from the past to the present, by highlighting certain events of progress whilst neglecting to mention the events that prevented progression. This trait of whig history is found, to a certain extent, within the commonly told story of antisepsis. The commonly told story does mention some of the hindrances to progress which Lister faced, such as the reluctance of many surgeons to accept the theory behind Lister's method of antisepsis.

However, it does so in a way that depicts Lister as the proponent of progress, which reinforces Lister as the hero of the story. Furthermore the road to the acceptance of antisepsis was a very long one, and the actual rate of progress made was much slower than commonly portrayed. The story also doesn't expose the range of compromises which Lister made in order to gain support for his method of antisepsis. He incorporated several practices from the method of cleanliness, and it has been said that the practise which resulted from this compromise, known today as asepsis, seems to have more in common with the method of cleanliness than antisepsis (Granshaw 1992). Although the omission of such obstacles to progress may make for a better story, this whiggish interpretation of the history of antisepsis creates a false impression of continuous scientific progress with the hero trying to convert others to his 'revolutionary' way of thinking.

The way in which the history of antisepsis is written also favours those who helped progress over those who were seen to prevent it. This division between the 'good guys' and the 'bad guys' in the development of antiseptic surgery is historically inaccurate, and is a characteristic of whig history. During the 1860s and 1870s, when Lister was attempting to implement antisepsis into surgery, there were those who supported his method and those who opposed it.

At the time, both of these groups believed that their opinions and actions were helping to progress science. It is only with hindsight, and the knowledge that the theory behind Lister's work was correct, that historians tend to side with the proponents of antisepsis. It is important, therefore, for a historian to attempt to see the past through the eyes of those who were living then, rather than to allow the present to cloud their judgement and introduce bias.

A further example of this in the commonly told story is the way in which the opponents of antisepsis are made to seem ignorant in their refusal of antisepsis, as they did not believe in germ theory (Granshaw 1992).

There is no consideration to the fact that, at that point in time, germ theory was a very new idea and was completely alien to how most scientists thought. This interpretation of the past with direct reference to the present is therefore another characteristic that makes the commonly told account of antisepsis' development more whiggish.

From this analysis of the commonly told story of antisepsis, it is evident that there are definitely elements of the story which are whiggish. However, despite this inaccurate representation of the development of antisepsis, it can be argued that this whiggish interpretation does have an important benefit. The creation of Lister as a scientific hero provides inspiration to current and future scientists. A completely accurate history of antisepsis would probably not have the same effect, as it would have shown that the progress made by Lister was not as spectacular because of the considerable concessions he made regarding his method of antisepsis. Furthermore the glory resulting from the success of antisepsis would have been shared among several individuals, and perhaps Lister would not have been seen as the scientific hero who revolutionised surgery. Therefore it becomes apparent that the role of the historian is not only to portray the past accurately, but also to create hero figures who can serve to inspire further progress.

Conclusion

In conclusion, it has been shown that the commonly told story of the development of antisepsis displays whiggish characteristics. This makes the story fairly inaccurate, mainly because it omits events which prevented scientific progress. Although whig history creates a readable and, at times, inspirational story, history should help serve as a template for the future, so that previous mistakes can be learned from and so that further progress can be made. Therefore, it is of greatest importance that history is documented accurately, even if it is at the expense of creating as many heroical figures.

Nevertheless, even if the commonly told story of antisepsis was not told whiggishly, Lister would most probably still be considered a scientific hero. The practice of asepsis, a combination of antisepsis and cleanliness, would not have been possible without the constant work and dedication of Lister. Not only did he make surgery safe, but he also made surgery 'scientific' (Worboys 2000) by applying Pasteur's germ theory to it. There is no doubt that Joseph Lister is indeed a hero of science, and although there were other individuals who played a key part in the development of asepsis, the contribution that Lister made to surgery was invaluable.

References

Blood and Guts: A History of Surgery (2008) [VHS video] BBC Four.

Butterfield, H. 1931 *The Whig Interpretation of History*. London: G. Bell.

Fisher, R. B. 1977 Joseph Lister, 1827-1912. London: MacDonald and Jane's.

Granshaw, L. 1992 "Upon this Principle I have based a Practice". The Development and Reception of Antisepsis in Britain, 1867-90.' In: *Medical Innovations in Historical Perspective*. ed. by Pickstone, J. V. Basingstoke: Macmillan, in association with the Centre for the History of Science, Technology, and Medicine, University of Manchester.

Guthrie, D. *1949 Lord Lister, his life and doctrine*. Edinburgh: Livingstone.

Smart, A., Khan, W. S. (2012). Is the commonly told story of Lister's antisepsis a whiggish one? *J. Perioper. Pract*. 22(3): 100-2.

Worboys, M. *2000 Spreading Germs: Disease Theories and Medical Practice in Britain 1865-1900*. Cambridge: Cambridge University Press.

In: Perioperative Practice in Trauma and Orthopaedic Surgery ISBN: 978-1-63483-325-7
Editor: Wasim S. Khan

Chapter 2

THE ROLE OF PERIOPERATIVE CARE IN REDUCING RATES OF METHICILLIN RESITANT STAPHYLOCCOCUS AUREUS

C. Byrne, A. Hazlerigg, W. S. Khan[*] and P. Smitham
University College London Institute of Orthopaedic and Musculoskeletal Sciences, Royal National Orthopaedic Hospital, Stanmore, Middlesex, UK

ABSTRACT

Methicillin Resistant *Staphylococcus aureus* (MRSA) is defined as any strain of *Staphylococcus aureus* resistant to beta-lactam antibiotics including the penicillin's and cephalosporins. Over the past ten years the UK has seen a dramatic increase in MRSA prevalence in healthcare facilities and the community with an estimated 30-50% of healthy adults thought to be colonised with MRSA. Surgical patients are among those at highest risk. With potential sequelae including septicaemia, septic shock, septic arthritis, osteomyelitis, meningitis, pneumonia or endocarditis, it is vital that all care facilities have up to date evidence-based guidelines to tackle this problem. The purpose of this chapter is to highlight the current evidence supporting some of the key perioperative measures which may be implemented in preventing MRSA.

Keywords: Perioperative care; MRSA; methicillin resistant *Staphylococcus aureus*; antibiotic resistance

INTRODUCTION

This chapter deals with the role of perioperative care in reducing Methicillin Resistant *Staphylococcus aureus* (MRSA) infection rates (Byrne et al. 2011).

[*] Corresponding author: Mr W. S. Khan, Clinical Lecturer, University College London Institute of Orthopaedics and Musculoskeletal Science, Royal National Orthopaedic Hospital, Stanmore, Middlesex, London, HA7 4LP, UK. Telephone number: +44 (0) 7791 025554, e-mail address: wasimkhan@doctors.org.uk.

MRSA is defined as any strain of *Staphylococcus aureus* resistant to beta-lactam antibiotics including the penicillins and cephalosporins (Livermore 2000). Strains of MRSA have acquired the mecA gene, which encodes an altered penicillin binding protein (PBP 2a) causing the resultant resistance, which occasionally causes resistance to other antibiotics as well (Ayliffe 1974).

MRSA prevalence in healthcare facilities and the community has increased dramatically in the UK over the past 10 years (Gemmell et al. 2006). In care settings, staff shortages, patient overcrowding, inadequate staff training, lack of isolation facilities, inattention to infection control procedures and the frequent relocation of staff and patients have been blamed for this rise (New Zealand Ministry of Health 2002). Risk factors for the development of MRSA include older age, previous hospitalisation, skin disease, intravenous drug abuse, ventilation, dialysis, prolonged hospitalisation or residence in long-term care facilities, and the presence of indwelling catheters or other medical devices (Waldvogel 1995, Laibl et al. 2005, Wyllie et al. 2005). In the community, acquisition from household contacts and 'silent' acquisition in healthcare settings associated with inpatient care lasting over five days in the previous year seem to be the most prominent causative factors (Calfee et al. 2003, Jernigan et al. 2003, Salgado et al. 2003, Tacconelli et al. 2004).

Patients may be colonised or infected with MRSA. Those colonised with MRSA are generally asymptomatic, while MRSA is being carried on or in the body without causing illness. Infection with MRSA means the patient is symptomatic, and this may range from a superficial wound infection to sepsis, bacteraemia and even death. It is possible to be colonised with MRSA, which does not progress to infection (Coello et al. 1997), however these patients may be at an increased risk of developing infection (Pujol et al. 1994). Risk factors for developing clinical infection with MRSA include staying in intensive care units, administration of three or more antibiotics, presence of ulcers, surgical wounds, nasogastric or endotrachial tubes, drains, and urinary or intravenous catheterisation.

Intravenous cannulation is an independent risk factor for the development of infection (Pujol et al. 1994). Once established, MRSA is difficult to control and its survival is increased by antibiotic use (Burnett et al. 1980, Boyce 1989, Schentag et al. 1998, Manian et al. 2003).

Changes in antibiotic prophylaxis and treatment may lead to selection of new clones of MRSA and subsequent resistance. However, the evolution and spread of resistance is not well described. Therefore, antibiotic use must adapt gradually with national and local changes in prevalence in order to avoid the selection of new clones (Gemmell et al. 2006).

MRSA infection has been shown to increase morbidity and mortality. Deaths mentioning MRSA are higher among males than females. In 2006 the office for National Statistics quoted male deaths with MRSA mentioned on their certificate at 26.8 per million population; for females in 2008 this was 10.3 per million. There is extensive guidance issued by the Department of Health (DoH), National Institute of health and Clinical Excellence (NICE) and the Association for Perioperative Practice (AfPP) that helps to guide current clinical practice. The added morbidity and prolonged hospital stay have a significant cost implication. Estimates have been quoted for the NHS spending an extra 1 billion pounds per year on Hospital Aquired Infections (HAI) (National Audit Office 2009). MRSA is the cause of a significant number of HAI, and has been isolated from nearly a quarter of all Surgical Site Infections (SSI) (AfPP 2007). Additional costs of SSI alone have been estimated to be between £814 and £6626 (NICE 2003), and this is increased to an estimated £9000 when the SSI has been caused by MRSA (Wernitz et al. 2005, Wendin 2008).

These additional costs incurred can be attributed to extra nursing care, barrier requirements, re-operation and medications. The potential litigation costs from patient dissatisfaction and reduced quality of life costs has not been fully established (NICE 2003). Since 2003-2004 The National Audit office estimates that the DoH and its associated bodies have spent £57 million on initiatives to tackle HAIs throughout the UK, and £63 million as a single payment for the deep clean in 2007-2008.

Areas commonly colonised include the nostrils, respiratory tract, urinary tract, wounds and sites of intravenous catheters. Presentation depends on the area affected. In the case of skin colonisation, patients may present with red, warm, tender skin with pus, boils, abscesses, styes, carbuncles, cellulitis or impetigo (Iyer and Jones 2004). Fever, increased peripheral white blood cell count, increased inflammatory markers e.g. C-reactive protein (CRP), ulcers and sores are also indicative of MRSA infection. However, MRSA is not limited to the skin and once the infection enters the blood stream septicaemia, septic shock, septic arthritis, osteomyelitis, meningitis, pneumonia or endocarditis may arise.

Screening for MRSA and Decolonisation Regimes

An estimated 30-50% of healthy adults are colonised with MRSA (Laibl et al. 2005). With an estimated 22% mortality rate from MRSA bacteraemia (Selvey et al. 2000), it is essential that we identify and treat those who are MRSA positive. Ideally all patients and staff should be routinely screened for MRSA. In reality this is rarely possible due to budget and staffing constraints, and staff turnover.

All patients awaiting an elective operation require preoperative screening. This may be carried out either by preadmission clinics or general practitioners. Ideally screening should be performed as close to the operation date as possible. Some hospital admission patients are not required to undergo screening e.g. those requiring termination, eye surgery or admission to mental health trusts (DoH 2006). Emergency admissions are screened on the ward at admission. Those patients known to be at high risk, for example care or residential home patients, patients who have had previous positive *Staphylococcus aureus* blood cultures, or those who have been transferred from another hospital, are put in a side room and barrier nursed until they have been screened and MRSA colonisation has been excluded (DoH 2007). Intravenous drug abusers, HIV positive patients and those involved in contact sports may also warrant regular screening (Coia et al. 2006).

Once MRSA has been isolated from the swab a decolonisation regime is adopted. This decolonisation regime is to reduce the MRSA to a sub detection level and should ideally be done five days prior to the operation as the regime is limited in its duration of effectiveness. The admitting ward should be notified to the preadmission candidate who has undergone a decolonisation regime as only suppression rather than complete eradication of MRSA may have been achieved. A typical decolonisation regime for a positive nasal swab would consist of topical application to the inner surface of each nostril of 2% mupirocin three times a day for five days. For the patient whom preoperative assessment has revealed they are a carrier of MRSA on their skin, a shampoo body wash of 4% chlorhexidine gluconate is applied to identified carriage sites e.g. axilla, groin or perineum.

Successful suppression is confirmed by three additional screens each taken a week apart, beginning at least two days after the regime has been completed (DoH 2007).

All high-risk patients should be screened on admission and at regular intervals during their hospital stay depending on local infection control protocols, unless they are being directly admitted to isolation with no plan to clear them of MRSA carriage. Samples should be taken from nostril, skin lesions, wounds, groin/perineum, sites of intravenous and urinary catheters, tracheostomy sites and the umbilicus in neonates.

In those with a productive cough, sputum may also be tested (Coia et al. 2006). This approach to the screening of surgical patients may decrease MRSA infections by facilitating the appropriate selection of antibiotic agents for preoperative prophylaxis (Zanetti et al. 2001, Stephan et al. 2008). Almost 70% of all cases of MRSA bacteraemia occur in surgical or emergency medical patients (Wyllie et al. 2005). SSIs may take two forms; colonisation of the operative field during surgery, the commonest form, or haematogenous seeding during sepsis/bacteraemia (Wilson et al. 1975). It comes as no surprise then that units deemed to carry a high risk of MRSA infections or colonisation include ICU, transplant wards, and cardiothoracic, vascular surgery, trauma and orthopaedic surgery.

These wards typically treat many patients with additional risk factors including over 60 years of age, diabetes, ulcers and urinary catheters; this group accounted for over 70% of cases (Gemmell et al. 2006). Oncology, haematology and renal care wards are also classed as high risk (Wyllie et al. 2005).

Treatment for MRSA

In an outbreak, surgical and intensive care patients should be prioritised. In order to prevent the development of MRSA infection in such patients it has been recommended that those who are colonised or have been identified as having one or more of the risk factors for progression to infection receive early treatment with vancomycin. This has been shown to decrease mortality (Coello et al. 1997). The decision of what to treat MRSA infection and colonisation with depends largely on local patterns of resistance. Current research supports the use of local guidelines, and an example is summarised in Figure 1.

However a UK multicentre study carried out in the period 2001-2003 found that:

- 92% and 72% of strains were respectively resistant to fluoroquinolones and macrolides.
- Most isolates were susceptible to tetracyclines, fusidic acid, rifampicin and gentamicin.
- 12% of tested strains were mupirocin-resistant 591.
- 50% of treatment regimens used included a glycopeptide alone or with other agents.
- In bacteraemic patients the rates of resistance to tetracyclines, macrolides and rifampicin appeared to be lower than previously reported.

Based on the current literature there is insufficient evidence to suggest whether topical, systemic or combination therapy is the best form of treatment to use (Speller et al. 1997, BSAC 2005).

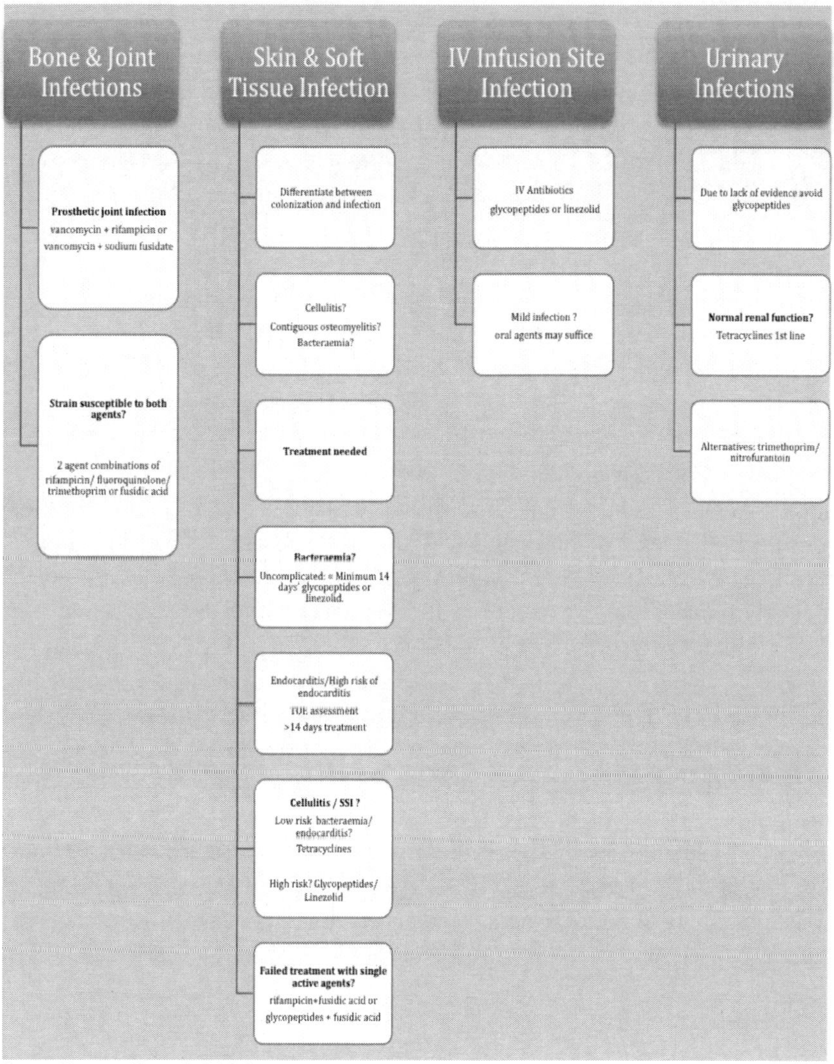

Adapted from Gemmell et al. 2006.

Figure 1. A summary of possible treatment options for common MRSA infections.

Drug resistant MRSA infections increase with increased exposure to antibiotics particularly at low concentrations (Ubukata et al. 1989). It has been shown that the efficacy of beta-lactam antibiotics is dependant on the length of time they remain above the minimum inhibition concentration (MIC) (Craig 1998). It is therefore advisable to administer such antibiotics at lower doses regularly e.g. every three hours, rather than once off at a higher dose to keep levels over their MIC (Kato et al. 2006).

Much debate surrounds when and for how long antibiotics should be administered. Nelson et al. (1983) conducted a study comparing the efficacy of administering antibiotics for one or seven days postoperatively and found no difference in infection rates between both regimens. Similarly another study found no difference in infection rates after one or three days of antibiotic treatment (Williams et al. 1984). It has therefore been recommended that postoperative antibiotic prophylaxis be limited to 24 hours after surgery (Kato et al. 2006).

PREVENTION OF MRSA

The primary form of MRSA spread is hand-borne transmission from the colonised hands of healthcare workers (Mulligan et al. 1993). Hand washing is the most effective way of preventing the spread of MRSA (AfPP 2007). MRSA can survive for months on surfaces such as equipment, floors and furniture. As such there is a transmission cycle of MRSA from the infected bedside cabinets surrounding the patient to healthcare workers hands and even those of the patients.

Standard principles for preventing hospital-acquired infections should be implemented to prevent the transmission of MRSA (Figure 2). The hospital environment must be clean, equipment should be thoroughly cleaned between patients, waste and laundry must be correctly handled and all staff must be adequately trained is hospital hygiene protocols particularly in relation to hand hygiene, the use of personal protective equipment and the safe use and disposal of sharps (NICE 2003).

While not intended to substitute good theatre practice, patient optimisation may aid in decreasing infection rates by optimising natural host defences against infection. As most pathogens originate from skin flora, decreasing the time a patient is exposed to pathogens in the hospital environment and, by screening and decontaminating surgical patients, infections rates could be further lowered (Dohmen and Konertz 2007).

An attempt should be made to reduce immunosuppressants preoperatively and discontinue if possible until after surgery (Dohmen and Konertz 2007). Diabetics have a markedly increased rate of SSIs. Blood glucose levels of > 300 mg/dL increase the odds of developing a SSI from 2.54 to 3.32 in comparison to those patients with blood glucose of <250mg/dL.

Therefore an attempt should be made to monitor and control all diabetic patients undergoing surgery (Dhinsa et al. 2010). Perioperatively the use of continuous insulin infusion was found to be superior to subcutaneous insulin (Dohmen and Konertz 2007).

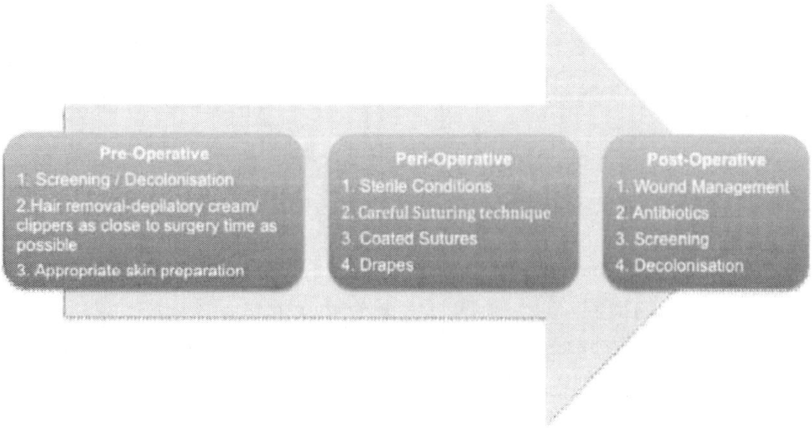

Figure 2. A summary of the measures suggested to prevent the transmission of MRSA in the preoperative, perioperative and post-operative settings.

Preoperative Strategies

There is evidence that preoperative showering 1-2 days before surgery, with soap decreases the skins bacterial burden however there is no evidence of a significant decrease in postoperative infections. NICE guidance advises that preoperative showering with chlorhexidine is not a cost-effective intervention to reduce SSI, and a Cochrane review showed there was no significant reduction in SSI after using chlorhexidine (Webster et al. 2011). In addition the authors recognise the risk that repeated chlorhexidine washing may encourage the development of resistant strains.

Preoperative hair removal is sometimes necessary in order to provide a clear operative field and allow a more effective seal from the surgical dressing. Shaving of surgical sites may increase the risk of infection due to the formation of micro-abrasions. Evidence has shown that patients who receive any form of preoperative hair removal suffer higher rates of SSIs than those patients who receive none (Winston 1992). It is therefore recommended that in cases where hair removal is necessary, electric clipping or depilatory cream be used as close to the time of surgery as possible to provide the best chance of decreasing SSIs (Cruse and Foord 1973, Ayliffe et al. 1983, Leigh et al. 1983, Ayliffe 1984, Masterson et al. 1984, Rotter et al. 1988).

Prior to the patient coming to theatre, theatre staff should have been notified of carriers and those who are infected with MRSA. Staff should be instructed on the appropriate procedures to minimise exposure. Typically the MRSA patient will be placed last on the list to cause the least disruption, and minimise cross contamination. If this is not viable then extra time for extra air exchanges before the next patient should be allowed (Association of Anaesthetists of Great Britain and Ireland 2008, Coia et al. 2006).

In the anaesthetic room, certain precautions must be carried out to reduce contamination or spread of MRSA, and to minimise the risk of infection. Prophylactic antibiotics have been shown to reduce SSI (Barker et al. 2002). The inclusion of this criterion on the World Health Organisation (WHO) 'Time Out Form' has increased administration compliance from 65% to 97% (Rosenberg et al. 2008).

Appropriate antibiotic prophylaxis should be administered between 30-60 minutes before the incision and before the tourniquet has been inflated. This is due to the effectiveness of the antibiotic being reliant on the need to have tissue levels of the antibiotic at the time of incision. Prophylactic antibiotics should be discontinued within 24 hours of the procedure, and typically for most outpatient procedures it will be a single dose administration.

Vancomycin 1g intravenously has been advocated if the patient is considered high risk. Special considerations surrounding the dosing of prophylactic antibiotics with the exception of vancomycin include cases where the duration of surgery exceeds four hours or where blood loss has exceeded 1500ml (Cosgrove 2011).

Typically the MRSA patient will be anaesthetised and recovered in theatre. To protect other patients, disposable anaesthetic circuits are used, and the disposal of these circuits is categorised as clinical waste. Equipment for terminal disinfection e.g. laryngoscope blades are also disposed. Intravenous cannulation, an independent risk factor for developing infection (Pujol et al. 1994), should be performed using the 'non touch' technique (Pratt et al. 2007). The theatre must be cleared of any surplus equipment. Reducing people traffic has been shown to reduce rates of infection (Babkin et al. 2007, Olsen et al. 2008).

Signs should be visible and doors shut to notify colleagues in order to reduce unnecessary thoroughfare through the operating theatre. The patient's trolley must remain inside the anaesthetic room, and all participating staff and portering staff in contact with the patient should be wearing protective clothing including donning gloves and plastic apron (AfPP 2007). A study showed that during routine patient care the rate of detection of MRSA on gowns and/or gloves was 18% (Snyder et al. 2008).

INTRAOPERATIVE STRATEGIES

1. Theatre Environment

Laminar airflow systems are used in many theatres to reduce the occurrence of infections. They are expensive to install and maintain (Kirkland et al. 1999, Merle et al. 2000, Coello et al. 2005). Their use is based on the assumption that they are successful in decreasing the number of SSIs. However, few controlled studies have been performed to back up this assumption. One recent study found an increase in the number of SSIs associated with the use of laminar flow theatres (Brandt et al. 2008). In order to justify their cost and to determine the efficacy of laminar airflow devices more randomised control trials are required.

Hypothermia results in vasoconstriction and decreased functioning of the immune system increasing the chance of developing an SSI. It has been shown that a decrease of 1.5 degrees centigrade from a patient's body temperature during surgery increases the risk of postoperative infection. Thus by monitoring a patient's temperature, using simple measures such as extra blankets and increasing the air temperature of theatres, infection rates may be lowered (Kurz et al. 1996, Mahoney and Odom 1999, Melling et al. 2001, Dohmen and Konertz 2007).

2. Hand Hygiene, Gloves and Facemasks

It is recommended that those scrubbing in hand wash for five minutes followed by three minutes of disinfection with alcohol disinfectant (Mangram et al. 1999). As surgical gloves are not totally fluid proof, wearing double gloves may be recommended in certain cases for the scrub team (Doyle et al. 1992).

There is no evidence that the use of surgical masks decreases infections. However, they do provide protection for the wearer and due to theoretical rationale it is not unreasonable for all those present in theatre to wear masks (Mangram et al. 1999).

The choice of aqueous surgical scrub has in many hospitals previously been left up to the surgeons' preference, with the main choice being between a water based solution containing chlorhexidine gluconate or a providone iodine scrub.

Chlorhexidine has been shown to be supcrior to iodine scrubs in reducing Colony Forming Units (Pereira et al. 1990, Furukawa et al. 2005). A Cochrane Review on surgical hand asepsis showed that alcohol rubs containing 60-90% ethanol, isoproanol or n-propanol were as effective as the aqueous scrubs in preventing SSI (Tanner et al. 2008).

3. Surgical Gowns, Drapes and Linens

All material should have a pore size of <20μm. Materials in the surgical field should be waterproof, sterile and preferably disposable (Mitchell et al. 1978). Antiseptic preparation of a patient's skin prior to surgery is an important aseptic precaution, however, antiseptic solutions can wash off during surgery potentially permitting bacterial re-growth. The use of plastic adhesive barrier drapes has been shown to reduce wound contamination but not to significantly reduce skin flora.

These drapes may be impregnated with iodine or other anti-septic agents (Dohmen and Konertz 2007). While there is no evidence of associated negative outcomes, there is some but insufficient evidence that the use of incisional drapes with or without iodine or other antiseptic products decreases infection rates (Fairclough et al. 1986, Dewan et al. 1987, Yoshimura et al. 2003, Segers et al. 2007, Parks et al. 2007, Kramer et al. 2010).

Agents used to prepare patients' skin preoperatively should ideally be broad-spectrum ready-to-use-dilutions in single use containers to avoid contamination. Alcohol based solutions have been found to be most effective.

While complete decontamination is impossible, such solutions can effectively reduce resident flora (Lilly et al. 1979, Kampf and Kramer 2004). Chlorhexidine Gluconate compares to iodine favourably in several studies showing a reduced SSI rate (Darouiche et al. 2010), and better elimination of bacteria (Ostrander et al. 2005).

4. Surgical Wound

Carefully sutured wounds seal with fibrin within 6-24 hours protecting them from moisture and bacterial contamination (Kato et al. 2006). Although more expensive, several studies have shown a decrease in the number of SSIs when antibiotic coated sutures are used (Fleck et al. 2007, Justinger et al. 2009). The use of such sutures in combating MRSA infection is supported by a study examining their ability to inhibit the colonisation of bacteria after direct *in vivo* inoculation with *Staphylococcus aureus*.

Although carried out on a guinea pig model, this study demonstrated a significant decrease ($p<0.05$) in infections when antimicrobial sutures where compared with standard sutures (Storch et al. 2004). Microbial sealants mechanically block the passage of pathogens into the surgical wound. While early clinical results are promising, particularly when combined with a topical iodine skin preparation, more studies are required before this method can be introduced into good surgical practice (Dohmen and Konertz 2007, Wilson 2008).

5. Operative Oxygenation

The most important immune defence against surgical pathogens are neutrophils. Neutrophils play a vital role in the immune defence against SSIs and are mediated by oxidative killing. They are dependent on the production of bactericidal superoxide radicals from molecular oxygen and on the partial pressure of oxygen to function adequately (Barbior 1978). The regulation of angiogenesis is also dependant on such factors (Hopf et al. 1997).

There is evidence that by using 80% oxygen instead of 30% oxygen during surgery and supplementary oxygen during recovery postoperative infection rates could be lowered by as much as 50% (Greif et al. 2000, Pryor et al. 2004, O'Connor 2004, Belda et al. 2005, Dohmen and Konertz 2007, Velazquez 2007).

POSTOPERATIVE STRATEGIES

The Health Protection Agency found that 44% of MRSA cases established while patients were staying in acute trusts between April 2006 and December 2009 were attributable to lines. 18% were from intravenous cannulas and 19% from central lines. Early removal of all surplus lines postoperatively is advised. Soft tissue infections and skin infections were found to be the source in a further 40% of cases. Antimicrobial gauze replacing sterile plain gauze reduced the MRSA SSI rate by 47% (Mueller et al. 2008). Commercially available silver coated dressings, such as Acticoat have been developed for the treatment and prevention of MRSA infection (Ulkur et al. 2005, Ip et al. 2006, Lee et al. 2010). More studies on their efficacy and how often the dressings need to be replaced along with cost analysis needs to be performed, and consideration needs to be given to the potential resistance these dressing may encourage.

CONCLUSION

In summary there is much controversy over the best approach to tackling the problem of MRSA. While targeted active surveillance is best reserved for high-risk patients or during times of an outbreak, adopting the simple perioperative practices discussed in this chapter can lower the incidence of MRSA infection and in turn its emergent resistance.

REFERENCES

Association for Perioperative Practice 2007 Standards and Recommendations for Safe Perioperative Practice Harrogate AfPP.

Association of Anaesthetists of Great Britain and Ireland 2008 Infection control in anaesthesia. *Anaesthesia* 63 1027-1036.

Ayliffe, G. 1974 Methicillin-resistant Staphylococcus aureus. *Lancet* 1:573.

Ayliffe, G. A. 1984 Surgical scrub and skin disinfection. *Infection Control* 5 23-27.

Ayliffe, G. A., Noy, M. F., Babb, J. R., Davies, J. G., Jackson, J. 1983 A Comparison of pre-operative bathing with chlorhexidine-detergent and non-medicated soap in the prevention of wound infection. *Journal of Hospital Infection* 4 237-244.

Babkin, Y., Raveh, D., Lifschitz, M., et al. 2007 Incidence and risk factors for surgical infection after total knee replacement. *Scandinavian Journal of Infectious Disease* 39 890-895.

Barbior, B. M. 1978 Oxygen-dependent microbial killing of phagocytes. *New England Journal of Medicine* 298 659-668.

Belda, F. J., Aguilera, L., Garcia de la Asuncion, J., et al. 2005 Spanish Reduccion de la Tasa de Infeccion Quirurigica Group. Supplemental perioperative oxygen and the risk of surgical wound infection: a randomised controlled trial. *Journal of the American Medical Association* 94 2035-2042.

Boyce, J. 1989 Methicillin-resistant Staphylococcus aureus: detection, epidemiology and control measures. *Infectious Disease Clinics of North America* 3 901-913.

BSAC 2005 Resistance Surveillance. Available at www.bsacsurv.org.uk.

Burnett, J., Gustilo, R., Williams, D., Kind, A. 1980 Prophylactic antibiotics in hip fractures: a double-blind, prospective study. *Journal of Bone and Joint Surgery of America* 62 457-462.

Brandt, C., Hott, U., Sohr, D., et al. 2008 Operating room ventilation with laminar airflow shows no protective effect on the surgical site infection rate in orthopedic and abdominal surgery. *Annals of Surgery* 248 695-700.

Byrne, C., Hazlerigg, A., Khan, W. S., Smitham, P. (2011). The role of perioperative care in reducing rates of methicillin resistant staphylococcus aureus. *J. Perioper. Pract.* 21(12): 410-7.

Calfee, D., Durbin, L., Germanson, T., et al. 2003 Spread of methicillin resistant Staphylococcus aureus (MRSA) among household contacts of individuals with nosocomially acquired MRSA. *Infection Control and Hospital Epidemiology* 24 422-426.

Coello, R., Charlett, A., Wilson, J., et al. 2005 Adverse impact of surgical site infections in English hospitals. *Journal of Hospital Infection* 60 93-103.

Coello, R., Glynn, J., Gaspar, C., Picazo, J., Fereres, J. 1997 Risk factors for developing clinical infection with methicillin-resistant staphylococcus aureus (MRSA) amongst hospital patients initially only colonized with MRSA. *Journal of Hospital Infection* 37 39-46.

Coia, J., Duckworth, G., Edwards, D., et al. 2006 Guidelines for the control and prevention of meticillin-resistant Staphylococcus aureus (MRSA) in healthcare facilities. *Journal of Hospital Infection* 63S S1 S44.

Cosgrove, S., Avdic, E. 2011 *Johns Hopkins Antibiotic Guidelines: Treatment Recommendations for Inpatients.* The John Hopkins Antibiotic Management Policy.

Craig, W. 1998 Pharmacokinetic/pharmacodynamic parameters: rationale for antibacterial dosing of mice and men. *Clinical Infectious Diseases* 261-12.

Cruse, P. J., Foord, R. 1973 A five-year prospective study of 23,649 surgical wounds. *Archives of Surgery* 107 206-210.

Darouiche, R. O., Wall, M. J., Itani, K. M., et al. 2010 CHG-Alcohol versus Providone-Iodine for Surgical Site Asepsis. *New England Journal of Medicine* 362 18-26.

Department of Health 2006 Screening for meticillin-resistant Staphylococcus aureus (MRSA) colonisation. *A strategy for NHS Trusts: a summary of best practice.*

Department of Health 2007 Isolating Patients with healthcare-associated infection. *A summary of best practice.* Available at www.clean-safe-care.nhs.uk.

Dewan, P. A., Van Rij, A. M., Robinson, R. G., Skeggs, G. B., Fergus, M. 1987 The use of an iodophor-impregnated plastic incise drape in abdominal surgery - a controlled clinical trial. *Australia and New Zealand Journal of Surgery* 57 859-863.

Dhinsa, B. S., Khan, W. S., Puri, A. 2010 Management of the diabetic patient in the perioperative period. *Journal of Perioperative Practice* 20 364-367.

Dohmen, P. M., Konertz, W. 2007 A review of current strategies to reduce intraoperative bacterial contamination of surgical wounds. *GMS Krankenhaushyg Interdiszip* 2(2) Doc 38.

Doyle, P. M., Alvi, S., Johanson, R. 1992 The effectiveness of double gloving in obstetrics and gynaecology. *British Journal of Obstetrics and Gynaecology* 99 3-84.

Fairclough, J. A., Johnson, D., Mackie, I. 1986 The prevention of wound contamination by skin organisms by the pre-operative application of iodophor impregnated plastic adhesive drape. *Journal of International Medical Research* 14 105-109.

Fleck, T., Moidl, R., Blacky, A., et al. 2007 Triclosan-coated sutures for the reduction of sternal wound infections: economic considerations. *Annals of Thoracic Surgery* 84(1) 232-236.

Furukawa, K., Tajiri, T., Sudzuki, H., Norose, Y. 2005 Are sterile water and brushes necessary for hand washing before surgery in Japan. *Journal of Nippon Medical School* 72 149-154.

Gemmell, C., Edwards, D., Fraise, A. 2006 Guidelines for the prophylaxis and treatment of methicillin resistant Staphylococcus aureus (MRSA) infections in the UK. *Journal of Antimicrobial Chemotherapy* 57 589-608.

Greif, R., Akca, O., Horn, E., et al. 2000 Supplemental perioperative oxygen to reduce the incidence of surgical-wound infection. *New England Journal of Medicine* 342161-169.

Hopf, H. W., Hunt, T. K., West, J. M., et al. 1997 Wound tissue oxygen tension predicts the risk of wound infection in surgical patients. *Archives of Surgery* 132 997-1004.

Ip, M., Lui, S. L., Poon, V. K., Lung, I., Burd, A. 2006 Antimicrobial activities of silver dressings; an in vitro comparison. *Journal of Medical Microbiology* 55 59-63.

Iyer, S., Jones, D. H. 2004 Community-acquired methicillin-resistant Staphylococcus aureus skin infection: a retrospective analysis of clinical presentation and treatment of a local outbreak. *Journal of the American Academy of Dermatology* 50(6) 854-858.

Jernigan, J., Pullen, A., Flowers, L., et al. 2003 Prevalence and risk factors for colonization with methicillin-resistant Staphylococcus aureus at the time of hospital admission. *Infection Control and Hospital Epidemiology* 24 409-414.

Justinger, C., Moussavian, M. R., Schlueter, C., et al. 2009 Antibiotic coating of abdominal closure sutures and wound infection. *Surgery* 145(3) 330-334.

Kampf, G., Kramer, A. 2004 Epidemiologic background of hand hygiene and evaluation of the most important agents for scrubs and rubs. *Clinical Microbiology Review* 17 863-893.

Kato, D., Maezawa, K., Yonezawa, I., et al. 2006 Randomized prospective study on prophylactic antibiotics in clean orthopedic surgery in one ward for 1 year. *Journal of Orthopaedic Science*. 11 20-27.

Kirkland, K. B., Briggs, J. P., Trivette, S. L., et al. 1999 The impact of surgical-site infections in the 1990s: attributable mortality, excess length of hospitalization, and extra costs. *Infection Control and Hospital Epidemiology* 20 725-730.

Kramer, A., Assadian, O. and Lademann, J. 2010 Prevention of postoperative wound infections by covering the surgical field with iodine-impregnated incision drape (Ioban® 2). *GMS Krankenhhyg Interdiszip* 5(2) Doc08.

Kurz, A., Sessler, D. I., Lenhardt, R. 1996 Perioperative normothermia to reduce the incidence of surgical-wound infection and shorten hospitalization. *New England Journal of Medicine*. 334 1209-1216.

Laibl, V., et al. 2005 Clinical Presentation of Community- Acquired Methicillin-Resistant Staphylococcus aureus in Pregnancy. *Obstetrics and Gynecology* 106(3) 461-465.

Lee, J. H., Chae, J. D., Kim, D. G., Hong, S. H., Lee, W. M., Ki, M. 2010 Comparison of the efficacies of silver-containing dressing materials for treating a full-thickness rodent wound infected by methicillin-resistant Staphylococcus aureus. *Korean Journal of Laboratory Medicine* 30 20-27.

Leigh, D. A., Stronge, J. L., Marriner, J., Sedgwick, J. 1983 Total body bathing with Hibiscrub (chlorhexidine) in surgical patients: a controlled trial. *Journal of Hospital Infection* 4 229-235.

Lilly, H. A., Lowbury, E. J., Wilkins, M. D. 1979 Limits to progressive reduction of resident skin bacteria by disinfection. *Journal of Clinical Pathology* 32 382-385.

Livermore, D. 2000 Antibiotic resistance in staphylococci. *International Journal of Antimicrobial Agents* 16 Suppl. 1 3-10.

Mahoney, C., Odom, J. 1999 Maintaining intraoperative normothermia: a meta-analysis of outcomes with costs. *AANA Journal* 67 155-164.

Mangram, A., Horan, T., Pearson, M., Silver, L., Jarvis, W. 1999 The Hospital Infection Control Practices Advisory Committee. Guideline for prevention of surgical site infection. *American Journal of Infection Control* 27 97-134.

Manian, F., Meyer, P., Setzer, J., Senkel, D. 2003 Surgical site infections associated with methicillin-resistant Staphylococcus aureus: do postoperative factors play a role? *Clinical Infectious Diseases* 36 863-868.

Masterson, T. M., Rodeheaver, G. T., Morgan, R. F., Edlich, R. F. 1984 Bacteriologic evaluation of electric clippers for surgical hair removal. *American Journal of Surgery* 148 301-302.

Melling, A. C., Ali, B., Scott, E. M., Leaper, D. J. 2001 Effects of preoperative warming on the incidence of wound infection after clean surgery: a randomised controlled trial. *Lancet* 358 876-880.

Merle, V., Germain, J. M., Chamouni, P., et al. 2000 Assessment of prolonged hospital stay attributable to surgical site infections using appropriateness evaluation protocol. *American Journal of Infection Control* 28 109-115.

Ministry of Health, New Zealand 2002. Methicillin-resistant Staphylococcus aureus (MRSA) in New Zealand. Available at www.moh.govt.nz/cd/mrsa.

Mitchell, N. J., Evens, D. C., Kerr, A. 1978 Reduction of skin bacteria in the theatre air with comfortable, non-woven disposable clothing for the operating-theatre staff. *British Medical Journal* 1 696-698.

Mueller, S. W., Le, K. 2008 Impact of an antimicrobial-impregnated gauze dressing on surgical site infections including methicillin-resistant Staphylococcus aureus infections. *American Journal of Infection Control* 36 651-655.

Mulligan, M., Murray-Leisure, K., Ribner, B., et al. 1993 Methicillin-resistant *Staphylococcus aureus*: a consensus review of the microbiology, pathegenesis and epidemiology with implications for prevention and management. *American Journal of Medicine* 94 313-328.

National Audit Office 2009. *Trends in rates of Healthcare Associated Infection in England 2004 to 2008*. Available at www.nao.org.uk/search/search.aspx?Schema=andterms=mrsa.

National Institute for Clinical Excellence 2003. *Infection control: prevention of healthcare associated infection in primary and community care*. London: NICE.

Nelson, C. L., Green, T. G., Porter, R. A., Warren, R. D. 1983 One day versus seven days of preventive antibiotic therapy in orthopedic surgery. *Clinical Orthopaedics* 176 258-263.

O'Connor, M. I. 2004 Wound healing problems in TKA: just when you thought it was over! *Orthopedics* 27 983-984.

Office for National Statistics. Available at www.statistics.gov.uk/hub/index.html.

Olsen, M. A., Nepple, J. J., Riew, K. D., et al. 2008 Risk factors for surgical site infection following orthopaedic spinal operations. *Journal of Bone and Joint Surgery* 90A 62-69.

Ostrander, R. V., Botte, M. J., Brage, M. E. 2005 Efficacy of surgical preparation solutions in foot and ankle surgery. *Journal of Bone and Joint Surgery* 87A 980-985.

Parks, P. J., Babadjanian, C., Johnson, E. J., Walters, S. A. 2007 Infection reduction with antimicrobial-impregnated incise foils. *European Bone and Joint Infection Society*, 26th annual meeting, Corfu, Greece, 20-22 Sep. 2007.

Perieira, L. J., Lee, G. M., Kade, K. J. 1990 The effect of surgical handwashing routines on the microbial counts of operating room nurses. *American Journal of Infection Control* 18 354-364.

Pratt, R. J., Pellowe, C. M., Wilson, J. A., et al. 2007 EPIC2; National Evidence-based Guidelines for Preventing Healthcare associated Infections in NHS Hospitals in England. *Journal of Hospital Infection* 65 S1-S64.

Pryor, K. O., Fahey, T. J. 3rd, Lien, C. A., Goldstein, P. A. 2004 Surgical site infection and the routine use of perioperative hyperoxia in a general surgical population: a randomized controlled trial. *Journal of the American Medical Association* 291 79-87.

Pujol, M., PeAa, C., Pallares, R., Ayats, J., Ariza, J., Gudiol, F. 1994 Risk factors for nosocomial bacteraemia due to methicillin-resistant Staphylococcus aureus. *European Journal of Clinical Microbial Infection and Disease* 13 96-102.

Rosenberg, A. D., Wambold, D., Kraemer, L., et al. 2008 Ensuring appropriate timing of antibiotic prophylaxis. *Journal of Bone and Joint Surgery* 90A 226-233.

Rotter, M. L., Larsen, S. O., Cooke, E. M., et al. 1988 A comparison of the effects of preoperative whole-body bathing with detergent alone and with detergent containing chlorhexidine gluconate on the frequency of wound infections after clean surgery. The European Working Party on Control of Hospital Infections. *Journal of Hospital Infection* 11 310-320.

Salgado, C., Farr, B., Calfee, D. 2003 Community-acquired methicillin resistant staphylococcus aureus: a meta-analysis of prevalence and risk factors. *Journal of Clinical Infection and Disease* 36 131-139.

Schentag, J., Hyatt, J., Carr, J., et al. 1998 Genesis of methicillin- resistant Staphylococcus aureus (MRSA), how treatment of MRSA infections has selected for vancomycin-resistant Enterococcus faecium, and the importance of antibiotic management and infection control. *Clinical Infection and Disease* 26 1204-1214.

Segers, P., de Jong, A. P., Spanjaard, L., Ubbink, D. T., de Mol, B. A. 2007 Randomized clinical trial comparing two options for postoperative incisional care to prevent poststernotomy surgical site infections. *Wound Repair and Regeneration* 15 192-196.

Selvey, L., Whitby, M., Johnson, B. 2000 Nosocomial methicillin resistant staphylococcus aureus bacteremia: is it any worse than nosocomial methicillin-sensitive Staphylococcus aureus bacteremia? *Infection Control and Hospital Epidemiology* 21 645-648.

Speller, D., Johnson, A., James, D. 1997. Resistance to methicillin and other antibiotics in isolates of Staphylococcus aureus from blood and cerebrospinal fluid England and Wales, 1989-95. *Lancet* 350 323-325.

Stephan, H., Carolina, F., Jacques, S. 2008 Universal Screening for Methicillin-Resistant Staphylococcus aureus at Hospital Admission and Nosocomial Infection in Surgical Patients. *Journal of the American Medical Association* 299(10) 1149-1157.

Storch, M. L., Rothenburger, S. J., Jacinto, G. 2004 Experimental efficacy study of coated VICRYL plus antibacterial suture in guinea pigs challenged with Staphylococcus aureus. *Surgical Infection* 5(3) 281-288.

Snyder, G., Thom, K., Furuno, J., et al. 2008 Detection of Methicillin-Resistant Staphylococcus aureus and Vancomycin-Resistant Enterococci on the Gowns and Gloves of Heathcare Workers. *Infection Control and Hospital Epidemiology* 29(7) 583-589.

Tacconelli, E., Venkataraman, I., De Girolami, P. C., et al. 2004 Methicillin- resistant Staphylococcus aureus bacteraemia diagnosed at hospital admission: distinguishing between community-acquired versus health- care-associated strains. *Journal of Antimicrobial Chemotherapy* 53 474-479.

Tanner, J., Swarbrook, S., Stuart, J. 2008 Surgical hand antiseptics to reduce surgical site infection. *The Cochrane Database of Systematic Reviews 4.*

Ubukata, K., Nonoguchi, R., Matsuhashi, M., Konno, M. 1989 Expression and inducibility in Staphylococcus aureus of the mecA gene, which encodes a methicillin-resistant S. aureus-specific penicillin- binding protcin. *Journal of Bacteriology* 171 2882-2885.

Ulkur, E., Oncul, O., Karagoz, H., et al. 2005 Comparison of silver coated dressing (Acticoat), chlorhexidine acetate 0.5% (Bactigrass) and fusidic acid 2% (Fusidin) for topical antibacterial effect on methicillin-resistant Staphylococci-contaminated, full-skin thickness rat burn wounds. *Burns* 31 874-877.

Velazquez, O. C. 2007 Angiogenesis and vasculogenesis: inducing the growth of new blood vessels and wound healing by stimulation of bone marrow-derived progenitor cell mobilization and homing. *Journal of Vascular Surgery* 45 A39-A47.

Waldvogel, F. 1995 Staphylococcus aureus. In: Mandell, G. L., Bennett, J. E., Dolin, R. editor(s). *Principles and Practice of Infectious Diseases.* 4th Edition. New York: Churchill Livingstone: 1754-1758.

Webster, J., Osborne, S. 2011 Preoperative bathing or showering with skin antiseptics to prevent surgical site infection. *The Cochrane Database of Systematic Reviews 3.*

Wendin, R. 2008 The economics of patient safety: can you afford not to be safe? *Report commissioned by The Royal College of Physicians*, London. Available at www.telegraph. co.uk/news/uknews/2194132/Every-MRSA-case-costs-NHS-an-extra-and1639,000.html.

Wernitz, M. H., Keck, S., Swidinski, S., Schulz, S., Veit, S. K. 2005 Cost analysis of a hospital-wide selective screening programme for methicillin-resistant Staphylococcus aureus (MRSA) carriers in the context of diagnosis related groups (DRG) payment. *Clinical Microbiology and Infections* 11 466-471.

Wilson, P., Salvati, E., Blumenfeld, E. 1975 The problem of infection in total prosthetic arthroplasty of the hip. *Surgical Clinics of North America* 55 1431-1437.

Wilson, S. E. 2008 Microbial sealing: a new approach to reducing contamination. *Journal of Hospital Infection* 70(Suppl. 2) 11-14.

Winston, K. R. 1992 Hair and neurosurgery. *Neurosurgery* 31 320-329.

Wyllie, D., Peto, T., Crook, D. 2005 MRSA bacteraemia in patients on arrival in hospital: a cohort study in Oxfordshire 1997-2003. *British Medical Journal* 331 7523.

Yoshimura, Y., Kubo, S., Hirohashi, K., et al. 2003 Plastic iodophor drape during liver surgery operative use of the iodophor-impregnated adhesive drape to prevent wound infection during high risk surgery. *World Journal of Surgery* 27 685-688.

Zanetti, G., Goldie, S., Platt, R. 2001 Clinical consequences and cost of limiting use of vancomycin for perioperative prophylaxis: example of coronary artery bypass surgery. *Emerging Infectious Disease* 7 820-827.

In: Perioperative Practice in Trauma and Orthopaedic Surgery ISBN: 978-1-63483-325-7
Editor: Wasim S. Khan

Chapter 3

Management of the Diabetic Patient in the Perioperative Period

B. S. Dhinsa, A. Puri and W. S. Khan*

University College London Institute of Orthopaedics and Musculoskeletal Science, Royal National Orthopaedic Hospital, Stanmore, Middlesex, London, UK

Abstract

With the ever increasing number of diabetic patients undergoing surgical procedures, the effective perioperative management of diabetes mellitus has become progressively more important. This article will discuss a number of approaches to improving the perioperative management of patient with this condition, and explore the fine balance of blood glucose management that should prevent hypo and hyperglycaemia. Also discussed will be the complications of diabetes mellitus, particularly where these directly compromise patient health and interventional outcomes.

Keywords: Diabetes mellitus, perioperative management, insulin, hypoglycaemia, sliding scale

Introduction

This chapter reviews the perioperative management of the diabetic patient (Dhinsa et al. 2010). With the worldwide prevalence of diabetes mellitus recorded at 171 million in 2000 and expected to more than double by 2030 (WHO 2010), knowledge of diabetes and the complications of diabetes mellitus in the surgical patients are best understood by appreciating the mechanisms of the disease as described below.

---

* Corresponding author: Mr Wasim S. Khan, Clinical Lecturer, University College London Institute of Orthopaedics and Musculoskeletal Science, Royal National Orthopaedic Hospital, Stanmore, Middlesex, London, HA7 4LP, UK. Telephone number: +44 (0) 7791 025554, fax number: +44 (0) 20 8570 3864, e-mail address: wasimkhan @doctors.org.uk.

WHAT IS DIABETES MELLITUS

Glucose is a necessary energy source for cells. Diabetes mellitus is a condition that causes derangement of glucose metabolism, resulting in hyperglycaemia (abnormally high blood glucose) and carbohydrate intolerance (inability to process the nutrient carbohydrates, including sugars into a source of energy). Hypoglycaemia (abnormally low blood glucose) occurs when blood glucose concentrations fall below a level necessary to properly support the body's need for energy and stability throughout its cells.

In the healthy individual, the blood glucose levels are tightly controlled to prevent states of hypo or hyperglycaemia and the associated complications (Gale et al. 2002). This regulation of blood glucose levels occurs in response to insulin, glucagon, epinephrine, cortisol and growth hormone release, from the major organs involved such as the liver, pancreas and peripheral tissue (Gale et al. 2002).

Insulin is synthesised in the pancreas and is responsible for the uptake of glucose by the liver, fat and muscles for storage as glycogen (Marks 2003). Many types of diabetes exist, with the most common being Types 1 and 2 (Expert Committee on the Diagnosis and Classification of Diabetes Mellitus 2003) and these are discussed below.

1. Type 1 Diabetes Mellitus

Type 1 or insulin-dependent diabetes mellitus is immune-mediated and leads to insulin deficiency through a loss of β-cells within the pancreas. While type 1 diabetes classically presents in children, it doesn't do so exclusively. For patients who suffer from type 1 diabetes mellitus and a lack of insulin production, artificial replacement is essential by means of a soluble biosynthetic human insulin product (Gale et al. 2002).

Multiple insulin injections are self administered on a daily basis, with rapid-acting varieties playing a role in glucose control before meals and long-acting varieties for night time (Cameron et al. 2009).

2. Type 2 Diabetes Mellitus

Type 2 or non-insulin independent diabetes mellitus results from either deranged insulin secretion from the pancreas or the resistance of cells in the body to insulin and, in contrast to type 1, tends to present within the adult population (Gale et al. 2002). Treatment for diabetes mellitus type 2 includes diet control and exercise.

Oral drugs are possibly indicated, where the first line treatment is biguanide (oral hypoglycaemic drugs that work by increasing insulin sensitivity e.g. metformin), followed by a sulphonylureas (oral hypoglycaemic drugs that work by increasing secretion of insulin e.g. gliclazide) (Gale et al. 2002). Insulin is added where diabetes is not controlled by oral drugs (National Collaborating Centre for Chronic Conditions 2008).

Complications of Diabetes Mellitus Relevant to the Surgical Patient

Poor blood glucose control, particularly over a prolonged time period is responsible for the complications often associated with diabetes. High blood sugar encourages glycosylation, (the binding of glucose to proteins) which impairs their function and is irreversible. The roles of proteins include building and repairing body tissues, regulation of body processes and formation of enzymes and hormones. When glucose binds irreversibly to proteins, proteins are unable to perform these roles. Osmotic swelling ensues, causing cell damage involving all systems in the body (Underwood 2002).

By means of these mechanisms, macro and microvascular damage occurs alongside nephropathies (renal complications) and neuropathies (nerve complications). Macrovascular damage describes a range of conditions including atherosclerotic vascular disease, myocardial infarction, cerebrovascular events and peripheral vascular disease (Hirsch et al. 1991). Complications directly relevant to the perioperative diabetic patient include the following:

1. Infection and Wound Complications

It is widely documented that diabetic patients suffer from infections, with surgical site infection rates two to three times higher in diabetic patients than their non-diabetic counterparts (WHO 2008). The poor peripheral vascularity prevents a good blood supply to the surgical site and the tissues become hypoxic. Because the blood supply is reduced, there is an impaired immune response at the site of the surgery increasing the risks of infection, and a delay in fibroblast (cells that repair tissue) action delaying wound healing. The additional presence of neuropathies can result in ulceration (Falanga 2005).

2. Nephropathy and Neuropathy

Nephropathies ultimately result in renal impairment or failure; a serious condition, which greatly impacts not only on the everyday life of the patient, but also on surgical procedures and drug treatment options. Decreased renal function places restrictions on the choice of drugs available for use in these patients e.g. the use of certain antibiotics that are excreted through the kidneys. Neuropathic complications include peripheral neuropathy (injury to peripheral nerves) resulting in them being unable to carry messages to the brain. This leads to altered sensation and an increased incidence of ulceration of the lower extremities (Hirsch et al. 1991), emphasising the perioperative role of careful patient positioning and vigilance with pressure areas (Hoogwerf 2006).

3. Diabetic Ketoacidosis

Acute diabetic emergencies include diabetic ketoacidosis that is associated with acidosis, hyperventilation, vomiting and abdominal pain as well as acute confusion.

Predominantly type 1 diabetics are affected, often as a result of prolonged disturbance of insulin therapy or due to the stress response evoked during surgery (Umpierrez and Kitabchi 2003). Management is with fluid resuscitation, initiation of insulin administration if not already in progress, and electrolyte replacement as required. Fluid resuscitation must be accurately monitored to prevent fluid overload in the circulation, lungs (pulmonary oedema) and the brain (cerebral oedema) (Marks et al. 1996).

Preoperative Considerations in Diabetes Mellitus

With approximately 25% of all hospital inpatients suffering from diabetes, rates of patients who have diabetes and have to undergo surgery are also inevitably rising (Patel 2008). The preoperative assessment of the diabetic patient includes a complete history, examination and investigations to look for evidence of renal and peripheral nerve complications, ulcers and infections (Marks 2003). Blood glucose levels and glycosylated haemoglobin (Hb1Ac) (laboratory blood test used to assess diabetic control) are measured. It is preferable to have diabetic patients placed in the earliest available slots on the theatre list to reduce fasting time (Hoogwerf 2006). The WHO Surgical Safety Checklist (Haynes et al. 2009) has been rolled out nationwide to provide a basic framework of surgical safety. These standards are being applied globally to try and decrease the number of surgical deaths and complications from preventable causes. This is particularly relevant in the context of elevated risk of surgical site infections in diabetic patients. Control of hyperglycaemia and administration of prophylactic antibiotics where appropriate will minimise bacterial colonisation at the surgical site (WHO 2008).

Perioperative Management of Diabetes Mellitus

Any surgical procedure will elicit a stress response in the patient to increase the circulating blood glucose levels by mechanisms previously described. In patients with diabetes mellitus this response is not as effective due to insulin resistance or deficiency and leads to hyperglycaemia.

Insulin administration may be required to counteract this rise in blood glucose levels and achieve normoglycaemia (Dagogo-Jack et al. 2002).

Patients on oral medication for the control of diabetes mellitus are advised to stop their medication on the day of surgery due to the risk of hypoglycaemia (Dagogo-Jack 2002). If the blood glucose levels are poorly controlled, or if the patient is undergoing major surgical procedures, intravenous insulin infusion should be commenced with regular monitoring of blood glucose levels (Marks 2003). Oral hypoglycaemics can generally be recommenced with the patient's first meal postoperatively. In patients that use subcutaneous insulin to manage their diabetes mellitus, the insulin is stopped on the day of surgery and an intravenous insulin infusion administered preoperatively with regular blood glucose monitoring. The key to good perioperative glycaemic control is to keep the patients blood glucose level within a pre-determined range to avoid sudden hyperglycaemia and hypoglycaemia.

The American Diabetes Association (2009) suggests a target range of 4.95-6.93 mmol/l in general surgical patients who are fasting. However a target range of 6.6-9.9 mmol/l has been suggested by Marks (2003). There is no standard target range in literature. The sliding scale infusion illustrated in Figure 1 is only an example and the choice of insulin infusion protocols utilised perioperatively will be dependant on local NHS Trust protocols developed in collaboration with the endocrinologists and anaesthetists. Potassium monitoring (on laboratory venous blood testing or arterial blood gas sampling) is important, as insulin stimulates cellular uptake of potassium. In a typical protocol patients with normal renal function are given 20mmol of potassium per litre of dextrose (Eldridge et al. 1996). Perioperatively it is important to be vigilant of diabetic emergencies such as diabetic ketoacidosis. Early warning signs such as drowsiness, abdominal pain and breathlessness should be noted (DOH 2007). Close monitoring of diabetics perioperatively with complete observations and blood glucose levels every 1-2 hours should also help to intercept any worsening patient states (Rehman et al. 2003). In recognising these emergencies promptly and bringing them to the attention of the anaesthetist, effective management can commence, potentially saving lives.

CONCLUSION

With the worldwide prevalence of diabetes mellitus increasing and more people falling victim to its associated complications, it is likely that surgery on diabetic patients will increase in the future.

Good blood glucose control remains the key to optimisation of the patient's health and prevention of postoperative complications, but must be monitored in addition to all the other perioperative measures discussed and in accordance with local policies and guidelines.

Insulin sliding scale infusion

50 units of Actrapid insulin in 50 mls of Normal saline should be infused at a rate adjusted according to the infusion table below.

Blood glucose (mmol/l)	Insulin infusion rate (mls/hr)
0-4	0.5 (Call doctor)
4.1-7	1
7.1-11	2
11.1-15	3
15.1-20	4
>20	6 (Call doctor)

If the blood glucose is less than 12 mmol/l dextrose can be infused with 20mmol of potassium, and normal saline is given if the blood glucose is greater than 12mmol/l with 20mmol of potassium.

Figure 1.

REFERENCES

American Diabetes Association: All about diabetes [online] Available from: http://www.diabetes.org/about-diabetes.jsp [Accessed December 2009].

Cameron, C. G., Bennett, H. A. 2009 Cost-effectiveness of insulin analogues for diabetes mellitus. *Canadian Medical Association Journal* 180 400-407.

Dagogo-Jack, S., Alberti, K. G. M. 2002 Management of diabetes mellitus in surgical patients. *Diabetes Spectrum* 15 44-48.

Dhinsa, B. S., Khan, W. S., Puri, A. (2010). Management of the diabetic patient in the perioperative period. *J. Perioper. Pract.* 20(10): 364-7.

DOH 2007. *National Service Framework for Diabetes*, London, DOH.

Eldridge, A. J., Sear, J. W. 1996 Perioperative management of diabetic patients: any changes for the better since 1985?. *Anaesthesia* 51 45-51.

Expert Committee on the Diagnosis and Classification of Diabetes Mellitus 2003 Report of the expert committee on the diagnosis and classification of diabetes mellitus. *Diabetes Care* 26 S5-S20.

Falanga, V. 2005 Wound healing and its impairment in the diabetic foot. *Lancet* 366 1736-1743.

Gale, E. A. M., Anderson, J. V. 2002 Diabetes mellitus and other disorders of metabolism. In: Kumar, P., Clark, M. 2002. *Clinical Medicine*, London, WB Saunders.

Golden, S. H., Peart-Vigilance, C., Kao, W. H., et al. 1999 Perioperative glycemic control and the risk of infectious complications in a cohort of adults with diabetes. *Diabetes Care* 22 1408-1414.

Haynes, A. B., Weiser, T. G., Berry, W. R., et al. 2009 A surgical safety checklist to reduce morbidity and mortality in a global population. *New England Journal of Medicine*. 360 491-499.

Hirsch, I. B., McGill, J. B., Cryer, P. E., et al. 1991 Perioperative management of surgical patients with diabetes mellitus. *Anaesthesiology* 74 346-359.

Hoogwerf, B. J. 2006 Perioperative Management of diabetes mellitus: how should we act on the limited evidence? *Cleveland Clinic Journal of Medicine* 73 95-99.

Marhoffer, W., Stein, M., Maeser, E., et al. 1992 Impairment of polymorphonuclear leukocyte function and metabolic control of diabetes. *Diabetes Care* 15 256-260.

Marks, J. B. 2003 Perioperative Management of Diabetes. *American Family Physician* 67 93-100.

Marks, J. B., Skyler, J. S. 1996 Complications of diabetics: diabetic ketoacidosis and hyperosmolar hyperglycaemic nonketotic coma. In: Hurst, J. W. 1996. *Medicine for the practicing physician*, Connecticut, Appleton and Lange.

National Collaborating Centre for Chronic Conditions 2008. *Type 2 Diabetes*, London, Royal College of Physicians.

Patel, K. L. 2008 Impact of tight glucose control on postoperative infection rates and wound healing in cardiac surgery patients. *Journal of Wound, Ostomy and Continence Nursing* 35 397-404.

Rehman, H., Mohammed, K. 2003 Perioperative management of diabetic patients. *Current Surgery* 60 607-611.

Umpierrez, G. E., Kitabchi, A. E. 2003 Diabetic ketoacidosis: risk factors and management strategies. *Treatments in Endocrinology* 2 95-108.

Underwood, J. C. E. 2002 Diabetes Mellitus. In: Underwood, J. C. E. 2002. *General and Systematic Pathology*, Sheffield, Churchill Livingstone.

WHO 2008. *Guidelines for Safe Surgery*, WHO Press.

WHO Diabetes Programme 2010 [online] Available from http://www.who.int/diabetes/facts/world_figures/en/ [Accessed April 2010].

In: Perioperative Practice in Trauma and Orthopaedic Surgery ISBN: 978-1-63483-325-7
Editor: Wasim S. Khan

Chapter 4

PERIOPERATIVE MANAGEMENT OF CARDIAC DISEASE

N. A. Aresti, A. A. Malik, K. M. Ihsan, S. M. Aftab and W. S. Khan*
University College London Institute of Orthopaedic and Musculoskeletal Sciences, Royal National Orthopaedic Hospital, Stanmore, Middlesex, UK

ABSTRACT

Cardiac pathologies are common and need to be managed well in the perioperative period to reduce complications. In this chapter we discuss the management of common cardiac pathologies including coronary artery disease, hypertension, arrhythmias and cardiac failure. We also discuss the management of anticoagulation.

Keywords: Perioperative, cardiac, hypertension, arrhythmias, cardiac failure

INTRODUCTION

In this chapter we discuss the management of common cardiac pathologies (Aresti et al. 2012). Pre-existing cardiac disease contributes significantly to morbidity and mortality amongst patients undergoing non-cardiac surgery. Patients with pre-existing cardiac disease or with risk factors for it, have as much as a 3.9% risk of suffering a major perioperative cardiac event (Devereaux et al. 2005, Lee et al. 1999).

Furthermore, the incidence of perioperative myocardial infarction (MI) is increased 10 to 50 fold in patients with previous coronary events (Jassal et al. 2008).

The pathology behind 'perioperative cardiac events' is not as well understood as that behind 'medical cardiac events.'

* Corresponding author: W. S. Khan, Clinical Lecturer, University College London Institute of Orthopaedics and Musculoskeletal Science, Royal National Orthopaedic Hospital, Stanmore, Middlesex, London, HA7 4LP, UK. Telephone number: +44 (0) 7791 025554, e-mail address: wasimkhan@doctors.org.uk.

Evidence suggests that myocardial oxygen supply-demand discrepancies and plaque ruptures are the end products of several contributory processes. Pain, bleeding and hypothermia inflicted by surgery as well as exposure to anaesthetic agents precipitate a stress reaction by activating the neuroendocrine system. This induces a hyper-coagulate hypoxic and inflammatory state. Furthermore, episodes of relative tachycardia and hypotension have been implicated in further increasing the risk of perioperative events.

Approximately 4.2 million operations are performed each year in the United Kingdom, costing the tax payer well over £1 billion (Hospital Episode Data 2012). Assuming half these patients have an existing cardiac pathology or risk factor, approximately 2 million patients in the country are at risk of a peri-operative cardiac event. A thorough understanding of the pathology and management of this large cohort of patients is therefore essential.

There are several aspects of cardiovascular physiology and pathology that must be considered. This includes myocardial ischaemia, hypertension, arrhythmias, anticoagulation, congestive heart failure and valvular heart disease. In this article we will look at each of these categories and identify key concepts in their management.

1. Myocardial Ischaemia

Myocardial ischaemia is the perhaps the biggest concern for patients undergoing surgery. Up to a quarter of patients with unstable angina develop MI after non-cardiac surgery (Shah et al. 1999). Post-mortem studies have demonstrated that around half of patients who die as a result of peri-operative myocardial ischaemia have pre-existing coronary artery disease (Darood et al. 1996). A higher proportion of deaths are as a result of a thrombus on a background of >50% stenosis as opposed to total occlusion of coronary arteries (Cohen et al. 1999, Ellis et al. 1996).

The American College of Cardiology and American Heart Association have issued guidelines on pre-operative risk stratification for cardiovascular morbidity depending on the severity of surgery, patient related clinical predictors and functional capacity of the patient (Eagle et al. 2002).

Cardiac Risk Stratification for non-cardiac procedures	
High Risk (reported cardiac risk often > 5%)	• Emergency major operations, particularly elderly patients • Aortic and major vascular surgery • Prolonged surgical procedures associated with large fluids shifts/loss.
Intermediate Risk (reported cardiac risk generally < 5%)	• Carotid endarterectomy • Head and neck surgery • Intra-peritoneal/intra-thoracic surgery • Orthopaedic surgery • Prostate surgery
Low Risk (reported cardiac risk generally < 1%)	• Endoscopic procedures • Superficial procedures • Cataract surgery • Breast surgery

<table>
<tr><th colspan="2">Clinical Predictors increased peri-operative cardiovascular risks (MI, congestive heart failure, death)</th></tr>
<tr><td>Major</td><td>• Unstable Coronary Syndromes:
o Acute or recent MI with evidence of important ischaemic risk by clinical symptoms or non-invasive study (acute <7days; Recent 7<days<30)
o Unstable or severe angina
• Decompensated heart failure
• Significant arrhythmias
o High grade atrioventricular block
o Symptomatic ventricular arrhythmias in the presence of underlying heart disease
o Supraventricular arrhythmias with uncontrolled ventricular rate
• Severe valvular disease</td></tr>
<tr><td>Intermediate</td><td>• Mild Angina Pectoris
• Previous MI by history of pathological Q waves
• Compensated or prior heart failure
• Diabetes Mellitus (particularly insulin dependant)
• Renal Insufficiency</td></tr>
<tr><td>Minor</td><td>• Advanced Age
• Abnormal ECG (left ventricular hypertrophy, LBBB, ST-T abnormalities)
• Rhythm other than sinus
• Low functional capacity
• History of stroke
• Uncontrolled systemic hypertension.</td></tr>
</table>

The ACC/AHA committee has devised a detailed algorithm in order to help manage cardiovascular morbidity. In summary, patients with major clinical predictors should have their surgery postponed until appropriate cardiac investigations and management has been instituted. If emergency surgery is absolutely necessary then both patients and family should be made aware of the high risks very clearly.

Patients with intermediate clinical predictors are evaluated according to their functional capacity (using the Duke Activity Status index and expressed at metabolic equivalents (MET) (Eagle et al. 2002). Depending on their functional capacity, tests are undertaken to help predict their cardiac risk and address management.

Low clinical predictor patients should have their necessary investigations if their functional capacity is poor and they are undergoing a high-risk procedure. However, these are not necessary in low or intermediate risk procedures.

Tests for risk stratification recommended by the ACC/AHA committee include:

- Dobutamine stress echocardiography
- Myocardial perfusion scans
- Coronary angiography

Pre-operative tests which induce myocardial ischaemia are the most reliable indicators of peri-operative risk, however positive results are not necessarily accurate at predicting cardiac events. The principle mode of intra-operative myocardial perfusion monitoring involves real-time ECG ST segment trend analysis. Perioperative ST segment changes indicative of myocardial ischaemia are the strongest independent predictor of perioperative cardiac events in high risk surgical patients. Patients experiencing myocardial ischaemia may also show fluctuations in blood-pressure, pulse and end organ perfusion.

2. Hypertension

An estimated 24% of the population are hypertensive and the problems is therefore commonly encounter in surgical practice (Burt et al. 1995). Even though uncontrolled systemic hypertension is considered a minor clinical predictor by the ACC/AHA committee, management of hypertension represents a common and an important challenge to surgical practice (Stewart et al. 1997, Goldman et al. 1977).

Several studies have demonstrated that hypertension increases the risk of perioperative events. One recent meta-analysis for example, analysed over 2000 patients in 30 studies and demonstrated an odds ratio of 1.35 (1.17-1.56) between hypertensive disease and perioperative cardiac outcomes (Howell et al. 2004). This suggests that in the presence of hypertension, there is approximately a 35% risk of perioperative cardiac morbidity.

This increased risk is not only caused by the increased risk of associated coronary artery disease and other hypertensive associated diseases, but also by significant fluctuations in peri-operative blood pressure. Hypertensive patients may experience exaggerated hypotensive responses at induction of anaesthesia. Conversely they are susceptible to heightened pressor responses, leading to hypertension and tachycardia, following intubation and extubation, or following pain caused by surgery itself. Furthermore hypertensive patients are more at risk of significant rises in blood pressure in the post-operative period following factors such as inadequate pain control. These exaggerated fluctuations in blood pressure are not only associated with myocardial ischaemia, but also of heart failure and stroke.

Several factors must be considered when managing hypertensive patients pre-operatively. First a diagnosis of the cause of hypertension must be ascertained. The majority of hypertensive patients have 'essential hypertension' (primary hypertension), i.e. there is no known primary factor causing the raised blood pressure. In a small proportion of hypertensive patients (secondary hypertension) there is a pathological cause.

These pathologies include phaeochromocytomas, renal artery stenosis and coarctation of the aorta. Any potential causes of secondary hypertension must be established as they have several anaesthetic implications. Consequences of hypertension must be predicated and prepared for. End organ damage such a kidney disease, left ventricular hypertrophy and coronary artery disease must be identified as they put the patient in the 'high risk' category.

Drug history must be determined and side effects expected. Diuretics for example may lead to hypokalaemia which may need to be corrected. Most anti-hypertensives may be continued leading up to surgery. ACE inhibitors and angiotensin II receptor agonists however have been shown to cause hypotension if given on the morning of surgery and so are emitted by some anaesthetists.

All hypertensive patients should be evaluated pre-operatively in the elective setting. Those with stage 3 disease (systolic BP >180mmHg or diastolic BP > 110mmHg) or those with stage 2 disease (systolic BP >160mmHg or diastolic BP > 100mmHg) with evidence of target organ disease, should receive pre-operative treatment.

The mode of intra-operative monitoring of blood pressure depends of the severity of surgery and the preference of the anaesthetist. Non-invasive monitoring generally involves the use of an intermittently inflated blood pressure cuff.

Disadvantages include lack of real-time readings, cuff failure and positioning which is often difficult to address intra-operatively in patients where the sterile surgical drapes cover the monitored limb. Invasive monitoring is often used in longer surgical cases or where there are likely to be significant haemodynamic stresses on the patient. This is centred around radial arterial lines which give real time, accurate readings.

However they are invasive and risk introducing infection, causing bleeding and vascular complications such as thromboses and pseudo-aneurysms.

3. Arrhythmias

Arrhythmias are a commonly encountered phenomenon in non-cardiac surgery and have been reported to occur in up to 89% of patients, depending on whether Holter monitors or intermittent ECG monitoring are used to asses for their presence (Katz et al. 1970, Bertrand et al. 1971). Various large studies have identified both ventricular and supraventricular arrhythmias as independent risk factors for perioperative cardiac events (Goldman et al. 1977). Furthermore, the presence of arrhythmias may be an indication of underlying cardiac abnormalities, metabolic issues or drug toxicity. It therefore stands to reason that management of these is important to safe surgical practice.

Supraventricular arrhythmias, in particular atrial fibrillation (AF) are one of the most common perioperative arrhythmias and are seen most often in the elderly. They may produce ischaemia, increasing myocardial oxygen demand, and may deteriorate in to life threatening rhythm disturbances as a result of metabolic disturbances or ischaemia.

Ventricular arrhythmias when not associated with haemodynamic compromise can be left untreated in the perioperative period, although their presence increases the risk of further peri and post operative arrhythmias. When they do occur they should be evaluated accordingly with quantification of ventricular function and presence of coronary artery disease.

The ACC/AHA guidelines incorporate arrhythmias in the clinical outcome predictors. These are considered along the following lines:

1) How serious is the arrhythmia?
2) Does the arrhythmia point to serious but unsuspected cardiopulmonary pathology
3) Whether there is a reversible cause for the arrhythmia (e.g. hypo or hyperkalaemia).

According to these guidelines, supra-ventricular arrhythmias, supra-ventricular arrhythmias with an uncontrolled ventricular rate, and high-grade atrioventricular blocks represent significant arrhythmias and are major clinical predictors (i.e. high risk). Significance is decided on the basis of whether patients are symptomatic.

Asymptomatic arrhythmias are classed as minor clinical predictors and further investigations depend on the functional capacity of the patient. Similar to ischaemia, decisions regarding further investigations and management are in line with the algorithm discussed above. Accordingly a high risk patient should have their surgery postponed unless essential.

Intra-operatively monitoring is also based around real time ECG use. If a patient were to develop an arrhythmia these would manifest in the ECG and may show signs of altered pulse rate, blood pressure fluctuations, poor end organ perfusion and even cardiac arrest.

When arrhythmias such as AF are detected in the community or in pre-assessment, treatment often constitutes cardioversion (DC or chemical) or rate control if this is not successful or appropriate. This is usually undertaken by cardiology in conjunction with the general practitioner. The risks of AF include intra-cardiac emboli leading to cerebrovascular accident (ischaemic stroke) and myocardial ischaemia among others.

4. ANTICOAGULATION

Patients who present for surgery on anticoagulation are at an increased risk of haemorrhage or, if the anticoagulation is stopped, of thrombosis. As a result the treating team must firstly decide on whether the risk is appropriate, easier perhaps in cases of life or limb threatening injury. The risk stratification must include a decision on whether anticoagulation must be stopped and whether to use a bridging agent. This is based on the clinical indication for anticoagulation. No risk stratification system has been validated, however the American College of Chest Physicians have issued guidelines separating patients into those at high, moderate or low risk (Lee et al. 2007).

	Mechanical Heart Valve	AF	VTE
High	• Mitral valves • Caged/tilting disc aortic valves • Recent (6 months) TIA/Stroke	• $CHADS_2$ of 5-6 • Recent (3 months) TIA/Stroke • Rheumatic valve disease	• Recent (3 months) VTE • Severe thrombophilia
Moderate	• Bileaflet aortic valve prosthesis AND either: AF, prior TIA/stroke, HTN, DM, CCF, >75 years	• $CHADS_2$ of 3-4	• VTE within past 3-12 months • Non-severe thrombophilic conditions • Recurrent VTE • Active cancer
Low	• Bileaflet aortic valve prosthesis without AF and no other risk factors	• $CHADS_2$ of 0-2	• Single VTE > 12 months prior

Table adapted from ACCP guidelines (Lee et al. 2007).

The guidelines recommend the following, as per the determined risk:

Risk	Recommendations
High	Bridging anticoagulation with therapeutic-dose SC LMWH or IV UH over no bridging during temporary interruption of VKA therapy
Moderate	Bridging anticoagulation with therapeutic-dose SC LMWH, therapeutic-dose IV UFH, or low-dose SC LMWH over no bridging during temporary interruption of VKA therapy
Low	Low-dose SC LMWH or no bridging over bridging with therapeutic-dose SC LMWH or IV UFH

UFH = Unfractioned heparin.
LMWH = Low molecular weight heparin.
VKA = Vitamin K antagonist.

Patients with coronary stents also pose a problem. The guidelines suggest that patients with bare metal stents within 6 weeks of placement should continue their anti-platelet therapy during the course of their surgery. Patients with drug eluding stents should continue their anti-platelet therapy within the first 12 months of their stent placement.

5. Congestive Heart Failure (CHF)

Heart failure is common and there are large bodies of evidence for its management. The New York Heart Association (NYHA) classification describes heart failure in four categories based on symptoms. This provides medical teams with rates of mortality and quality of life (Lee et al. 2007). The ACC/AHA also offers a four part classification which highlights the progressive course of heart failure and helps identify those at risk.

Perioperative heart failure has not only been identified as a major risk factor for surgery itself, but medication used to treat heart failure has important anaesthetic considerations. Postoperative heart failure occurs in 1-6% of patients, but this figure rises to 6-25% if there is a history of existing heart failure, valvular heart disease or coronary artery disease (Goldman et al. 1977, Charlson et al. 1991, Mangano et al. 1990).

Medical optimisation prior to surgery is of paramount importance.

Diuretics, beta blockers and ACE inhibitors form the bulk of drugs used to do so. Evidence suggests however that perioperative use of ACE inhibitors may lead to significant hypotension at induction after all modalities of anaesthesia (Groban et al. 2006). Many anaesthetists therefore omit the dose of ACE inhibitor on the day of surgery.

Intraoperative management of heart failure includes preserving cardiac output, based around the availability of adrenaline, care over the use of vasopressors and use of inotropes such as dobutamine or phosphpdiasterase inhbitors.

Furthermore myocardial work must be minimised. This is achieved through adequate analgesia, consideration during factors which precipitate tachycardia, e.g. intubation, hypovolaemia, anaemia etc. and the reduction of afterload.

New York Heart Association Classification		
I	No limitation of physical activity. Ordinary physical activity does not cause undue fatigue, palpitation, or dyspnoea (shortness of breath)	
II	Slight limitation of physical activity. Comfortable at rest, but ordinary physical activity results in fatigue, palpitation, or dyspnoea.	
III	Marked limitation of physical activity. Comfortable at rest, but less than ordinary activity causes fatigue, palpitation, or dyspnoea.	
IV	Unable to carry out any physical activity without discomfort. Symptoms of cardiac insufficiency at rest. If any physical activity is undertaken, discomfort is increased.	
ACC / AHA		
A	At risk for heart failure but without structural heart disease or symptoms of HF	e.g. patients with HTN, CAD, DM or patients using cardiotoxins or with a family history
B	Structural heart disease without symptoms of HF	e.g. patients with previous MI, LV dysfunction, asymptomatic valvular disease
C	Structural heart disease with prior or current symptoms of HF	e.g. patients with known structural death disease, SOB and fatigue, reduced exercise tolerance
D	Refractory HF requiring specialized interventions	e.g. Patients who have marked symptoms at rest despite maximal medical therapy

Adapted from: Hunt SA et al. ACC/AHA Guidelines for the Evaluation and Management of Chronic Heart Failure in the Adult: An Executive Summary. *J. Heart Lung Transplant.* 2003;21:189–203.

6. Aortic Stenosis (AS)

Aortic stenosis is another risk factor for cardiac complications of non-cardiac surgery. The risk is considerably increased when in the presence of arrhythmias and heart failure (Goldman et al. 1977). The prevalence of aortic stenosis in the general population is approximately 2% (Stewart et al. 1997). The normal aortic valve area is 2.6 - 3.5cm^2 in adults and significant haemodynamic obstruction occurs when the area approaches 1.0cm^2. As the stenosis increases, so does the work of the left ventricle and consequentially its size. The ventricle initially hypertrophies in response to increased systolic pressure and eventually stiffens causing diastolic dysfunction in the aid of maintaining systolic function and cardiac output. As diastolic function further deteriorates and leads to lower aortic pressures and a reduction in myocardial oxygen demand. In the latter stages of the disease, cardiac output, stroke volume and valvular pressure gradients all fall. This leads to the symptoms of angina, dyspnoea and syncope. The pathology of aortic stenosis is such that atrial work load becomes more significant in maintaining systolic function and the heart relies on preload and hence systemic vascular resistance. Intraoperative maintenance of heart rate and sinus rhythm, and preventing variations in blood pressure are thus imperative in maintaining cardiac output.

If a patient presents for surgery with asymptomatic or low - moderate aortic stenosis, they should be evaluated and treated for concomitant coronary artery disease prior to surgery. If a patient has symptomatic or severe aortic stenosis they should, where possible, have their valvular disease treated prior to undergoing their non-cardiac surgery.

Conclusion

There are multiple factors one must consider when dealing with perioperative cardiac disease. Thorough preoperative evaluation and preparation of patients for surgery is paramount. Decisions on which investigations and treatments should be initiated are made easier through the use of various published guidelines, however one must always fully understand the pathologies and evidence behind these decisions, particularly when dealing with emergency cases. Where there is any doubt in whether an investigation should be conducted, we refer the reader to the NICE "CG3 Preoperative tests" guideline, which gives a comprehensive guide as to what tests should be requested, based on the ASA and type of surgery (Reynolds et al. 2006). We would recommend a low threshold for contacting a cardiologist for further management of patients with coronary stents, undiagnosed arrhythmias, and patients with structural heart disease of NYHA grade IV or complex valvular disease. Furthermore, local guidelines and/or haematologists should be contacted to discuss reversing anticoagulants or bridging agents.

Whereas much of the research cited in this article is British in origin, the majority of large clinical trials and guidelines produced are from overseas. This may introduce problems due to discrepancies between our health care systems, but the quoted guidelines are the most commonly employed in the UK and as such we recommend their use.

Furthermore, many of the larger clinical trials, although dated demonstrate the basic science of cardiovascular disease with relevance to anaesthetic particularly well. Given many of the disease associations were made several decades ago, newer clinical trials along those lines have not been conducted as they have been deemed unnecessary.

References

Aresti, N. A., Malik, A. A., Ihsan, K. M., Aftab, S. M., Khan, W. S. (2014). Perioperative management of cardiac disease. *J. Periop. Pract.* 24(1-2): 9-14.

Bertrand, C. A. 1971 Disturbances of cardiac rhythm during anesthesia and surgery. *JAMA* 216 1615-17.

Burt, V. L. 1995 Prevalence of hypertension in the US adult population. Results from the Third National Health and Nutrition Examination Survey, 1988-1991. *Hypertension* 25 (3) 303-4.

Charlson, M. E. 1991 Risk for postoperative congestive heart failure. *Surg. Gynecol. Obstet.* 172(2) 95.

Cohen, M. C. 1999 Histological analysis of coronary artery lesions in fatal postoperative myocardial infarction. *Cardiovascular Pathology* 8 133-9.

Dawood, M. M. 1996 Pathology of fatal perioperative myocardial infarction: implications regarding pathophysiology and prevention. *International Journal of Cardiology* 57 37-44.

Devereaux, P. J. 2005 Perioperative cardiac events in patients undergoing noncardiac surgery: a review of the magnitude of the problem, the pathophysiology of the events and methods to estimate and communicate risk. *Canadian Medical Association Journal* 173 627-34.

Eagle, K. A. 2002 ACC/AHA Guideline Update for Perioperative Cardiovascular Evaluation for Noncardiac Surgery--Executive Summary. A report of the American College of Cardiology/American Heart Association Task Force on Practice Guidelines (Committee to Update the 1996 Guidelines on Perioperative Cardiovascular Evaluation for Noncardiac Surgery). *Anesth. Analg.* 94(5)1052-64.

Ellis, S. G. 1996 Angiographic correlates of cardiac death and myocardial infarction complicating major nonthoracic vascular surgery. *American Journal of Cardiology* 77 1126-8.

Goldman, L. 1977 Multifactorial index of cardiac risk in noncardiac surgical procedures. *N. Engl. J. Med.* 297 845-50.

Groban, L. 2006 Perioperative management of chronic heart failure. *Anesth. Analg.* 103(3) 557-75.

Hospital Episode Data, Department of Health.

Howell, S. J. 2004 Review: hypertension, hypertensive heart disease and perioperative cardiac risk. *Br. J. Anaesth.* 92 570-83.

Jassal, D. 2008 Perioperative cardiac management. *eMedicine* 285328.

Katz, R. L. 1970 Cardiac arrhythmias during anaesthesia and operation. *Anesthesiology* 33 193-213.

Lee, A. 2007 ACC/AHA 2007 Guidelines on Perioperative Cardiovascular Evaluation and Care for Noncardiac Surgery: Executive Summary: A Report of the American College of Committee to Revise the 2002 Guidelines on Perioperative Cardiovascular Evaluation for Cardiology/American Heart Association Task Force on Practice Guidelines (Writing Noncardiac Surgery). *Circulation* 116 1971-1996.

Lee, T. H. 1999 Derivation and prospective validation of a simple index for prediction of cardiac risk of major noncardiac surgery. *Circulation* 100 1043-49.

Mangano, D. T. 1990 Association of perioperative myocardial ischemia with cardiac morbidity and mortality in men undergoing noncardiac surgery. The Study of Perioperative Ischemia Research Group. *N. Engl. J. Med.* 323(26) 1781.

Reynolds, T. M. 2006 *National Institute for Health and Clinical Excellence guidelines on preoperative.*

Shah, K. B. 1990 Angina and other risk factors in patients with cardiac disease undergoing noncardiac operations. *Anesth. Analg.* 70(3) 240-247.

Stewart, B. F. 1997 Clinical factors associated with calcific aortic valve disease. Cardiovascular Health Study. *J. Am. Coll. Cardiol.* 29(3) 630-4.

In: Perioperative Practice in Trauma and Orthopaedic Surgery ISBN: 978-1-63483-325-7
Editor: Wasim S. Khan

Chapter 5

Perioperative Management of Respiratory Disease

Wasim S. Khan*[*] and Jonathan J. E. White
University College London Institute of Orthopaedics and Musculoskeletal Sciences, Royal National Orthopaedic Hospital, Stanmore, London, UK

Abstract

Respiratory disease contributes significantly to the perioperative challenges of surgery. Pre-existing pulmonary comorbidities and respiratory complications can have profound effects on patient outcomes. Knowledge of these conditions and the potentially deleterious effects of anaesthesia and surgery can enable clinicians to optimize lung function, reduce complications and improve results.

Keywords: Surgery, respiratory disease, anaesthesia

Introduction

This chapter deals with the perioperative management of respiratory disease (Ihsan et al. 2012). A large number of procedures take place worldwide and up to 25% of perioperative complications are associated with the respiratory system (Mark 2009). Respiratory management is therefore a vital part of any surgical procedure.

Even in healthy patients, anaesthetic and surgical intervention can cause significant respiratory compromise. Anaesthesia and medications used for it affect both the mechanics of breathing and the neurochemical drive to breathing.

[*] Corresponding author: Mr Wasim S. Khan, Clinical Lecturer, University College London Institute of Orthopaedic and Musculoskeletal Research, Royal National Orthopaedic Hospital, Stanmore, London, HA7 4LP, UK. Telephone number: +44 (0) 77791 025554, fax number: +44 (0) 1707 655059, e-mail address: wasimkhan@doctors.org.uk.

Deep vein thrombosis and subsequent pulmonary embolism is not going to be considered in this discussion as it is not generally considered a respiratory side-effect and is outside the remit of this article. Quiet breathing involves diaphragmatic and intercostal contraction with passive expiration due to elastic recoil of the lungs and chest wall.

Accessory structures in respiration include neck, shoulder and abdominal muscles and are involved in active or distressed breathing (Cuschieri et al. 2001). Muscle relaxants and anaesthesia paralyses the diaphragm and reduces the compliance of the respiratory system.

Other anaesthetic and analgesic techniques such as intercostal nerve blocks also reduce activity of important respiratory structures. There is an overall reduction in lung volume, ventilation and gas exchange with resultanttelectasis and ventilation perfusion mismatch (Mark 2009). Surgery on the abdomen or chest further impairs function of the respiratory muscles and compliance of the chest wall and lungs. Anaesthetic and opiate drugs also inhibit the respiratory drive perioperatively, reducing the hypercapnic and hypoxic responses. The net effect compromises respiratory function and leads to complications such as hypoxia, hypercapnia, dyspnoea, infection, pneumonia, pleural effusion and respiratory failure.

Respiratory disease such as asthma and COPD (Chronic Obstructive Pulmonary Disease) is extremely prevalent worldwide. It is predicted that up to 17% of over 65s worldwide will have some form of obstructive airways disease (Diaz-Guzman and Mannino 2010).

These significantly increase the risk of perioperative respiratory complications. Careful management of the respiratory system in the perioperative period is therefore essential. The respiratory system must be assessed carefully preoperatively, optimised, monitored and managed in the intraoperative and postoperative period with great vigilance.

Preoperative Assessment

A thorough history and examination is essential to safe and effective perioperative respiratory management. History of any respiratory disease and recent symptomatology should be actively sought, including hospital attendances and admissions. Shortness of breath, exercise intolerance, cough and history of smoking are important. History of asthma, COPD, obstructive sleep apnoea, or any other respiratory illness should be considered. Examination should include inspection, auscultation and special tests looking for wheeze, crackles, decreased breath sounds or a prolonged expiratory phase. A general examination must also be performed on the patient. The patient's general health status, obesity, alcohol consumption, age, other medical history including interstitial lung disease, neurological impairment and immunosuppression should be given great importance.

A preoperative chest radiograph is a very commonly ordered radiological examination. However evidence suggests that unless there are risk factors a routine chest radiograph should not be performed (Munro et al. 1997). The Association of Anaesthetists of Great Britain and Ireland recommend that anyone scheduled for admission to critical care should have a preoperative chest radiograph (Verma et al. 2010). In a systematic review of the literature, Joo et al. (2005) found that postoperative complications were similar between patients who had a preoperative chest radiograph and those who did not. Preoperative chest radiographs findings led to a change in management of 10% of patients who had radiographs for established cardio-pulmonary disease. Pulmonary function tests may also be considered.

However, the results are not predictive of postoperative complication rate (Smetana 2006) unless the patient is undergoing lung resection (Mark 2009). These tests should be considered only if a patient is to undergo lung resection surgery or there is unexplained shortness of breath or respiratory symptoms found on preoperative assessment. Even in abdominal surgery, spirometry is not predictive of complication rates (Lawrence et al. 1989). Spirometry is therefore not to be performed routinely in preoperative assessment.

Other investigations such as arterial blood gas have not been found to be useful in predicting postoperative respiratory complications (Fisher et al. 2002) unless there is existing acute or chronic respiratory disease. Patients with obstructive lung disease such as asthma should have their function optimised preoperatively. This may be defined as an absence of symptoms and a FEV_1 of greater than 80% predicted or personal best (Mark 2009).

Asthma is known to increase respiratory complications such as atelectasis and infection (NAEPP 2007). Similarly COPD must also be optimised before surgery. Patients with COPD are also known to be at increased risk of pulmonary complications including mortality (Fuster et al. 2006). Optimisation includes use of bronchodilators, steroids and antibiotics as necessary. Chest infections or infective exacerbations of COPD are a relative contraindication to anaesthesia or surgery and the merits of surgery must be weighed against the risks on an individual basis by the anaesthetist and the surgeon.

The clinician must also have a high index of suspicion for conditions such as obstructive sleep apnoea (OSA). OSA can cause can lead to significant perioperative complications such as hypoxia, hypercapnia, need to re-intubate, difficult airway, difficult intubation, obstructed airway and respiratory arrest with opioid usage (Cullen 2001, Gupta et al. 2001). Often patients themselves are unaware of OSA. Clinicians should suspect OSA in patients with a history snoring, daytime somnolescence and sleep disturbance. OSA is commoner in obese patients as adipose tissue deposits in the pharyngeal tissue.

To anticipate difficulties that may be experienced during intubation of a patient with OSA the Mallampati score has been used (Mallampati et al. 1985). This grades the oropharynx visually into 4 classes based on what structures are easy to see. A high score is associated with OSA and precautionary measures should be used accordingly.

It is also important to identify smokers. Smoking is associated with significant complications in the respiratory system (Moores 2000). Smoking reduces mucociliary clearance and the immune response. Therefore infections are more common in smokers than those who have never smoked. Smoking cessation is recommended before all surgical and anaesthetic procedures but it is unclear as to the optimal time frame for smoking cessation.

It seems that at least four to eight weeks of smoking cessation is required for significant reductions in smoking related complications (Nakagawa et al. 2001). However there is some evidence to suggest that there is also a paradoxical effect if smoking is ceased a short time before surgery only. This may be due to increased mucous production or possibly due to the abrupt end of the irritant effect of smoke and therefore a reduced cough response for mucous clearance (Mark 2009).

Despite these considerations, it is still recommended that smoking cessation is pursued before surgery (Theadom and Cropley 2006) as patients given support for smoking cessation with pharmacological or psychological means do better than those who do not.

Furthermore, patients who quit smoking 6 months before surgery have a risk similar to those who have never smoked although there are still slight increases in risk until 1 year after smoking cessation in terms of postoperative pneumonia (Arozullah et al. 2003).

Long term corticosteroid usage before surgery is associated with a risk of respiratory complications (Mark 2009). However, patients receiving steroids should have their therapy continued to avoid the effects of adreno-cortical suppression.

Patient education is also known to be of significant benefit particularly in high risk surgery. This includes inspiratory muscle training by physiotherapists aimed at strengthening muscles of respiration and teaching patient deep breathing and coughing exercises (Dronkers et al. 2008).

RISK STRATIFICATION

The American Society of Anaesthesiologists (ASA) classification system is the most commonly used risk stratification system. It is based on history, examination and preoperative findings. A patient with a higher ASA class has a higher risk of postoperative complications (Clague at al. 2002). The ASA class is as follows:

Class I: normal, healthy patient without organic, physiological, or psychiatric disturbance (e.g., healthy with good exercise tolerance).

Class II: controlled medical conditions without significant systemic effects (e.g., controlled hypertension or controlled diabetes without systemic effects, cigarette smoking without COPD, anaemia, mild obesity, age younger than 1 year or older than 70 years, pregnancy).

Class III: medical conditions with significant systemic effects, intermittently associated with significant functional compromise (e.g. controlled heart failure, stable angina, old myocardial infarct, poorly controlled hypertension, mild obesity, bronchospasm with intermittent symptoms, chronic renal failure).

Class IV: medical condition that is poorly controlled, associated with significant dysfunction and is a potential threat to life (e.g. Unstable angina, symptomatic COPD, symptomatic heart failure, hepato-renal failure).

Class V: critical medical condition that is associated with little chance of survival with or without the surgical procedure (e.g., multi-organ failure, sepsis syndrome with haemodynamic instability, hypothermia, poorly controlled coagulopathy).

Class VI: brain dead and undergoing anaesthesia for the purposes of organ retrieval and donation.

Other risk indices have been developed such as the Goldman Cardiac risk index but their predictive ability is uncertain (Melendez and Carlon 1998).

INTRAOPERATIVE MANAGEMENT

Once the patient is prepared and ready for surgery, they will in most cases receive either local, regional or general anaesthesia with additional analgesia. Respiratory management in cases of local and regional anaesthesia usually include oxygen administration (with relative contraindications such as COPD kept in mind), pulse oximetry, and clinical assessment of the rate of breathing.

Often talking to the patient and gauging their response is sufficient to confirm that the airway is patent and the patient is sufficiently alert to maintain an airway, breathe and communicate. In cases of general anaesthesia, the patient is pre-oxygenated and either a laryngeal mask airway (LMA) or a more secure airway is placed carefully by the anaesthetist during induction of anaesthesia. Adequate placement is confirmed by inspecting the chest for bilaterally equal chest movements and auscultation of air entry to both lungs or as deemed appropriate. Oxygen saturation is carefully monitored with pulse oximetry. A carbon dioxide monitor (capnograph) is also placed near the airway to measure the concentration of expired carbon dioxide and ensure that sufficient gas exchange is taking place in the lungs. Blood gas analysis can be performed intermittently to measure blood pH, partial pressures of oxygen or carbon dioxide and bicarbonate levels. Adjustments are made as necessary.

There are myriad factors which influence the respiratory outcome in surgery and all must be kept in consideration. Distance of the surgical site from the diaphragm is known to be inversely related to respiratory complications (Arozullah et al. 2003). Similarly, the longer the operation and anaesthesia time, the higher the rates of respiratory complications. Minimally invasive surgery (such as laparoscopic cholycystectomy versus open cholecystectomy) is also known to carry a lower incidence of respiratory complications (Torrington et al. 1996).

The method of anaesthesia employed is also thought to significantly affect respiratory morbidity. Even though it is generally thought that spinal or epidural anaesthesia is better than general anaesthesia, evidence suggests that it is the addition of a spinal or epidural anaesthesia to the general anaesthetic that contributes to the lower rate of respiratory complications rather than the avoidance of general anaesthesia alone (Rodgers et al. 2000). The effects of regional versus general anaesthesia in patients with obstructive airways disease is less clear (Warner 2000), although it is generally accepted that regional is recommended over general anaesthesia in order to avoid oral airway involvement (Haeck et al. 2009). Regional anaesthesia may also reduce the activity of respiratory muscles leading to further compromise. In addition, specific drugs used during anaesthesia also affect respiratory complication rates. Intermediate-acting neuromuscular blockers (such as atracurium or vecuronium) for example, seem to be less detrimental than longer-acting blockers (such as Pancuronium). Opioids are relatively well tolerated in asthmatics (Groeben 2004).

Patients known to have COPD or asthma may benefit from prophylactic beta-2 adrenergic agonists (such as salbutamol) to reduce the risk of bronchospasm. The administration of corticosteroids should also be considered depending on the patient's functional status, lung function tests, type of surgery and/or history of previous usage (Silvanus et al. 2004). Volatile anaesthetic drugs are generally preferred due to their inhibitory effect on bronchospasm (e.g. halothane and sevoflurane) (Groeben 2004).

Patients with OSA may benefit from pre- and postoperative continuous positive airway pressure management (CPAP). Intubation is performed carefully with the patient in the sniffing position to aid visualisation of oropharyngeal structures. A fibre optic scope may be used to aid intubation. Full reversal of neuromuscular blockade is required before extubation.

The administration of sedatives and opioid analgesics in OSA and COPD patients has to be undertaken with great caution (Haeck et al. 2009). These drugs cause respiratory depression, inhibit airway muscle activity and depress pharyngeal tone, increasing the risk of apnoeic events. A regional or local anaesthesia is preferred generally. Narcotic analgesics should also be substituted for other drugs such as non-steroidal anti inflammatory drugs

(NSAIDS), where appropriate. If unavoidable, use should be carefully titrated to pain and the patient monitored closely. CPAP should be available at all times.

Pneumothorax is a complication worthy of mention. This can occur as a results of barotrauma after general anaesthetic, other trauma (which may also be iatrogenic) or spontaneous. It leads to accumulation of air in the pleural space and can cause significant morbidity in otherwise well patients. Rates of pneumothorax are higher in cardio-thoracic surgery for obvious reasons and in patients who have COPD, possibly to due perforation of pulmonary bullae.

A pneumothorax can rapidly progress to a tension pneumothorax if a one-way valve mechanism becomes established. Therefore one must be vigilant and continuously monitor chest wall movements, tracheal position, oxygen tension and the general state of the patient. Prompt action has to be taken (e.g. needle thoracostomy with subsequent chest drain) if necessary (Haeck et al. 2009).

Postoperative Management

In general anaesthesia, once the neuromuscular blocking agents are reversed, the patient is extubated once airway maintenance is ensured. In general, a patient who coughs and pulls out their own airway their airway is safe to extubate. Whether a regional or general anaesthesia is used, respiratory monitoring postoperatively is important to ensure the patient is adequately maintaining an airway and has adequate gas exchange.

This is measured again by pulse oximetry and capnography, ensuring oxygenation and ventilation respectively (Haeck et al. 2009). Inspection of the patient, monitoring chest movements and listening for snoring are equally important. If there are any concerns, a simple manoeuvre such as a chin-lift or jaw thrust may be used with airway adjuncts such as an orophayngeal or a nasopharyngeal tube.

Early mobilisation is essential all cases postoperatively. Lung expansion manoeuvres, guided by physiotherapists and nursing staff and continuous positive airway pressure (CPAP) in selected cases are all useful methods to avoid respiratory complications (Overend et al. 2001, Kindgen-Milles et al. 2005).

Pain must be well controlled, especially if surgery involves the abdomen and thorax where pain will inhibit respiratory muscle activity, thereby further reducing tidal volume, promoting atelectasis and causing infection (Cuschieri et al. 1985). This can be achieved by patient controlled analgesia, epidural analgesia, oral analgesia with, local anaesthesia administered at the end of surgery or any other analgesic modality. Paracetamol, narcotic drugs, NSAIDS or neuromodulators such as gabapentin may be used as appropriate.

References

Arozullah, A. M., Conde, M. V., Lawrence, V. A. 2003 Preoperative evaluation for postoperative pulmonary complications. *The Medical Clinics of North America* 87(1) 153-173.

Clague, J. E., Craddock, E., Andrew, G., Horan, M. A., Pendleton, N. 2002 Predictors of outcome following hip fracture. Admission time predicts length of stay and in-hospital mortality. *Injury* 33(1) 1-6.

Cullen, D. J. 2001 Obstructive sleep apnea and postoperative analgesia - a potentially dangerous combination. *Journal of Clinical Anesthesia* 13(2) 83-85.

Cuschieri, A., Steele, R. J., Moossa, A. R. 2001 Essential surgical practice: basic surgical training London, Hodder Arnold.

Cuschieri, R. J., Morran, C. G., Howie, J. C., McArdle, C. S. 1985 Postoperative pain and pulmonary complications: comparison of three analgesic regimens. *The British Journal of Surgery* 72(6) 495-498.

Diaz-Guzman, E., Mannino, D. M. 2010 Airway obstructive diseases in older adults: from detection to treatment. *The Journal of Allergy and Clinical Immunology* 126(4) 702-709.

Dronkers, J., Veldman, A., Hoberg, E., van der Waal, C., van Meeteren, N. 2008 Prevention of pulmonary complications after upper abdominal surgery by preoperative intensive inspiratory muscle training: a randomized controlled pilot study. *Clinical Rehabilitation* 22(2) 134-142.

Fisher, B. W., Majumdar, S. R., McAlister, F. A. Predicting pulmonary complications after nonthoracic surgery: a systematic review of blinded studies. *The American Journal of Medicine* 112(3) 219-225.

Fuster, R. G., Argudo, J. A., Albarova, O. G., et al. Prognostic value of chronic obstructive pulmonary disease in coronary artery bypass grafting. *European Journal of Cardio-thoracic Surgery* 29(2) 202-209.

Groeben, H. 2004 Strategies in the patient with compromised respiratory function. *Best Practice and Research. Clinical Anaesthesiology* 18(4) 579-594.

Gupta, R. M., Parvizi, J., Hanssen, A. D., Gay, P. C. 2001 Postoperative complications in patients with obstructive sleep apnea syndrome undergoing hip or knee replacement: a case-control study. *Mayo Clinic Proceedings* 76(9) 897-905.

Haeck, P. C., Swanson, J. A., Iverson, R. E., Lynch, D. J. 2009 Evidence-based patient safety advisory: patient assessment and prevention of pulmonary side effects in surgery. Part 1. Obstructive sleep apnea and obstructive lung disease. *Plastic and Reconstructive Surgery* 124(4 Suppl.) 45S-56S.

Ihsan, K. M., Nannaparaju, M. R., Aftab, S., Khan, W. S., Malik, A. A., White, J. J. E. (2012). Perioperative management of chronic respiratory disease. *J. Periop. Pract.* 22 (10): 324-7.

Joo, H. S., Wong, J., Naik, V. N., Savoldelli, G. L. 2005 The value of screening preoperative chest x-rays: a systematic review. *Canadian Journal of Anaesthesia* 52(6) 568-574.

Kindgen-Milles, D., Muller, E., Buhl, R., Bohner, H., Ritter, D., Sandmann, W., Tarnow, J. 2005 Nasal-continuous positive airway pressure reduces pulmonary morbidity and length of hospital stay following thoracoabdominal aortic surgery. *Chest* 128(2) 821-828.

Lawrence, V. A., Page, C. P., Harris, G. D. 1989 Preoperative spirometry before abdominal operations. A critical appraisal of its predictive value. *Archives of Internal Medicine* 149 (2) 280-285.

Mallampati, S. R., Gatt, S. P., Gugino, L., Desai, S. P., Waraksa, B., Freiberger, D., Liu, P. L. 1985 A clinical sign to predict difficult tracheal intubation: a prospective study. *Canadian Journal of Anaesthesia* 32(4) 429-434.

Melendez, J. A., Carlon, V. A. 1998 Cardiopulmonary risk index does not predict complications after thoracic surgery. *Chest* 114(1) 69-75.

Moores, L. K. 2000 Smoking and postoperative pulmonary complications: an evidence-based review of the recent literature. *Clinics in Chest Medicine* 21(1) 139-146.

Munro, J., Booth, A., Nicholl, J. 1997 Routine preoperative testing: a systematic review of the evidence. *Health Technology Assessment* 1(12) 1-62.

Nakagawa, M., Tanaka, H., Tsukuma, H., Kishi, Y. 2001 Relationship between the duration of the preoperative smoke-free period and the incidence of postoperative pulmonary complications after pulmonary surgery. *Chest* 120(3) 705-710.

National Asthma Education and Prevention Program (NAEPP) 2007 Expert Panel Report 3 (EPR-3): Guidelines for the Diagnosis and Management of Asthma – Summary Report 2007. *The Journal of Allergy and Clinical Immunology* 120(5 Suppl.) S94-S138.

Overend, T. J., Anderson, C. M., Lucy, S. D., Bhatia, C., Jonsson, B. I., Timmermans, C. 2001 The effect of incentive spirometry on postoperative pulmonary complications: a systematic review. *Chest* 120(3) 971-978.

Rodgers, A., Walker, N., Schug, S., et al. 2000 Reduction of postoperative mortality and morbidity with epidural or spinal anaesthesia: results from overview of randomised trials. *British Medical Journal* 321(7275) 1493.

Silvanus, M. T., Groeben, H., Peters, J. 2004 Corticosteroids and inhaled salbutamol in patients with reversible airway obstruction markedly decrease the incidence of bronchospasm after tracheal intubation. *Anesthesiology* 100(5) 1052-1057.

Smetana, G. W. 2006 Preoperative pulmonary evaluation: identifying and reducing risks for pulmonary complications. *Cleveland Clinic Journal of Medicine* 73(Suppl. 1) S36-S41.

Theadom, A., Cropley, M. 2006 Effects of preoperative smoking cessation on the incidence and risk of intraoperative and postoperative complications in adult smokers: a systematic review. *Tobacco Control* 15(5) 352-358.

Torrington, K. G., Bilello, J. F., Hopkins, T. K., Hall, E. A. Jr 1996 Postoperative pulmonary changes after laparoscopic cholecystectomy. *Southern Medical Journal* 89(7) 675-678.

Verma, R., Wee, M. Y. K., Hartle, A., et al. 2010. *Pre-operative Assessment and Patient Preparation: The Role of the Anaesthetist* [online] Available from: http://www.aagbi.org/publications/guidelines/docs/preop_2010.pdf [Accessed March 2011].

Warner, D. O. 2000 Preventing postoperative pulmonary complications: the role of the anaesthesiologist. *Anaesthesiology* 92(5) 1467-1472.

Yoder, M. A., Sharma, S. 2009. *Perioperative Pulmonary Management* [online] Last updated 11/03/2009 Available from: http://emedicine.medscape.com/article/284983-overview [Accessed March 2011].

In: Perioperative Practice in Trauma and Orthopaedic Surgery ISBN: 978-1-63483-325-7
Editor: Wasim S. Khan

Chapter 6

MANAGEMENT OF ANTICOAGULATION THERAPY IN THE PERIOPERATIVE PATIENT

Baljinder S. Dhinsa, Hiteshkumar Tailor and Wasim S. Khan*

University College London Institute of Orthopaedics and Musculoskeletal Science, Royal National Orthopaedic Hospital, Stanmore, Middlesex, London, UK

ABSTRACT

With the increasing use of oral anticoagulation therapy the appropriate management of perioperative anticoagulation is of surgical importance. There is a delicate balance between the risk of a perioperative thromboembolic event and the risk of operative bleeding from anticoagulation. Whilst there are a range of options available to the clinician, there appears to be no precise agreement as to how to best manage this problem.

Keywords: Anticoagulation, surgery, warfarin, unfractionated heparin, low molecular weight heparin

INTRODUCTION

This chapter deals with the management of perioperative anticoagulation (Dhinsa et al. 2011), that is becoming an increasingly important surgical dilemma as the prevalence of people requiring oral anticoagulation therapy rises. Vital to the management of this is an understanding of the risk of a perioperative thromboembolic event from inadequate anticoagulation versus the risk of excessive bleeding from anticoagulation.

---

* Corresponding author: Mr W. S. Khan, Clinical Lecturer, University College London Institute of Orthopaedics and Musculoskeletal Science, Royal National Orthopaedic Hospital, Stanmore, Middlesex, London, HA7 4LP, UK. Telephone number: +44 (0) 7971 190720, fax number: +44 (0) 20 8570 3864, e-mail address: wasimkhan @doctors.org.uk.

Both thromboemboli and excessive bleeding can cause significant morbidity and mortality, and also have significant implications on resources (Chimutengwende-Gordon et al. 2010). Oral anticoagulation therapy, commonly Warfarin in the United Kingdom, is usually given for atrial fibrillation, venous thromboembolism, mechanical heart valves and thrombophilia states such as patients with antiphospholipid antibody syndrome, antithrombion III deficiency, and protein C and protein S deficiency.

Those taking oral anticoagulation may be at risk of having a thromboembolic event if this therapy was stopped preoperatively without any cover during the perioperative period. Unfractionated intravenous heparin (UFH) and subcutaneous low molecular weight heparin (LMWH) are commonly used perioperative anticoagulation agents, as well as being used in the intensive care setting and in medical patients.

The problem that perioperative teams encounter is that there is no agreement on the optimal perioperative anticoagulation management of patients receiving oral anticoagulants partly due to the individuality of each case, and the perioperative team need to be guided by haematology departments who are involved with the care of the patient.

HOW ANTICOAGULANTS WORK

The coagulation cascade is part of a series of events that leads to haemostasis after a vascular injury and is illustrated in Figure 1. With a vascular injury there is exposure of sub-endothelial tissue factor and collagen, as well as vasoconstriction. A platelet plug then forms at the site of injury, as a result of platelet adherence and aggregation to the sub-endothelial collagen. Then the coagulation cascade is activated with fibrin production which acts to stabilise the platelet plug. There are four main groups of anticoagulants as described below.

1. Warfarin

This class of drugs works by blocking the synthesis of the vitamin K dependent factors. The fat soluble vitamin K, absorbed in the small intestine, is involved in the production of factors II, VII, protein C and protein S that are involved in the extrinsic pathway of the coagulation cascade (Figure 1).

Warfarin is monitored by measuring the prothrombin time (PT), measured in seconds, and this is generally expressed as an international normalised ratio (INR). This ratio should be around 1.0 in patients not on oral anticoagulants and without any coagulopathy.

In patients at risk of thromboemboli, the efficacy of warfarin is monitored by measuring this ratio and generally needs to be kept between 2.0 and 3.5 depending on the indications for anticoagulation.

2. Unfractionated Heparin

Unfractionated heparin (UFH) acts by binding to antithrombin III and activating it, which in turn inactivates thrombin, as well as factors VIIa, IXa, Xa and XIa.

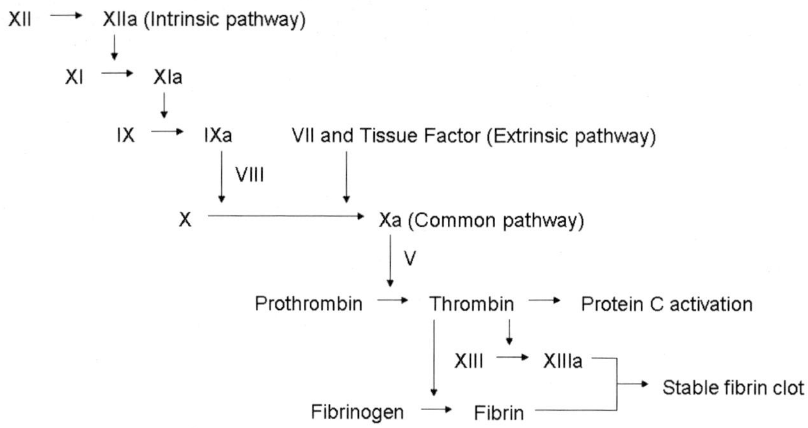

Figure 1. Illustration of the factors involved in the coagulation cascade.

These factors are primarily involved in the intrinsic pathway of the coagulation cascade (Figure 1). This results in reduced fibrin formation. It requires monitoring of the therapeutic level by measuring the activated partial thromboplastin time (aPTT) measured in seconds.

This too can be expressed as a ratio to enable better monitoring. UFH non-specifically binds to a number of proteins and cells, such as macrophages and endothelial cells, which results in a limitation of its affect, which can be variable and unpredictable. It has a relatively short half life of between thirty minutes and an hour.

It can be used in patients with renal impairment as it is cleared primarily by the reticuloendothelial system. It needs to be administered intravenously and requires frequent monitoring. As the clearance is relatively fast, the therapeutic level can be easily and frequently adjusted (Arbit et al. 2006). It can be reversed using protamine sulphate and 1 mg of protamine neutralises approximately 100 units of UFH.

3. Low Molecular Weight Heparin

Low molecular weight heparin (LMWH) is a class of heparin produced by controlled depolymerisation of unfractionated heparin. This preparation has become more popular than UFH due to its more predictable pharmokinetic profile. The actions of LMWH have greater predictability and reliability compared with UFH due to substantially less non-specific binding to proteins and cells. They can be administered subcutaneously and do not require laboratory monitoring (Arbit et al. 2006). Compared with UFH, they have an increased half life of between four to six hours, and this does vary with renal function (Hirsh et al. 1998). Due to the smaller size of LMWH, compared to UFH, they are unable to form the same complex with antithrombin III and thrombin, as described above. Consequently, there is minimal thrombin inhibition with LMWH. The anticoagulant affect of LMWH occurs almost entirely due to factor Xa inactivation and some factor IIa inhibition (Hirsh et al. 1998).

LMWH generally requires no monitoring but in renal failure and pregnancy, monitoring can be performed with anti-Xa levels. Although UFH and LMWH are frequently used for thromboprophylaxis in hospitalised surgical patients, these agents are not ideal for out-patient use due to their mode of administration.

Some hospitals are able to arrange a service for patients to come to the wards for injections or for community nurses to administer LWMH at home.

4. New Oral Anticoagulants

Newer oral anticoagulants are continually being developed, and the main difference compared to warfarin is their direct modes of action against one clotting factor e.g. factor IIa in dabigatran and factor Xa in rivaroxaban (Harbrecht 2011). Although these new anticoagulants have much shorter half lives, specific antidotes are not available. These also benefit from oral bioavailability and need for minimal to no monitoring (Knepper et al. 2011). Although many study patients have already been treated, further information is required on safety and efficacy, and interactions with other drugs before they are considered to replace the more established therapies (Harbrecht 2011). Whilst early studies have shown dabigatran to be comparable to LMWH with regards to safety and prevention of venous thromboembolism, further information is required to assess the efficacy and safety balance of a range of doses (Eriksson et al. 2005). Another direct thrombin inhibitor, ximelagatran, did not show advantages over other anticoagulants and it was withdrawn from the market. New drugs however are being developed (Lazo-Langner et al. 2009).

COMPLICATIONS

A major disadvantage of both UFH and LMWH is that they are administered parenterally, which is a requirement due to the size and charge of the molecules. Other documented side-effects are bleeding, heparin induced thrombocytopenia (HIT), and osteoporosis. Their use is contraindicated in those with pre-existing thrombocytopenia, platelet defects, acute peptic ulcer disease, acute cerebrovascular injury, spinal anaesthesia and lumbar puncture (Arbit et al. 2006). A meta-analysis performed by Rocha et al. (2000) showed a significantly lower incidence of major bleeding with LMWH compared with UFH.

Heparin induced thrombocytopenia (HIT) is a well documented complication of heparin use, and is caused by platelet activating antibodies that recognise chemokine platelet factor 4 when it is bound to heparin (Warkentin et al. 2007). Although it had previously been thought that LMWH use conferred a lower incidence of HIT, a meta-analysis by Morris et al. (2007) failed to support this and showed no significant difference between the use of LMWH and UFH. This study however included medical as well as surgical patients.

In studies looking at venous thromboprophylaxis in orthopaedic surgery, Warkentin et al. (2003) and Walenga et al. (2004) found a greater incidence of HIT in those using UFH compared to LMWH.

INDICATIONS FOR ANTICOAGULANTS

The main reasons for patients being on warfarin are atrial fibrillation, arterial and venous thromboemboli and prosthetic heart valves. Atrial fibrillation is associated with an increased risk of strokes and thromboembolic complications especially if associated with risk factors including congestive cardiac failure, hypertension, age greater than 75 years, diabetes mellitus and a history of stroke or transient ischaemic attacks (Singer et al. 2004). Patients who have had a recent arterial or venous thrombus are at a higher risk of a recurrent thromboembolism (Kearon and Hirsh 1997). The risks of thromboemboli in patients with prosthetic heart valves reduce significantly with anticoagulant therapy. Prosthetic valves in the mitral position have a greater risk of thrombus than aortic valves due to the increased vascular stasis. Older prostheses such as the caged-ball valves pose a greater risk than newer bileaflet valves (Cannegieter et al. 1995).

Risk Assessment

Perioperative anticoagulation planning should begin in the preoperative assessment clinic and should include input from the surgical, anaesthetic and haematology teams. NICE (2007) and SIGN (2002) have both published guidelines for peri-operative thromboprophylaxis in surgical patients. However, these guidelines do not include management of patients who are already on oral anticoagulation. They do recommend the risk assessment of patients preoperatively. This is often done at the preoperative assessment clinic, but can also be done on admission by nurses or doctors. Although no specific risk assessment tool was recommended by NICE, there are tools available. Autar (2003) devised a Risk Assessment Scale for stratifying the DVT risk of a patient as low, moderate or high risk. More recently, the Department of Health has also published a screening tool (DH 2008). Risk assessment, therefore, is an important guide to using the correct resources for the correct patient risk category. If alterations are to be made to a patient's perioperative anticoagulation, it is important to discuss these risks and benefits with them.

Management of Perioperative Anticoagulation

As with all surgical patients, mechanical adjuncts should be offered, such as graduated compression stockings from the point of admission, unless contraindicated (NICE 2007). A systematic review by Dunn and Turpie (2003) found that patients taking oral anticoagulation rarely suffered with major bleeding whilst undergoing dental procedures, arthrocentesis, cataract surgery, ureterorenoscopy, and upper endoscopy and colonoscopy with or without biopsy. Thus, for these procedures oral anticoagulants need not be ceased preoperatively, however the INR must not be greater than 2.5 (Turna et al. 2008). Low, intermediate and high risk procedures are outlined in Figure 2.

The majority of authors suggest that those patients at intermediate and high risk of a thromboembolic event should have the oral anticoagulant stopped four to five days preoperatively, and restarted postoperatively when the surgeon feels it is safe to, with heparin administered whilst the INR is sub-therapeutic. Most surgical procedures can be performed safely if the INR is less than 1.5. The last preoperative dose of heparin should be no later than twelve hours prior to surgery with LMWH, and six hours before surgery with UFH. The heparin can be recommenced postoperatively once the surgeon agrees that it is safe to do so.

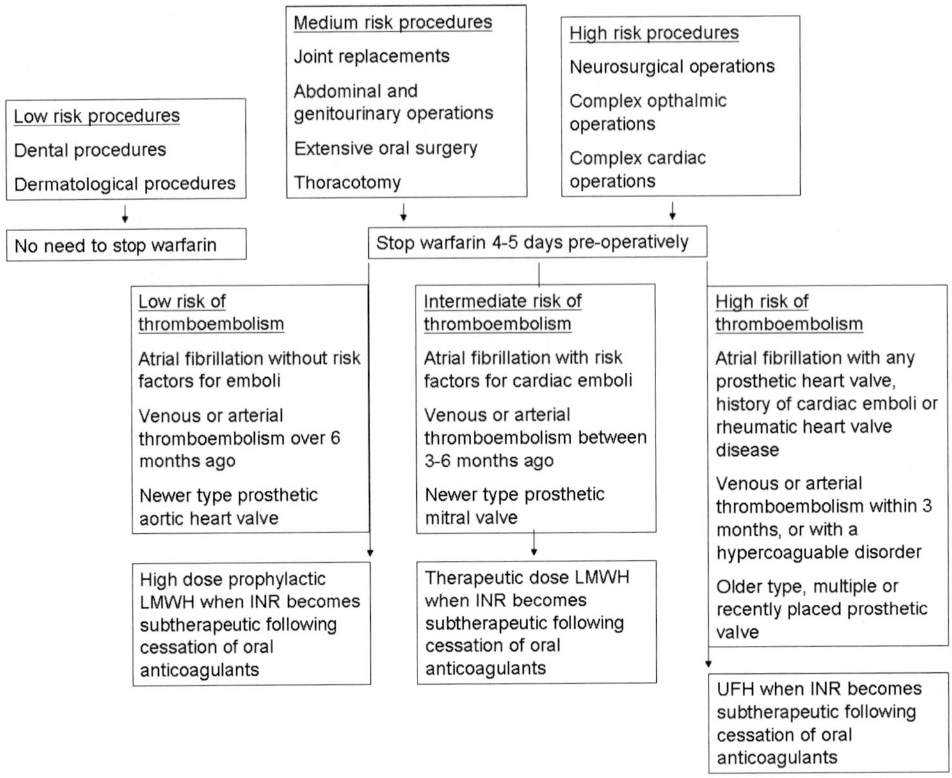

Figure 2. Summary of guidelines for patients on oral anticoagulant therapy undergoing surgery, and the criteria for low, high and very high risks for thromboemboli.

The oral anticoagulant can be restarted on the evening of surgery, dependent on the surgeon's opinion of its safety, and the heparin is stopped once the INR is in therapeutic range. The general opinion is that in surgical procedures with moderate to low risk of postoperative bleeding the oral anticoagulant can be restarted on the evening of surgery, whilst in procedures with a high risk of bleeding it may be recommenced the day after depending on the risk of further bleeding.

Hewitt et al. (1999) suggested that the use of LMWH had been observed to have advantages over the use of UFH in terms of safety and efficiency. It was found that the perioperative use of UFH was justified in those who had an acute venous thromboembolic event within the last month. UFH use was also justified in the postoperative period if venous thromboembolic event occurred in the previous two to three months.

However, the use of UFH was not justified, in light of the potential complications, in those who had a venous thromboembolic event more than three months prior to surgery. Insertion of a vena caval filter may be considered if the patient is at high risk of bleeding, recurrent thromboembolic event or surgery is planned within two weeks of an acute venous thromboembolic event. Insertion should follow discussion with the haematologist and interventional radiologist. A temporary filter is preferable as it can be removed following the procedure.

Cheng et al. (2009) looked at patients on oral anticoagulation therapy for mechanical heart valves undergoing pacemaker implantation.

They found that excessive bleeding and haematoma formation was associated with preoperative cessation of oral anticoagulation less than three days before surgery and the use of heparin postoperatively. They came to the conclusion that oral anticoagulants should be stopped more than three days prior to surgery, with therapeutic LMWH bridging until twelve hours preoperatively, and oral anticoagulants restarted immediately after surgery without LMWH. It has been shown that if the INR is between 2.0 and 3.0, it falls to less than 1.5 within 4-5 days of the last dose (White et al. 1995), but INR testing is recommended preoperatively. LMWH injections can commence 31-2 days following the last warfarin dose without checking the INR.

If the patient had an arterial thromboembolic event within a month of planned surgery, the surgery should be deferred beyond a month if possible due to the potential increased risk of a recurrent event (Hewitt et al. 1999). In those patients who are at high risk of bleeding, LMWH is preferred to UFH, until the INR becomes therapeutic and the heparin can be ceased. Some clinicians may consider antiplatelets (e.g. Aspirin) as thromboprophylaxis, as indeed, many patients are on such therapy for secondary myocardial infarction and stroke prevention. It has been shown to reduce the risk of thromboemboli in patients, especially when used as an adjunct with heparin (APT 1994). However, the risk of operative bleeding is increased, albeit small. In addition, NICE (2007) have not recommended the use of antiplatelets alone as prophylaxis.

A summary of management of perioperative anticoagulation is given in Figure 2. In brief, oral anticoagulants need not be stopped preoperatively in low risk procedures but should be stopped four to five days preoperatively for all other surgical procedures. The management following cessation of oral anticoagulants depends on the risk of thromboemboli; whether this is low, intermediate or high risk. Although LMWH can be given in low and intermediate risk patients, UFH should be given in high risk patients. The criteria for thromboembolism risk assessment are also outlined in Figure 2. The authors' hospital protocol coincides with the recommendations mentioned in this article. However, in other Trusts, it likely that there are other protocols specific to surgery-type that will take precedence over any other guidelines. There is also a mutual agreement between nursing staff and the surgical teams where an individual's anticoagulation regime is allowed to deviate from the guidelines; this again highlights patient-specific management. Nevertheless, liaising with the local haematology department in managing patients' anticoagulation is invaluable.

Emergency Surgery

In emergency cases, the anticoagulation needs to be reversed. This can be achieved with prothrombin complex concentrate (PCC), fresh frozen plasma (FFP) or recombinant factor VII. PCC contains concentrated factors II, VII, IX and X. It can be administered rapidly in a smaller volume and avoids the need for blood group matching.

The coagulation factors contained in it are more predictable. These agents however have a short half-life and require the simultaneous administration of vitamin K. Vitamin K can also be considered in cases where the INR remains high preoperatively despite the cessation of oral anticoagulants. Oral vitamin K administration offers similar efficacy and better safety than intravenous administration.

Conclusion

With increased experience with perioperative anticoagulation, the management of patients with significant risk of perioperative thromboembolic events will improve and become more precise. For medium and high risk invasive surgical procedures, oral anticoagulation needs to be ceased, however the use of UFH, LMWH and retrievable inferior vena cava filters depends on the individual case and the clinicians own experience (Thakur et al. 2010). Of importance is that the period of time that the patient's INR is sub-therapeutic should be kept to a minimum in those at high risk of further thromboembolic events. There is limited information in literature to aid this decision process, thus further research studies are required to make an informative decision. More audits should be performed to correlate patients' demographics, management and outcome with regards to anticoagulation via local governance teams. Nevertheless, the best strategy for perioperative management of anticoagulation involves an individual assessment of the patient taking into account the procedure they are undergoing and the reasons for their anticoagulation, and closely liaising with the haematologists.

References

Antiplatelet Trialists' Collaboration 1994 Collaborative overview of randomised trials of antiplatelet therapy - III: Reduction in venous thrombosis and pulmonary embolism by antiplatelet prophylaxis among surgical and medical patients. *British Medical Journal* 308 235-246.

Arbit, E., Goldberg, M., Gomez-Orellana, I., Majuru, S. 2006 Oral heparin: status review. *Thrombosis Journal* 10 6.

Autar, R. 2003 The management of deep vein thrombosis: The Autar DVT Risk Assessment Scale re-visited. *Journal of Orthopaedic Nursing* 7 114-124.

Cheng, M., Hua, W., Chen, K., Pu, J., et al. 2009 Perioperative anticoagulation for patients with mechanic heart valve(s) undertaking pacemaker implantation. *Europace* 11 1183-1187.

Brathwaite, C. E., Mure, A. J., O'Malley, K. F., Spence, R. K., Ross, S. E. 1993 Complications of anticoagulation for pulmonary embolism in low risk trauma patients. *Chest* 104 718-720.

Cannegieter, S. C., Rosendaal, F. R., Wintzen, A. R., et al. 1995 Optimal oral anticoagulant therapy in patients with mechanical heart valves. *New England Journal of Medicine* 333 11-7.

Chimutengwende-Gordon, M., Khan, W. S., Maruthainar, N. (2010). Perioperative blood transfusion: The role of allogenous, autologous transfusions and pharmacological agents. *J. Perioper. Pract.* 20(8): 283-87.

Department of Health 2008 Risk Assessment for Venous Thromboembolism [online] Available from http://www.dh.gov.uk/en/Publicationsandstatistics/Publications/PublicationsPolicyAndGuidance/DH_088215 [Accessed Dec. 2009].

Douketis, J. D 2002 Perioperative anticoagulation management in patients who are receiving oral anticoagulant therapy; a practical guide for clinicians. *Thrombosis Research* 108 3-13.

Dunn, A. S., Turpie, A. G. G. 2003 Perioperative management of patients receiving oral anticoagulants. A systematic review. *Archives of Internal Medicine* 163 901-908.

Eriksson, B. I., Dahl, O. E., Büller, H. R., et al. 2005 A new oral direct thrombin inhibitor, dabigatran etexilate, compared with enoxaparin for prevention of thromboembolic events following total hip replacement or knee replacement: BISTRO II randomised trial. *Journal of Thrombosis and Haemostasis* 3 103-111.

Garcia, D. A., Regan, S., Henault, L. E., et al. 2008 Risk of thromboembolism with short-term interruption of warfarin therapy. *Archives of Internal Medicine* 168 63-69.

Harbrecht, U. 2011 Old and new anticoagulants. *Hamostaseologie* 31 21-27.

Hewitt, R. L., Chun, K. L., Flint, L. M. 1999 Current clinical concepts in perioperative anticoagulation. *The American Surgeon* 65 270-273.

Hirsh, J., Warkentin, T. E., Raschke, R., et al. 1998 Heparin and low molecular-weight heparin. Mechanisms of action, pharmokinetics, dosing considerations, monitoring, efficacy and safety. *Chest* 114 S489-S510.

Hirsh, J., Raschke, R. 2004 Heparin and low-molecular-weight heparin: the Seventh ACCP Conference on Antithrombotic and Thrombolytic Therapy. *Chest* 126 S188-S203.

Jafri, S. M. 2004 Periprocedural thromboprophylaxis in patients receiving chronic anticoagulation therapy. *American Heart Journal* 147 3-15.

Kearon, C., Hirsh, J. 1997 Management of anticoagulation before and after elective surgery. *New England Journal of Medicine* 336 1506-1511.

Knepper, J., Ramacciotti, E., Wakefield, T. W. 2011 Novel anticoagulants: a discussion of clinical use in the treatment and prevention of venous thromboembolism. *Phlebology* 26 3-7.

Lazo-Langner, A., Rodger, M. A., Wells, P. S. 2009 Lessons from ximelagatran: issues for future studies evaluating new oral direct thrombin inhibitors for venous thromboembolism prophylaxis in orthopedic surgery. *Clinical Application in Thrombosis and Hemostasis* 15 316-326.

Madura, J. A., Rookstool, M., Wease, G. 1994 The management of patients on chronic Coumadin therapy undergoing subsequent surgical procedures. *The American Surgeon* 60 542-547.

Morris, T. A., Castrejon, S., Devendra, G., et al. 2007 No difference in risk for thrombocytopenia during treatment of pulmonary embolism and deep venous thrombosis with either low-molecular-weight-heparin or unfractionated heparin: A meta-analysis. *Chest* 132 1131-1139.

National Institute for Health and Clinical Excellence 2007 The reduction of venous thromboembolism (deep vein thrombosis and pulmonary embolism) in patients undergoing orthopaedic surgery and other high-risk surgical procedures. *NICE*, London.

O'Donnell, M., Kearon, C. 2006 Perioperative management of oral anticoagulation. *Clinics in Geriatric Medicine* 22 199-213.

Rocha, E., Martinez-Gonzalez, M. A., Montes, R., Panizo, C. 2000 Do the low molecular weight heparins improve the efficacy and safety of the treatment of deep venous thrombosis? A meta-analysis. *Haematologica* 85 935-942.

Scottish Intercollegiate Guidelines Network 2002 Guidelines 62: Prophylaxis Of Venous Thromboembolism. *SIGN*, Edinburgh.

Singer, D. E., Albers, G. W., Dalen, J. E., et al. 2004 Antithrombotic therapy in atrial fibrillation: the Seventh ACCP Conference on Antithrombotic and Thrombolytic Therapy. *Chest* 126 S429-S456.

Thakur, N. A., Czerwein, J. K., Butera, J. N., Palumbo, M. A. 2010 Perioperative management of chronic anticoagulation in orthopaedic surgery. *Journal of the American Academy of Orthopaedic Surgeons* 18 729-738.

Turna, B., Stein, R. J., Smaldone, M. C., et al. 2008 Safety and efficacy of flexible ureterorenoscopy and holmium:YAG lithotripsy for intrarenal stones in anticoagulated cases. *The Journal of Urology* 179 1415-1419.

Walenga, J. M., Jeske, W. P., Prechel, M. M., Bacher, P., Bakhos, M. 2004 Decreased prevalence of heparin-induced thrombocytopenia with low-molecular-weight heparin and related drugs. *Seminars in Thrombosis and Haemostasis* 30 69-80.

Warkentin, T. E., Roberts, R. S., Hirsh, J., Kelton, J. G. 2003 An improved definition of immune heparin-induced thrombocytopenia in postoperative orthopedic patients. *Archives of Internal Medicine* 163 2518-2524.

Warkentin, T. E., Greinacher, A. eds. 2007 *Heparin-induced thrombocytopenia* 4th Ed. Informa Healthcare US, New York.

White, R. H., McKittrick, T., Hutchinson, R., Twitchell, J. 1995 Temporary discontinuation of warfarin therapy: changes in the international normalized ratio. *Annals of Internal Medicine* 122 40-42.

In: Perioperative Practice in Trauma and Orthopaedic Surgery ISBN: 978-1-63483-325-7
Editor: Wasim S. Khan

Chapter 7

PSYCHOSOCIAL CONSIDERATIONS OF PERIOPERATIVE CARE IN CHILDREN, WITH A FOCUS ON EFFECTIVE MANAGEMENT STRATEGIES

Kishan Rajdev, Avnita L. D. Amin, Emeka Oragui, Ansuya Puri and Wasim S. Khan*

University College London Institute of Orthopaedics and Musculoskeletal Science, Royal National Orthopaedic Hospital, Stanmore, Middlesex, London, UK

ABSTRACT

Children are not just 'small adults.' They have specific physical, psychological and social requirements that must be identified and addressed to optimise their well-being in the perioperative period. The health care practitioner should be trained to understand the needs of the paediatric patient in hospital, such as the potential triggers for anxiety and distress, in addition to the ever-increasing need to take into account cultural differences.

Hospital policy should include a preoperative preparation programme, specially aimed at the paediatric population, where parental involvement is encouraged throughout, with a structured care plan continuing into the post-operative period. Factors involved the success of these preoperative programmes include their early commencement, orientation tours and role-play over potentially distressing points of care, along with appropriate resources to inform the child and parents. While day-case surgery is associated with improved outcomes and decreased anxiety, care must be taken to ensure parents are adequately placed to manage their children's needs after discharge.

Keywords: Children, preparation programme, parents, day-case surgery, analgesia

* Corresponding author: Mr Wasim S. Khan, Clinical Lecturer, University College London Institute of Orthopaedics and Musculoskeletal Science, Royal National Orthopaedic Hospital, Stanmore, Middlesex, London, HA7 4LP, UK. Telephone number: +44 (0) 7971 190720, fax number: +44 (0) 20 8570 3864, e-mail address: wasimkhan @doctors.org.uk.

INTRODUCTION

This chapter deals with psychosocial considerations of perioperative care in children with a particular focus on effective management strategies (Amit et al. 2010). Surgery is a stressful event for many children, leading to negative emotional behaviours and distress which can extend beyond the perioperative period into adolescence (Ahmed et al. 2011; Brewer et al. 2006). Such responses have led to the development of preoperative preparation programmes to decrease anxiety and improve satisfaction for both the child and their parents. However, these are heterogeneous in their structure and adoption across trusts. Clear guidance exists about the responsibilities of NHS organisations in the provision of care for children (DOH 2006, 2007; RCS 2013), though some healthcare practitioners still lack a fundamental understanding of these differing healthcare requirements. The pre- and post-hospital care provided to children has also been found to differ from hospital to hospital.

In addition, our increasingly multicultural society has raised a greater need to address the trans-cultural issues that may arise in the perioperative care of children (Royaltey 1988). The implementation of guidance in perioperative care, tailored to the local population and coupled with education of healthcare professionals across the multidisciplinary team, may help to ensure that the physical, psychological and social requirements of children presenting for surgery are accommodated for. This chapter briefly summarises the emotional and psychological impact hospitalisation has on children and describes the main triggers of anxiety faced. We discuss the benefits of a preoperative preparation programme and the increasing popularity of day case procedures, as well as looking into difficulties that may arise cross-culturally and exploring the methods that may be used to overcome them.

ANXIETY AND DISTRESS IN THE PAEDIATRIC PATIENT

Since the early twentieth century, there has been a growing recognition of the potentially adverse psychological impact of hospitalisation on children, including the negative effect anxiety can have on health (Forsyth 1934, Platt 1959). Between 40-60% of paediatric patients report apprehension at being in hospital, regardless of the country, surgical procedure or healthcare system in question (Bortone and Picetti 2002, Brophy and Erickson 1990, Justus et al. 2006). Anxiety can be detrimental to procedures in the perioperative period, delay anaesthetic induction and hinder the postoperative recovery (Bar-Mor 1997, Justus et al. 2006, Kain et al. 2006, Voepel-Lewis et al. 2003).

In particular, it can be responsible for later behavioural problems such as bed wetting, nightmares, food rejection, anxiety and negativity (Wollin et al. 2004). An individual child's reaction to surgery can vary based on their temperament, ability to cope with change, age, any past negative experiences in healthcare, and their parents' levels of anxiety before surgery, in addition to biological vulnerabilities such as developmental delay (Ahmed et al. 2011).

Five aspects of hospitalisation that pose as potential triggers of distress in the paediatric patient (Visintainer and Wolfer 1975) have been identified as:

1. Physical harm or injury in the form of pain, mutilation or death
2. Fear of the unknown and unfamiliar

3. Uncertainty about acceptable behaviour in a hospital setting
4. Loss of control, autonomy and competence
5. Separation from parents and the absence of trusted adults

Below we discuss these triggers of distress in paediatric patients and discuss how the perioperative experiences of these patients might be improved.

1. Experiencing Pain

Differences surrounding the experience, expressions and behaviours of children in pain exist and need to be recognised (Zeltzer et al. 1992, McGrath andFrager 1996). Schechter (1989) reported that 'the management of pain in children is not addressed with the same vigour and enthusiasm as is the management of pain in adults', a statement that seems to be echoed in more recent times with the lack of experimental and clinical studies exploring this issue (Anderson et al. 2009). The Association of Paediatric Anaesthetics released updated evidence-based guidelines in 2012 on pain management in children, highlighting the importance of early recognition and assessment of pain with consideration of their developmental age and ability to communicate.

Measurement of pain is difficult, especially in younger children or those with cognitive impairment. The guidelines suggest the use of the COMFORT and FLACC scales in infants, the faces pain scale (FPS) in children over 3, and the visual analogue scale (VAS) in children over 7, alongside effective communication with the family. The NCCPC-R has been validated in children with severe cognitive impairments (Breau et al. 2002).

Medical staff should be well-trained in pre-emptive and early administration of analgesia appropriate to the level of pain experienced. Novel strategies have been developed to help children better understand and express their pain, such as the Painbusters Guide (Alder Hey 2013) which is given to children as part of a preoperative preparation programme and outlines the potential treatment options for pain and as well as tools the family can use in its assessment. For minimally invasive procedures the application of EMLA (eutectic mixture of lidocaine and prilocaine) cream one hour prior has been shown to be beneficial.

Alternatives to EMLA such as vapocoolant sprays have been considered, due to their rapid onset and decreased cost, however results in children have been mixed (MacLaren and Cohen 2007). Nitrous oxide can also be considered in combination with EMLA or on its own, particularly in older children (Hee et al. 2003; Kennedy and Luhrmann 2001). In patients who are not nil-by-mouth, paracetamol and ibuprofen are commonly used to reduce preoperative and postoperative pain. The use of Feldene Melt (piroxicam) in patients who are nil-by-mouth is favourable to children, given its sherbert-like taste (Woodhead and Wicker 2005).

2. Unfamiliar Settings

Anxiety often arises from exposure to unfamiliar locations and uncertainty surrounding medical procedures. LeRoy et al. (2003) identified particularly stressful points for children to include venepuncture, separation from parents outside the operating theatre and induction of anaesthesia.

Much of this anxiety can be mitigated by consistently providing factual information and emotional support prior to each stress point. A study with intervention consisting of continual supportive care in combination with information rehearsal proved to be 'significantly superior to the control group on most outcome variables.' Information rehearsal incorporated descriptions of hospital routine, event sequences and staff roles. It also aided parents in successfully communicating all this information to their child (Visintainer and Wolfer 1975). Additional techniques to improve children's coping strategies within the hospital setting include familiarising the child with surgical and anaesthetic equipment in 'medical play' (Moushey et al. 1988) and the use of information films and leaflets (Bar-Mor 1997). Children's books may be a useful starting point for individual hospital-based programmes, while older children may appreciate computer- or web-based programs specific to the treatment they are to receive, with a further opportunity of viewing the operating theatre and equipment they are likely to see (Justus et al. 2006). Such experiences provide a grounding for questions and elaboration about the procedures which may not have otherwise been explored (Litke et al. 2012). Techniques used to reduce anxiety in the anaesthetic room before surgery include distraction using bubbles, books and DVDs, and familiarisation using the child's own toys or teddy bears. Distress due to unfamiliarity of the hospital setting can be diminished both by ensuring referral to a hospital close to the child's home (Hatch and Rollin 2000) and by preadmission visits to the ward. Allowing children to bring their own possessions to hospital also strengthens the feeling of familiarity to some extent.

Day case surgery has a role in alleviating some of the stresses associated with the hospital stay and is discussed later.

3. Uncertainty about Appropriate Behaviour for a Hospital Setting

The impact of hospitalisation and surgery in children goes beyond the single experience and can influence future interactions with healthcare professionals, trust in the healthcare system and responsibility for their own health (Bar-Mor 1997). Preoperative anxiety behaviour is not solely modelled around present interactions but also in relation to their past experiences and the sensed anxiety levels of the guardian(s) present (Justus et al. 2006).

Anxiety at anaesthetic induction has been associated with negative behaviour postoperatively such as rebellion against authority, difficulty sleeping and psychological upset (Kain et al. 1999, Bortone and Picetti 2002). In a further attempt to minimise anxiety perioperatively, play specialists may be involved early on; an approach that has been shown to be effective for both the child and parent alike (Thornes 1991, Bortone and Picetti 2002).

Behavioural techniques such as distraction of the child are shown to have great benefit over reassurance such as telling the child not to worry, as the latter has been shown, counterintuitively, to increase distress during procedures such as venepuncture (McMurtry et al. 2010).

4. Loss of Control

Children should be encouraged to have a sense of control over their healthcare as this has been shown to reduce anxiety and lead to greater compliance with treatment (Miller 2009).

This can be supported by giving them choices where possible, ranging from informing then about their illness and planned treatment, through to shared and autonomous decision making (McCabe et al. 1996).

Providing children with opportunities for choice during the perioperative period, such as deciding which arm to have their blood pressure taken, helps to foster a sense of control (Bayne and Kirkland 2012). While parents and healthcare professionals are the main decision makers for their treatment, children value being able to voice their preferences (Coyne et al. 2014). In addition, it is important to elucidate any false beliefs children may have about the procedure, as they form their own explanations for illness, even if their concepts are flawed (Williams and Binnie 2002), for example perceiving the need for surgery as a punishment for wrongdoing (Felder-Puig et al. 2003). The healthcare provider should explain procedures to both the guardians and patient in a manner suitable for their developmental age, encouraging a two-way dialogue and thus including them in their care plan.

5. Separation from Parents

The adverse effect of parental separation in the hospitalisation of children was elucidated in the early twentieth century. Platt (1959) recommended that parents be allowed to remain with children in hospital with suitable accommodation provisions. Separation anxiety can be observed in children from 7-8 months old, peaking at around 1 year of age (Litke et al. 2012). Many paediatric wards are able to provide an additional bed for one parent to stay with their child in some bays or siderooms. However, given the practicalities, cost implementation and viability of parental accommodation for all paediatric patients in hospitals nationwide, the step towards increasing the day case surgery load has largely avoided this issue.

Parental Presence at Induction of Anaesthesia (PPIA)

Anaesthetic induction is a particularly stressful period for children and parental presence reduces the anxiety of being in an unfamiliar environment as well as decreasing the need for premedication. Studies suggest that most parents wish to be present at induction to assert their role as primary caregivers and feel helpful in their child's experience (O'Conner-Von 2000, Kam et al. 1998). Wolf (2009) comments on a number of RCTs indicating that routine parental presence is not beneficial, however the parent has a right to be present. The role of premedication is well established, with behavioural techniques utilised, for example, by play specialists gaining wider acceptance (Sullivan and Wong 2013). However, a randomised controlled trial has shown that combined parental presence with cognitive preparation methods, is equally as effective as premedication (Fortier et al. 2011). This intervention system requires considerable funding due to specialist training with psychologists and as a result is difficult to implement, however the benefits of family-centred care are encouraging. Lack of evidence to support a long-term benefit of parental presence during anaesthetic induction is reiterated elsewhere, however the combined effects of increasing parental participation and decreasing anxiety suggest the importance of active parental involvement in children's healthcare in hospital (Thornes et al. 1991, Piira et al. 2005, Alsop-Shields 2000). Though once again, this benefit is not universal and does depend on the personality of the parent (Wolf 2009). Exploring parental anxiety concerning induction may enable a better-informed decision about PPIA.

In the UK the majority of children are accompanied to theatre by one or more parents, and The Association of Anaesthetists of Great Britain and Ireland recommend that this is offered to the parents as a standard of care.

Theatre staff can play a pivotal role in supporting the parent allowing them in turn to reduce the child's anxieties, though parents should leave the anaesthetic room before the child falls asleep as this moment often arouses negative emotions in parents (Litke et al. 2012). Certain events in particular, such as seeing their child in distress, going limp or rolling their eyes, can be stressful for parents, though the majority prefer PPIA for subsequent surgeries regardless of their first experience (Ahmed et al. 2011).

Preoperative Preparation Programmes

Preparation programmes for children have been shown to reduce patient distress, improve compliance with treatment and recovery, and increase parental satisfaction of healthcare (Bar-Mor 1997). Specific preparation programmes should be implemented in all hospitals caring for children and use a mixture of factual information in various formats including role play and emotional support to restore some sense of control and independence into the child's mindset. Familiarity with the ward, anaesthetic induction room and equipment will decrease anxiety, and a preadmission visit will enable parents and children to ask questions in a warm and supportive atmosphere (Woodhead and Wicker 2005).

While there is no standard procedure, certain elements are common to many preoperative programmes and have been shown to be useful in reducing anxiety and increasing satisfaction in both children and their parents preoperatively (AAP 2014; Bayne and Kirkland 2008; Fortier et al. 2011; Hatava et al. 2000; Kain et al. 1996; O'Sullivan and Wong 2013; Perry et al. 2012; RCS 2013):

- Consideration of each patient individually taking into account their developmental age, past experiences and comorbidities
- Commencement of the programme at least 5 days before the procedure, especially in children over 6 years old, to allow adequate time to process the information
- Offering a tour of the department and operating theatre to familiarise the child with these surroundings
- Role play of potentially stressful procedures, for example practice with an anaesthesia mask in the days leading up to the surgery
- Use of materials such as colouring books, leaflets, films and video games to educate the child about the events involved in the preoperative period and the feelings that they might experience
- Use of distraction in the waiting area and in the anaesthetic room by trained theatre nurses and play specialists, with bubbles, dolls and other toys, including allowing the child to bring in their own possessions if appropriate
- Teaching parents techniques to manage their children's anxiety in the perioperative period and offering parental presence at induction if appropriate
- Ensuring parents are given sufficient information on assessment of pain and how to administer analgesics after discharge

EMERGENCE AGITATION

The phenomenon of emergence agitation including thrashing, unsettled behaviour and distress upon recovery from anaesthesia has an impact on both psychological and physical recovery (Voepel-Lewis et al. 2003). We recommend that parents be informed of the possible post-anaesthetic behavioural changes and prepare them for how their child will look following surgery, to avoid parental distress. The healthcare team should also be aware of these behaviours and have a plan for dealing with particularly difficult behaviour in the postoperative period. Some of the possible causes include anxiety in the young child, midazolam premedication and sevoflurane anaesthesia. A meta-analysis of management strategies found that propofol, ketamine, fentanyl, and preoperative analgesia have a prophylactic effect in preventing emergence agitation, and that the analgesic properties of these drugs do not seem to have a role in this effect (Dahmani et al. 2010). Prevention of preoperative anxiety, using premedication and psychological techniques, is also important in reducing the risk of emergence agitation (Dahmani et al. 2014).

Postoperative agitation may be due either to postoperative pain or emergence agitation. Although differentiating the cause of postoperative agitation may be difficult, it also may be unnecessary as treatment with opioids is recommended as the primary strategy for the safe recovery of child (Manworren et al. 2004).

DAY-CASE SURGERY

There has been a continued drive to allocate more procedures to day-case units for a multitude of reasons, including reduction in the chance of any negative outcomes from surgery (Justus et al. 2006) and to decrease financial spending. Further advantages of day-case surgery include less child-parent separation and decreased risk of nosocomial infections (Zuckerberg 1994). This increasing trend towards day-case surgery, where possible, requires a specific day-case protocol tailored to the paediatric patient.

The document 'Just for the day' outlines 12 quality standards which serve as a practical guide to caring for paediatric day-cases and state the necessity of a preadmission visit, written information for parents to help outline their important role in their child's care, separation of children's from adult cases and elective day-case from acute cases, and the importance of staff trained in day-case and paediatric care (Thornes 1991).

Care should be consultant led, with a clear pain management policy and advice on "take-home" analgesia (RCS 2007). More recent guidelines in 2013 from the Royal College of Nursing echo these themes, outlining the need for a suitable pre-admission programme and appropriate facilities for play, as well as appropriate tools for pain assessment.

Prolongation of day cases into overnight admission usually results from a complaint of nausea or actual vomiting. The subjective symptom of nausea must be explored in the child's words prior to admission so that optimum relief can be provided.

In 2009, the Association of Paediatric Anaesthetists published guidelines on the prevention of postoperative vomiting in children. Optimal control of symptoms can be achieved with a mixture of pharmacological and non-pharmacological management (Keller 1995).

Observation of fluid balance, intravenous anaesthetic induction with propofol, avoidance of opioids and use of dexamethasone, ondansetron or droperidol as an antiemetic have also been shown to be effective (Kova 2007, Patil 2007, Woodhead and Wicker 2005).

Routine checks of physical health, weight and age, combined with the exploration of psychosocial issues, are also important for assessing suitability of paediatric day-surgery unit admission to ensure their needs can be sufficiently met.

Post-Hospital Care and Pain Management

It is important that sufficient information is provided to the parents or guardians to support them when the child is at home.

Pain is the most commonly cited problem following the discharge of children from hospital, with 50% of children reported to have clinically significant pain post-discharge (Rawal 2001). A combination of poor communication and misunderstanding between healthcare professionals and parents may be the reason only 8.3% of these children are receiving the full dose of analgesia prescribed. Inadequate delivery of medication within the home setting may also result from underestimation of pain by the child's parent (Wolf 1999).

Therefore there is a need to educate parents on the role of medication and to elucidate any parental concerns about administering analgesia. Prescribing analgesia according to weight rather than age, as is common practice (Girgis and Sanders 2004; Litke et al. 2012), should overcome any significant episodes of postoperative pain in children if the maximum dose has been prescribed and administered. Simple instructions should be given to both the guardians and, if appropriate, the child.

This should accompany basic education of pain assessment and effective administration of analgesia, where the benefits of simple analgesics such as paracetamol and NSAIDS are often underestimated. Pain assessment tools and pain scores can be used by parents as a more formal means of quantifying pain levels and medicating accordingly. Resources containing this information, such as the Painbusters guide (Alder Hey 2013) and the My Child Is In Pain website, have been developed recently by individual NHS trusts as part of preoperative preparation programmes and should be considered for widespread adoption.

It is important that for those undergoing more extensive surgery as a day-case, provisions are made to extend their stay in hospital if post-discharge pain management is forecast to be an issue. A pain service operating in a hospital may also be of use in managing acute pain with the utilisation of extended duration regional analgesia (Wolf 1999; APA 2012).

Discharge plans should be discussed with the carers and be in keeping with hospital and community policy to ensure a smooth transition from secondary to community care. Children under the age of five are attended by a health visitor and those older than five are under the care of the district or school nurse (Woodhead and Wicker 2005).

Socioeconomic Considerations

The socioeconomic impact of a hospital stay on the family is great, including days taken off work to stay with the child and the knock-on effects that other members of the family face. Adequate support must be given, either through automatic hospital follow-up appointments or referral to a community practice. Healthcare professionals should be intimately acquainted with the needs of the individual child and their family, ideally with input from social services. Once a child is discharged from hospital, the responsibilities of care come to lie with the parents and family of that child. In addition to financial and healthcare backing that may be on offer it is also vital that psychosocial support is made available to the family as a whole, not only post-discharge but throughout the medical journey. Counselling services for parents are often a useful means of forming a trusting relationship with the healthcare providers and can be a form of healthcare education (Bar-Mor 1997).

Cultural Requirements

The transcultural context of healthcare has been widely documented and the healthcare practitioner should understand that the patient's view of healthcare care may be heavily influenced by their personal beliefs. These accounting factors should be reflected in patient management and hospital protocol as far as is practical (Royaltey 1988). The increasingly multicultural environment of hospitals in the United Kingdom means that staff awareness and sensitivity to cultural needs and constraints are paramount and must be actively promoted. Recognition that cultural and ethnic differences can influence a child's behaviour is also necessary (Woodhead and Wicker 2005). Differences in parents' belief systems concerning the role of medication can greatly affect whether or not a child receives their medication postoperatively, and so care must be taken to ascertain what worries families may have and to take into account variations in beliefs across cultures (Carter 2015).

A balance between cultural constraints and hospital policy must be sought and individual hospitals are best placed to implement a policy sensitive to their serving community. Culinary differences in a transcultural context can be looked into, exploring the child's likes and dislikes, so that allowances can be made where possible, further fostering a feeling of familiarity within the hospital. On a further practical note, hospitals should ensure that all forms of preoperative preparation are widely available in a number of languages and formats, with the possibility of interpreters or translators to aid communication when English is not the first language of choice (Justus et al. 2006). It may be the case that foreign nationals coming to reside in the UK bring ideas and traditions with them which are at odds with medicine as practiced here, and they may be somewhat resistant to Western input. Health education in such cases must be approached with care and the realistic expectation made that while these individuals may be responsive to the knowledge on offer, their practices are unlikely to change in the short term, if ever (Royaltey 1988).

Conclusion

Anxiety and other negative emotions are common in children undergoing surgery and their parents. The child's physical, psychological and social requirements must be carefully considered to minimise the impact on their short- and long-term wellbeing.

Parental involvement is beneficial to child outcomes and strategies to encourage this must be reflected in hospital policy. Well-structured preoperative preparation programmes can help allay the fears and anxieties of both the child and responsible guardian, improve compliance with treatment and result in a higher service satisfaction rate. Post-hospital care programmes should facilitate a seamless continuum of high quality care after discharge from hospital, with community and outreach services continuing a patient-specific care package which incorporates parental education. A comprehensive hospital protocol for day case surgery in children should also exist, providing the same standard of care as for paediatric inpatients.

REFERENCES

Ahmed, M. I., et al., 2011. Preoperative anxiety in children risk factors and non-pharmacological management. *Middle East Journal of Anesthesiology*, 21(2), pp. 153-170.

Alder Hey Children's NHS Foundation Trust, 2013. Painbusters,

Alsop-Shields, L. 2000 Perioperative care of children in a transcultural context. *AORN Journal* 71 1004-1020.

American Academy of Pediatrics, 2014. The Pediatrician's Role in the Evaluation and Preparation of Pediatric Patients Undergoing Anesthesia. *Pediatrics*, 134(3), pp. 634-641. Available at: http://pediatrics.aappublications.org/cgi/doi/10.1542/peds.2014-1840.

Amin, A. L. D., Oragui, E., Khan, W. S., Puri, A. (2010). Psychological considerations of perioperative care in children, with a focus on effective management strategies. *J. Perioper. Pract.* 20(6): 198-202.

Anderson, T., Khan, N. K., Tassinari, M. S., Hurtt, M. E. 2009 Comparative juvenile safety testing of new therapeutic candidates: relevance of laboratory animal data to children. *Journal of Toxicology Science* 34 209-215.

Association of Paediatric Anaesthetists 2009. *The Recognition and Assessment of Acute Pain in Children*, London, UK, RCN.

Association of Paediatric Anaesthetists 2009. *Guidelines on the Prevention of Postoperative Vomiting in Children*, London, UK, RCN.

Association of Paediatric Anaesthetists of Great, B. and Ireland, 2012. Good practice in postoperative and procedural pain management, 2nd edition. *Paediatr. Anaesth.*, 22 Suppl. 1(July), pp. 1-79. Available at: http://www.ncbi.nlm.nih.gov/pubmed/22817132. Bar-Mor, G. 1997 Preparation of children for surgery and invasive procedures: Milestones on the way to success. *Journal of Pediatric Nursing* 12 252-255.

Bortone, L., Picetti, E. 2002 Preparation, premedication and parental presence. *Minerva Anestesiologica* 68 396-401.

Breau, L. M., et al., 2002. Validation of the Non-communicating Children's Pain Checklist-Postoperative Version. *Anesthesiology*, 96(3), pp. 528-35. Available at: http://www.ncbi.nlm.nih.gov/pubmed/11873023 [Accessed April 26, 2015].

Brophy, C. J., Erickson, M. T. 1990 Children's self-statements and adjustment to elective outpatient surgery. *Journal of Developmental and Behavioral Pediatrics* 11 13-16.

Carter, B., 2015. Parents' and children's beliefs and concerns about taking medicines. Journal of Child Health Care, 19(1), pp. 3-4. Available at: http://chc.sagepub.com/cgi/doi/10.1177/1367493515572694.

Coyne, I., et al., 2014. Children's participation in shared decision-making: Children, adolescents, parents and healthcare professionals' perspectives and experiences. *European Journal of Oncology Nursing*, 18(3), pp. 273-280. Available at: http://www.ejoncologynursing.com/article/S1462-3889(14)00015-5/abstract.

Dahmani, S., Stany, I., Brasher, C., et al. 2010 Pharmacological prevention of sevoflurane- and desflurane-related emergence agitation in children: a meta-analysis of published studies. *British Journal of Anaesthesia* 104 216-223.

Dahmani, S., Delivet, H. and Hilly, J., 2014. Emergence delirium in children: an update. *Current opinion in anaesthesiology*, 27(3), pp. 309-15. Available at: http://www.ncbi.nlm.nih.gov/pubmed/24784918 [Accessed April 26, 2015].

Department of Health 1984. *Hospital Accommodation for Children, Health Building Note 23*, London, UK, HMSO.

Department of Health 1991. *The Welfare of Children and Young People in Hospital*, London, UK, HMSO.

Department of Health 1996. Services for Children and Young People London, UK, HMSO.

Department of Health 2006. *Working Together to Safeguard Children*, London, UK, HMSO.

Department of Health 2007. *Statutory Guidance on Making Arrangements to Safeguard and Promote the Welfare of Children Under Section 11 of the Children Act 2004*, London, UK, HMSO.

Felder-Puig, R., et al., 2003. Using a children's book to prepare children and parents for elective ENT surgery: Results of a randomized clinical trial. *International Journal of Pediatric Otorhinolaryngology*, 67(1), pp. 35-41.

Forsyth, D. 1934 Psychological effects of bodily illness on children. *Lancet* 227 15-18.

Fortier, M. a., et al., 2011. Analysing a family-centred preoperative intervention programme: A dismantling approach. *British Journal of Anaesthesia*, 106(5), pp. 713-718.

Girgis, M., Sanders, D. 2004 Are we Giving our Children the Right Dose? An Audit of Paediatric Day Surgery: Post-operative Analgesia Prescribing. *Journal of One-day Surgery* 3 65-68.

Hatava, P., Olsson, G. L. and Lagerkranser, M., 2000. Preoperative psychological preparation for children undergoing ENT operations: A comparison of two methods. *Paediatric Anaesthesia*, 10(5), pp. 477-486.

Hatch, D. J., Rollin, A. M. 2000 Quality in paediatric anaesthesia. *Current Anaesthesia and Critical Care* 11 239-244.

Hee, H. I., Goy, R. W. L. and Ng, A. S. B., 2003. Effective reduction of anxiety and pain during venous cannulation in children: A comparison of analgesic efficacy conferred by nitrous oxide, EMLA and combination. *Paediatric Anaesthesia*, 13(3), pp. 210-216.

Justus, R., Wyles, D., Wilson, J., et al. 2006 Preparing children and families for surgery: Mount Sinai's multidisciplinary perspective. *Pediatric Nursing* 32 35-43.

Kain, Z. N., Wang, S. M., Mayes, L. C., Caramico, L. A., Hofstadter, M. B. 1999 Distress during the induction of anaesthesia and postoperative behavioural outcomes. *Anaesthesia and Analgesia* 88 1042-1047.

Kain, Z. N. et al., 2006. Preoperative Anxiety, Postoperative Pain, and Behavioral Recovery in Young Children Undergoing Surgery. *Pediatrics*, 118(2), pp. 651-658. Available at: http://pediatrics.aappublications.org/content/118/2/651.abstract.

Kain, Z. N., et al., 2000. Social adaptability, cognitive abilities, and other predictors for children's reactions to surgery. *Journal of Clinical Anesthesia*, 12(7), pp. 549-554.

Kain, Z. N., Mayes, L. C. and Caramico, L. A., 1996. Preoperative preparation in children: A cross-sectional study. *Journal of Clinical Anesthesia*, 8(6), pp. 508-514.

Kam, P., Voss, T., Gold, P., Pitkin, J. 1998 Behaviour of children associated with parental participation during induction of general anaesthesia. *Journal of Paediatric Child Health* 34 29-31.

Keller, V. 1995 Management of nausea and vomiting in children. *Journal of Paediatric Nursing* 10 280-286.

Kennedy, R. M. and Luhmann, J. D., 2001. Pharmacological management of pain and anxiety during emergency procedures in children. *Paediatric drugs*, 3(5), pp. 337-354.

Kovac, A. L. 2007 Management of postoperative nausea and vomiting in children. *Paediatric Drugs* 9 47-69.

LeRoy, S., Elixson, E. M., O'Brien, P., et al. 2003 Recommendations for preparing children and adolescents for invasive cardiac procedures: A statement from the American Heart Association Pediatric Nursing Subcommittee of the Council on Cardiovascular Nursing in collaboration with the Council on Cardiovascular Diseases of the Young. *Circulation* 108 2550-2564.

Litke, J., Pikulska, A. and Wegner, T., 2012. Management of perioperative stress in children and parents. Part I--the preoperative period. *Anaesthesiology intensive therapy*, 44(3), pp. 165-9. Available at: http://www.ncbi.nlm.nih.gov/pubmed/23110295.

Manworren, R. C., Paulos, C. L., Pop, R. 2004 Treating children for acute agitation in the PACU: differentiating pain and emergence delirium. *Journal of Perianaesthesia Nursing* 19 183-193.

MacLaren, J. E. and Cohen, L. L., 2007. Interventions for paediatric procedure-related pain in primary care. *Paediatrics and Child Health*, 12(2), pp. 111-116.

McCabe, M. a, 1996. Involving children and adolescents in medical decision making: developmental and clinical considerations. *Journal of pediatric psychology*, 21(4), pp. 505-516.

McGrath, P. J., Frager, G. 1996 Psychological barriers to optimal pain management in infants and children. *Clinical Journal of Pain* 12 135-141.

McMurtry, C. M., et al., 2010. When "don't worry" communicates fear: Children's perceptions of parental reassurance and distraction during a painful medical procedure. *Pain*, 150(1), pp. 52-8. Available at: http://www.ncbi.nlm.nih.gov/pubmed/20227831 [Accessed April 26, 2015].

Miller, V. A., 2009. Parent–child collaborative decision making for the management of chronic illness: A qualitative analysis. *Families, Systems, and Health*, 27(3), pp. 1-17. Available at: http://psycnet.apa.org/journals/fsh/27/3/249/.

Moushey, R., Sinacore, M. L., Diomede, B. 1988 A perioperative teaching program: A collaborative process. *Journal of Pediatric Nursing* 3 40-45.

O'Conner-Von, S. 2000 Preparing children for surgery: An integrative research review. *AORN Journal* 71 334-343.

O'Sullivan, M. and Wong, G. K., 2013. Preinduction techniques to relieve anxiety in children undergoing general anaesthesia. *Continuing Education in Anaesthesia, Critical Care and Pain*, 13(6), pp. 196-199.

Patil, V. 2007 Day surgery for children. *Anaesthesia and Intensive Care Medicine* 8 176-179.

Perry, J. N., Hooper, V. D. and Masiongale, J., 2012. Reduction of Preoperative Anxiety in Pediatric Surgery Patients Using Age-Appropriate Teaching Interventions. *Journal of Perianesthesia Nursing*, 27(2), pp. 69-81. Available at: http://dx.doi.org/10.1016/j.jopan.2012.01.003.

Piira, T., Sugiura, T., Champion, G. D., Donnelly, N., Cole, A. S. 2005 The role of parental presence in the context of children's medical procedures: a systematic review. *Child: Care, Health and Development* 31 233-243.

Platt 1959. Central Health Services Council (Great Britain). *The Welfare of Children in Hospital: Report of the Committee*, London, UK, HMSO.

Rawal, N. 2001 Analgesia for day-case surgery. *British Journal of Anaesthesia* 87 73-87.

Robertson, J. 1955 Young children in long-term hospitals. *Nursing times* 23 63-65.

Royal College of Nursing, 2013. *Guideline 3: Day Surgery Information Children and young people in day surgery*, pp. 1-7.

Royal College of Surgeons, 2013. *Standards for Children's Surgery*. Children's Surgical Forum.

Royaltey, H. H. 1988 The information needs of health care professionals and consumers in developing countries. *Bulletin of the Medical Librarians Association* 76 35-43.

Schechter, N. L. 1989 The undertreatment of pain in children: an overview. *Pediatric Clinics of North America* 36 781-794.

Thornes, R. 1991. *Just for the day: Caring for children in the health service*, London, UK, NAWCH.

Visintainer, M. A. Wolfer, J. A. 1975 Psychological preparation for surgical pediatric patients: the effect on children's and parents' stress responses and adjustment. *Paediatrics* 56 187-202.

Voepel-Lewis, T., Malviya, S., Tait, A. R. 2003 A prospective cohort study of emergence agitation in the paediatric postanaesthesia care unit. *Anaesthesia and Analgia* 96 1625-1630.

Williams, J. M. and Binnie, L. M., 2002. Children's concepts of illness: an intervention to improve knowledge. *British journal of health psychology*, 7(Pt 2), pp. 129-47. Available at: http://www.ncbi.nlm.nih.gov/pubmed/14596705 [Accessed April 26, 2015].

Wollin, S. R., et al., 2004. Anxiety in children having elective surgery. *Journal of Pediatric Nursing*, 19(2), pp. 128-132.

Wolf, A. R. 1999 Tears at Bedtime: a pitfall of extending paediatric day-case surgery without extending analgesia. *British Journal of Anaesthesia* 82(3) 319-320.

Wolf, A. R. 2009 Pro-Con Debate; the place of premedication in pediatric practice. *Pediatric Anesthesia* 19 817-828.

Woodhead, K., Wicker, P. 2005. *A textbook of perioperative care London*, UK, Churchill Livingstone.

Zeltzer, L., Barr, R. G., McGrath, P. A., Schechter, N. L. 1992 Pediatric pain: interacting behavioral and physical factors. *Pediatrics* 90 816-821.

Zuckerberg, A. L. 1994 Perioperative approach to children. *Pediatric Clinics of North America* 41 15-29.

In: Perioperative Practice in Trauma and Orthopaedic Surgery ISBN: 978-1-63483-325-7
Editor: Wasim S. Khan

Chapter 8

DIATHERMY IN PERIOPERATIVE PRACTICE

A. G. Potty, H. D. Tailor and W. S. Khan*
University College London Institute of Orthopaedics and Musculoskeletal Science, Royal National Orthopaedic Hospital, Stanmore, Middlesex, London, UK

ABSTRACT

Diathermy has revolutionised modern surgery and is an important tool for efficient and safe surgical practice. It has evolved to become the modern day scalpel, cutting and coagulating tissues. This article aims to elicit the functioning and safe usage of diathermy in the perioperative setting. The various precautionary checks before surgery, which are prerequisite for safe usage, are highlighted along with the necessary safety drills taken during and after operation. A specific note is included about the usage of electrical equipment when used in specialised surgeries like cardiac and laparoscopic surgery. A quick insight to issues regarding the maintenance and repair and finally, the anticipation for a future with precise and safer cutting and coagulation devices is addressed.

Keywords: Diathermy, perioperative practice, safety, electrodes, laparoscopic surgery

This chapter reviews the principles and practicalities of the use of diathermy in operative practice (Potty et al. 2010). Existence of electrodes for medical uses, such as removing skin lesions, dates back to over 100 years (Rivière 1900). Over the century, its usage has evolved and diathermy electrical devices are now a valuable tool in modern surgery to facilitate cutting of tissues and to prevent bleeding from small vessels during operative procedures (Kirk 2010, Meeker & Rothrock 1999). It is therefore important to understand how it works, and the principles and precautions involved with its safe use in the perioperative setting.

* Mr Wasim S Khan, Clinical Lecturer, University College London Institute of Orthopaedics and Musculoskeletal Science, Royal National Orthopaedic Hospital, Stanmore, Middlesex, London, HA7 4LP, UK; Telephone number: +44 (0) 7791 025554; Fax number: +44 (0) 20 8570 3864; E-mail address: wasimkhan@doctors.org.uk.

TECHNICAL CONCEPTS OF DIATHERMY DEVICES

Diathermy electrosurgical devices work by converting electrical current to a high frequency alternating current (HFAC). The current used is in the range of 200kHz to 3MHz which is much higher than the frequency that would cause neuromuscular stimulation or electrocution (Covidien 2009). Electrical currents passing through diathermy circuits generate localised heat due to the resistance of the tissues to the flow of current. In addition to other variables, altering the frequency waveform can cause three different effects on tissues resulting from a rise in temperature. It can cut the tissue by generating heat and destroying cells, it can coagulate vessels by contracting the tissues, and it can fulgurate or dehydrate cells (Covidien 2008, Phippen & Wells 1999). There are two different types of diathermy devices which are commonly used depending on how the electrical circuit is completed, monopolar and bipolar.

1. Monopolar Diathermy

device and is emitted via an active electrode controlled by the operator. The active electrode is commonly in the form of a diathermy pen, with various tips, such as balls and spatulas, available for the desired procedure. Forceps may also be used where the surgeon requires grasping in haemostasis. It can be operated using either finger switches at the active electrode site or remotely with two pedals attached to the diathermy machine. The blue finger switch or pedal activates coagulating and the yellow switch or pedal activates cutting. It is often used for haemostasis at the surgical wound site. However, the potential of monopolar diathermy as a dissecting tool is under-appreciated, and is facilitated by the use of the foot control and the round-tipped spatula end (Beasley 2008). The current then passes through the patient's body tissues and then returns back to the diathermy machine via a dispersive electrode or patient return pad. Hence, the patient is an important part of the circuit. The large area of the patient return pad results in a lower current density than that of the active electrode (Hay 2007); the significance of this is explained later.

2. Bipolar Diathermy

In contrast to monopolar diathermy, forceps are more frequently used. HFAC generated by the diathermy electrosurgical device passes down one tine of the forceps and then through the patient's tissue placed between the tips before returning to the diathermy machine through the second tine (Hay 2007). Common use for bipolar diathermy is securing haemostasis in peripheral tissues. Cutting is also possible with the use of bipolar scissors and graspers (Jones et al.. 2006).

Maintenance and General Considerations

Maintenance checks should be done by a qualified and experienced engineer annually. This is usually done by the biomedical engineering department who can then mark the equipment as safe for usage (AORN 2005). There should be labels on all electrical equipment with clear documentation of safety testing. The date of testing, the due date for next test, the testing authority seal and testers signature should be checked before usage. All faulty equipment should be taken off the theatre premises and repaired before further use (Wicker & O'Neill 2010). In addition, manufacturers should be updated with faults and performance of the equipment.

Only manufacturer recommended and quality assured electrical equipment should be used. Diathermy should only be set up by an experienced and competent practitioner who has had prior training with the equipment and must use the equipment according to the manufacturer's guidelines. All the necessary safety precautions and checks should be carefully followed as advised in the instruction manual. The equipment should be inspected and safety features tested before every use (AfPP 2007). The volume of the activation sound indicator should be turned on and tested so any malfunctioning can be heard when the device is switched on. Failure to pass the necessary preoperative safety tests should be taken seriously and reported to the hospital biomedical engineering department immediately for repairs or replacements (Wicker & O'Neill 2010).

If the operator reports any inaccuracies or any malfunctioning during the procedure, unscrubbed theatre staff should check the entire electrosurgical circuit to rectify the problem and, if necessary, reset the unit. If sterility is an issue, the active electrode should be disconnected from the main unit with the lead, and the whole system should be replaced with a new sterile set. Capacitive coupling occurs when alternating current is transferred from an insulated instrument to a non-insulated instrument through a capacitor. Therefore, intraoperatively, care should be taken to keep non-insulated metal objects at a safe distance from an activated electrode to avoid short-circuit. This can cause a spark and result in serious injuries in theatres (Hay 2007). Capacitance in relation to the cables and laparoscopic procedures is discussed later.

Any injury or burns to patient or staff, and any equipment failure with the active or dispersive electrode must be managed according to the recommendations of the Safe Medical Devices Act (FDA 2000). An incident form should be completed and evidence of injury should be documented in the patient's notes. The device identification, maintenance and service information and the adverse event information should be included in this report (AORN 2005).

Components of the Diathermy Set-up

The typical diathermy set-up consists of the diathermy generator unit, cables and electrodes (Covidien 2008). Each of these components is discussed below.

1. Diathermy Unit

The unit should be placed on a stand with wheels so that it can be moved easily around the theatre without any problems. It should be kept as far as possible from highly inflammable liquids and gases. Fluids, especially alcoholic preparation, should never be placed on top of the diathermy unit as these units pose a potential fire hazard (Beesley & Taylor 2006).

Power settings should be adjusted in conjunction with the manufacturers' guidelines, type of surgery, patient's weight and body surface area. The diathermy should be set to the lowest effective energy setting for desired cutting and coagulation to reduce the potential of burns and injuries (AORN 2005). Power setting should be confirmed verbally.

2. Cables and Electrodes

All cables and electrodes must be checked prior to use to ensure insulation is intact. All knots and twists in the electrode cable must be removed before plugging in the electrode. The electrode cable should not be wrapped around metal objects as metal is a conductor of electricity and may cause burns (AfPP 2007, AORN 2005, Coviden 2008). All cables should be completely insulated, of adequate length and without any stress. Active electrodes should be within easy reach of surgeons and secured to drapes with non-metal clips to maintain sterility. When not in use the active electrode should be placed in a clean well-insulated holster to prevent burns to the patients and drapes (AfPP 2007, Wicker & O'Neill 2010). The build up of eschar on the electrode tips is a potential fire hazard (Covidien 2008). Therefore, a scratch card should be used to clean off any eschar to ensure efficiency and safety of the electrode (AORN 2005). Availability of specially-coated tips are said to reduce the build-up of eschar (Covidien 2008). It is the responsibility of the operating surgeon to activate the electrode (AORN 2005). After all the necessary checks and final count, the disposable active electrode tip should be discarded into a sharps bin.

If two or more electrical units are used concurrently during an operation, the manufacturers' instructions for compatibility of differing equipment must be adhered to. If this is not followed, there is a risk of short circuits and burns to the staff and the patient (AORN 2005).

Surgical plume, the large amount of smoke generated when diathermy is used on tissue, should be constantly sucked off to prevent inhalation of toxic chemical by-products like toluene, formaldehyde, benzene and hydrogen cyanide (Ulmer 2008). These plumes also contain intact cells, cell parts, intact viral DNA, viable bacteria, including Mycobacterium tuberculosis (Woodhead & Wicker 2005). Further protection is achieved through specially designed smoke evacuation systems and surgical filtration masks donned for all surgical procedures (AORN 2005, NATN 2004).

3. Dispersive Electrode

An important aspect of effective diathermy functioning is the proper placement and sizing of the dispersive electrode when using the monopolar setup. Choose an appropriate size dispersive electrode based on the patient's weight. After safely positioning the patient on the operating table, the dispersive electrode should be placed on a dry intact skin surface overlying a large, well-perfused muscle tissue to allow optimal dissipation of energy. Ideally, this should be as close to the operative site as possible (AfPP 2007). This could be at the buttock, posterior or anterior thigh, mid or lower back, upper calf or abdomen (Wicker 2010). Dispersive electrodes should not be placed over scar tissue, hairy skin, bony prominences, metal prosthesis and areas distal to a tourniquet. Hair should be shaved if necessary as imperfect bonding of a dispersive electrode to skin caused by moisture or hair can lead to failure of the equipment (Phippen & Wells 1999, Wicker 2010). However, if an electrode does not adhere satisfactorily, a new dispersive plate should be repositioned at a different site. In the cases of existing skin conditions such as epidermolysis bullosa, a bipolar diathermy should be used instead of dispersive electrodes.

The dispersive electrode should never be cut or trimmed as it can cause serious malfunctioning by reducing surface area, increase the impedance of the electrical current, and increases the risk of burns. This concept can understood by the equation stated by Covidien (2008) where

Burn = Current x Time / Area of electrode

Therefore, larger patient return electrodes will minimize the risk of burns.

Dispersive electrodes that have been removed from a patient's skin should be discarded. The surgeon should ensure that the dispersive electrode is removed carefully without denuding the surface of the skin, and any breach in skin or burns identified should be documented. The surgeon should be informed of all injuries and necessary treatment commenced immediately. An incident form should be completed by the practitioner who removed the electrode or the nurse in charge, and accurate documentation and handover to recovery and ward should be done. The surgeon or anaesthetist should finally inform the patients and relatives of any adverse events and the likely management and prognosis. It is also important to evaluate and document the skin quality and integrity in the perioperative care plan before and after the use of diathermy (AfPP 2007).

SPECIAL PRECAUTIONS

Special precautions need to be taken in certain circumstances. These include procedures on patients with pacemakers, and cardiac and cochlear implants. There are also special considerations in laparoscopic and arthroscopic surgery and they are outlined below.

1. Pacemaker and Cardiac Implants

There is an increasing number of patients who are now being fitted with cardiac pacemakers and Automatic Cardioverter Implantable Defibrillators (ACID) (Allen 2006). Especially with monopolar diathermy, it is understandable that there is severe risk of malfunctioning of the cardiac device or even fatal arrythmias. Many of these patients will be identified at a pre-surgical assessment clinic. If identified, it should be clearly documented in the patient's casenotes for the attention of the operating surgeon. Precautionary checks should be performed prior to surgery. Knowing when the device should be disabled or reprogrammed requires careful consideration and consultation between the cardiologist, anaesthetist and surgeon.

The Medicines Healthcare products Regulatory Agency (MHRA) have published guidelines (MHRA 2006) on the management of patients with implantable cardiac devices in the presence of surgical diathermy. They advise not to use any diathermy device, but if necessary, bipolar diathermy should be used. The ACID will need to be deactivated before diathermy is used. It is important that a cardiac resuscitation team and functioning external defibrillators are available (MHRA 2006). The anaesthetist should ensure continual ECG monitoring is set up and that all cables are kept away from the pacemaker. They should also connect the leads to a defibrillator for any intraoperative emergencies. The overall aim is to obtain an accurate history and use bipolar diathermy in any doubts.

2. Cochlear Implants in ENT Surgery

As with implanted cardiac devices, certain precautions should be observed for patients with cochlear implants. Ideally, bipolar diathermy should be used. If monopolar diathermy has to be used, the distance between the active electrode and the dispersive electrode should be kept as short as possible. This is to ensure the current path between the surgical site and dispersive electrode does not pass through the vicinity of the implant stimulator or leads (Smith & Smith 2001).

3. Laparoscopic and Arthroscopic Surgery

Similar risks and precautions that apply to open surgery are also applicable to laparoscopic and arthroscopic surgery. Current can escape from crevices or cuts in the insulation and can result in burns to the exposed areas. For example, there is a risk of unintentional bowel perforation. Therefore, all insulated laparoscopic and arthroscopic equipment must be checked before and after use to ensure there are no defects (AfPP 2007). A non-conducting trocar used at a low voltage will substantially reduce the risk of capacitive coupling. If using a metal trocar (conducting trocar) the surgeon should ensure a good contact with the abdominal wall (*HSE 2002*) to further reduce the risk of capacitive coupling. It is important to be aware of other laparoscopic instruments, especially metal ones, in the vicinity to avoid direct coupling. Laparoscopic active electrodes which are damaged should be disposed safely and disposable single use laparoscopic active electrodes should never be re-used or autoclaved (Hay 2007, HSE 2002). Laparoscopic bipolar diathermy instruments should be used to keep the current spatially as minimal as possible (AfPP 2007, Jones et al. 2006). In arthroscopic surgery extreme care should be taken whilst irrigating the joint and the saline irrigation should be kept on the opposite side of diathermy machine to prevent spillage of liquid. Diathermy pedals should be well-insulated and waterproof.

Developments in Haemostasis

With research and developments in electrical and surgical sciences, highly precise and safer devices are becoming available, but they come at a high financial cost. With evolution of endoscopic and reconstructive surgery there has been a high demand for new technology to achieve precise vascular control. Suture ligation can be time-consuming and cumbersome during laparoscopic dissection. Titanium and plastic clips have been used for haemostasis, but more recently energy sources such as ultrasonic coagulating shears and bipolar thermal energy devices have become popular (Harold et al. 2003). Torsional mode ultrasonic coagulating shears have recently been developed for endoscopic and conventional surgery. The torsional mode shears had the extended ability to coagulate larger-sized vessels up to 7.4 mm diameter with good results (Ching & McMahon 2007). The invention of the gamma knife is exploited in neurosurgery to operate on small brain tumours and arterio-venous malformation by stereotactically directing high doses of radiation to destroy or coagulate the target (Siegfried et al. 1998). This accuracy and safety will drive newer technological discovery which will be the future of today's diathermy.

Conclusion

Diathermy should be used safely and judiciously. Staff should be adequately trained and supported to set it up. It is important that practitioners are aware of the risks associated with diathermy and take steps to avoid any complications. All necessary equipment safety checks must be performed preoperatively. Any adverse event should be recognised early and dealt with according to local protocol. With constantly emerging new technological advances, the future of diathermy is entering into an exciting era where cutting and coagulation will be achieved with fewer risks and greater precision. Safety will however continue to be one of the most important considerations in its use.

References

Allen M 2006 Pacemakers and implantable cardioverter defibrillators Anaesthesia 61 883-890.

Association for Perioperative Practice (AfPP) 2007 Standards & Recommendations for safe perioperative practice Harrogate, UK.

Association of Peri Operative Registered Nurses (AORN) 2005 Recommended practices for electrosurgery. *AORN Journal* 81 616-642.

Beesley J, Taylor L 2006 Reducing the risk of surgical fires: are you assessing the risk? *Journal of Perioperative Practice* 16 591-597.

Beasley SW 2008 Monopolar diathermy dissection made easy. *ANZ Journal of Surgery* 78 1119-1121.

Ching SS, McMahon MJ 2007 Comparison of linear and torsional mode ultrasonic coagulating shears for the sealing of medium- to large-sized arteries. *Surgical Endoscopy* 21 1165-1169.

Covidien 2008, *Principles of Electrosurgery*, Colorado, USA.

Covidien 2009 Electrosugery Continuing Education Module. Available: http://www.valleylabeducation.org/esself-2a/pages/esself2-08.html. Last accessed 19 April 2010.

Food and Drug Administration (FDA) 2000 Medical device reporting: Manufacturer reporting, importer reporting, user facility reporting, distributor reporting. *Federal Register* 65 4112-4121.

Harold KL, Pollinger H, Matthews BD et al. 2003 Comparison of ultrasonic energy, bipolar thermal energy, and vascular clips for the hemostasis of small-, medium-, and large-sized arteries. *Surgical Endoscopy* 17 1228-1230.

Hay DJ 2007 Electrosurgery Surgery (Oxford) 26 66-69.

Health and Safety Executive (HSE) 2002 COSHH Health and Safety, Norwich, UK.

Jones CM, Pierre KB, Nicoud IB et al. 2006 *Electrosurgery Current Surgery* 63 458-463.

Kirk RM 2010, *Basic Surgical Techniques*, Sixth Edition Churchill Livingstone, Edinburgh.

Medicines and Healthcare products Regulatory Agency (MHRA) 2006 Guidelines for the perioperative management of patients with implantable pacemakers or implantable cardioverter defibrillators, where the use of surgical diathermy/electrocautery is anticipated London, UK.

Meeker MH, Rothrock JC 1999 Alexander's care of the patient in surgery, Ninth Edition Mosby, Saint Louis, MO, USA.

National Association of Theatre Nurses (NATN) 2004 NATN Position Statement-Management of Electrosurgical Smoke and Laser plume. *British Journal of Perioperative Nursing* 14 414.

Phippen ML & Wells MP 1999 Patient Care During Operative and Invasive Procedures WB Saunders Company, Philadelphia.

Potty AG, Khan WS, Tailor HD (2010). Diathermy in perioperative surgery. *J. Perioper Pract.* 20(11): 402-5.

Rivière AJ 1900. Action des courants de haute fréquence et des effleuves du résonateur Oudin sur certaines tumeurs malignes. J*ournal de Médecine Interne* 4 776-7.

Ulmer BC 2008 The hazards of surgical smoke. *AORN Journal* 87 721-734.

Siegfried J, Haller D, Heinzel F et al. 1998 Gamma knife radiosurgery in neurosurgery Schweizerische medizinische Wochenschrift 128 115-122.

Smith TL & Smith JM 2001 Electrosurgery in Otolaryngology-Head and Neck Surgery: Principles, Advances, and Complications. *The Laryngoscope* 111 769-780.

Wicker P & O'Neill J 2010 Caring for the Perioperative Patient, Second edition Wiley-Blackwell, West Sussex, UK.

Woodhead K, Wicker P 2005. *A Textbook of Perioperative Care*. Churchill Livingstone, Edinburgh, UK.

In: Perioperative Practice in Trauma and Orthopaedic Surgery ISBN: 978-1-63483-325-7
Editor: Wasim S. Khan

Chapter 9

CORRECT PATIENT POSITIONING IN THEATRES

***Emeka Oragui*[1], *Wasim S. Khan*[2,*] *and Nimalan Maruthainar*[3]**

[1]Department of Trauma & Orthopaedics, West Middlesex University Hospital NHS Trust, London, UK

[2]Department of Trauma & Orthopaedics, Royal Free Hampstead NHS Trust, London, UK

[3]Department of Trauma & Orthopaedics, Royal Free Hampstead NHS Trust, London, UK

ABSTRACT

Patient positioning in theatre pertains to how a patient is transferred and positioned for a specific procedure. Patient safety is a central focus of care within the NHS and every healthcare practitioner must ensure that patients are protected from harm where possible. Mal-positioning of the patient has important implications in terms of associated problems of pressure sores, nerve compressions, deep vein thromboses and compartment syndrome, and should be avoided.

Keywords: Patient positioning, safety, pressure sores, nerve compression, deep vein thromboses, compartment syndrome

This chapter deals with correct patient positioning in theatre to optimize the surgical procedure and reduce complications (Oragui et al. 2010). Patient positioning in theatre pertains to how a patient is transferred and positioned for a specific procedure. A number of different positions can be adopted depending on the exposure required for the procedure, but must ensure the comfort and safety of the patient at all times. Careful planning must consider not only the procedure itself, but also the type of anaesthesia or sedation that needs to be administered, the duration of the procedure and any co-morbidities the patient may have. The

* Corresponding Author: Mr WS Khan, Clinical Lecturer, University College London Institute of Orthopaedics and Musculoskeletal Science, Royal National Orthopaedic Hospital, Stanmore, Middlesex, London, HA7 4LP, UK; Telephone number: +44 (0) 7971 190720; Fax number: +44 (0) 20 8570 3864; E-mail address: wasimkhan@doctors.org.uk.

importance of patient positioning can often be overlooked and underestimated, despite the evidence that proper patient positioning can prevent immediate problems and reduce the risk of long-term pain and disability (Warner 2004). In this chapter, we discuss the importance of correct patient positioning and associated problems, look at common positions adopted in theatre and highlight important considerations.

WHY PATIENT POSITIONING IS IMPORTANT

Patient safety is a central focus of care within the NHS framework (Carruthers & Philip 2006) and every healthcare practitioner must ensure that patients are protected from harm where possible. Proper positioning reduces the risk of pressure-related damage to nerves, muscle, skin, and joints. The anaesthetised or sedated patient is unable to communicate if they have been placed in a compromising or dangerous position, hence a proactive approach should be taken to prevent the deleterious effects of patient mal-positioning.

Correct positioning of a patient allows optimum exposure of the operative field (Millsaps 2006). Positioning must also take into account the degree of movement that maybe necessary during the procedure, for example knee and shoulder arthroscopy require significant movement of the lower and upper limbs respectively during the procedure and the surgical field must be setup accordingly. Additional equipment e.g. fluoroscopy, may also be required during the procedure and the method by which it will access the operative site whilst maintaining a sterile field should be planned for. The effects of patient transfer and positioning on any equipment attached to the patient such as intravenous access lines and catheters must be catered for. The anaesthetic requirement for maintaining the respiratory and circulatory function of the patient must also be considered.

Poorly executed patient transfer and positioning may also negatively impact on the health of theatre staff and be costly to the affected individual both in terms of suffering and time off work. Videman et al. (1985) have shown that back injuries may be prevented by teaching correct patient-handling skills. It may be necessary to provide hoisting equipment with special beds for the lifting and transfer of the morbidly obese patient to prevent injuries to the health care worker (Kaffarnik & Utzolino 2009).

PROBLEMS WITH POOR PATIENT POSITIONING

Complications with patient positioning can occur in transit when moving the patient into and out of theatre, or during the procedure itself. Problems may arise when the patient is poorly placed for a prolonged period of time. Four of the commonest complications are discussed below.

1. Skin pressure sores: Skin pressure sores can result in sepsis which may be fatal. Stevens et al. (2004) have shown that ‘patients with longer operative times were at greater risk of skin breakdown and required greater care during preoperative positioning.’ Theatre staff should ensure that pressure points around bony prominences such as the iliac crest, sacrum and heels, are well padded with pillows, ankle pads etc. and if necessary, the patient moved slightly in lengthy procedures. Theatre staff should also be proactive in checking for

signs of skin breakdown such as redness or bruising after the procedure. This allows appropriate measures to be taken to avoid pressure sores developing. The right equipment to prevent damage e.g. soft pads, pillows, axillary or chest rolls should be used. Ideally they should 'absorb compressive force, redistribute pressure, prevent excessive stretching and provide support for optimum stability' (Rothrock 2003).

2. Nerve compression: Theatre staff must be aware of the potential risk of nerve injury in a poorly positioned patient. Parks (1973) reviewed 50,000 surgical procedures and reported 0.14% of cases were linked with peripheral nerve complications. Rothrock (2003) noted that it only takes minutes for neurological complications to arise, but they have long-lasting effects on the patient.

Ulnar nerve palsy arises from compression of the ulnar nerve. The injury may result in a 'claw hand' deformity and the inability of the fingers of that hand to abduct and adduct, as well as a loss of sensation to the medial aspect of the hand. This can occur when the patient's arm slips off the mattress unnoticed by the theatre staff and the ulnar nerve becomes compressed by the medial epicondyle at the elbow and the table (Millsaps 2006). Brachial plexus injuries can occur in either the prone or supine position where the head is rotated and laterally flexed, or the arm is extended posteriorly. The complications that arise depend on which nerves in the plexus are damaged. Radial nerve damage will result in a wrist drop, whereas median nerve damage may result in an 'ape hand' deformity with a loss of the ability to grasp with that hand (Winfree & Kline 2005). Common peroneal nerve damage results in a foot drop and a loss of sensation over the lateral leg and dorsum of the foot (Winfree & Kline 2005).

3. Deep vein thrombosis: Improving patient safety is an important priority for the National Health Service. Patient safety initiatives aimed at creating a safe operating theatre culture are increasingly being adopted and reliable means of measuring their impact are being developed (Pronovost et al. 2005, Makary et al. 2006), and these include rates of deep vein thrombosis (DVT).

DVT can result from prolonged periods of immobility causing blood stasis, and is associated with the potential life threatening complication of pulmonary embolic phenomenon. They can arise particularly in long procedures where the patient has suffered fluid loss. Prophylactic anti-embolism stockings should be worn and consideration given to the use of external pneumatic compression applied to the lower legs. Early mobilisation of the patient in the postoperative period and prophylaxis with low molecular weight heparin should be encouraged unless contraindicated (NICE 2007, Pearse et al. 2007).

4. Compartment syndrome: This is a life- and limb-threatening complication associated with patient mal-positioning and has been covered in detail in an earlier review by the authors (Malik et al. 2009, Mabvuure et al. 2012, Donaldson et al. 2014). Prolonged compression of the vessels of a limb may impede circulation to the appendage and cause a compartment syndrome resulting in muscle necrosis and loss of function. Roher et al. (2008) noted that 'Long-lasting operations in the Lithotomy position are accompanied by the risk of an acute compartment syndrome of the lower extremities.' Safe positioning must allow for adequate blood flow to all four limbs

DIFFERENT PATIENT POSITIONS USED IN SURGICAL PRACTICE

Millsaps (2006) describes the four most common surgical positions as supine, prone, lateral and the lithotomy position and these are discussed below. The choice is based primarily on the procedure to be carried out, for example the prone position allows access to the spine for epidurals and spinal surgery whereas the lithotomy position is used in gynaecological procedures to permit access and clear visualisation of the internal and external female genitalia.

1. Prone position: The patient is placed lying flat face down on the operating table with arms placed either on the side of the body or forward with the elbows flexed and palms down. The face is either facing down into a specially designed headrest or turned to the side. The patient is generally anaesthetised in the supine position and moved into the prone position by a safe log roll. Movements of the spine should be minimised. A minimum of six theatre staff, including the anaesthetist, should be employed in the safe log-rolling of the patient. When placing patients in this position, it is important to support the head and neck and this is usually done by the anaesthetist. It is also important to have sufficient staff to support the patient along the length of their body whilst performing the log roll. If the arms are to be brought forwards, both arms should be moved into position at the same time, and similarly returned to the side simultaneously at the end of the operation.

Potential risks are brachial plexus injury if the head is rotated and laterally flexed or the arms hyper-extended during the transfer. Shoulder dislocations and other arm injuries have also been reported in the literature (Edgecombe et al. 2008). There are well documented adverse physiological effects to the respiratory and cardiovascular system in the prone position. Primarily these are the domain of the anaesthetist who should be well trained in optimising the patient and reducing the risk of these occurring. An increased risk of ophthalmic injury is well established in patients operated in a prone position (Lee 2003). The mechanism of injury is believed to be central retinal artery occlusion and ischaemic optic neuropathy (Kamming & Clark 2005).

Theatre staff should be aware of the existence of and correct use of aids used to optimise the prone patient positioning. These include the Montreal mattress where central hollow helps prevent abdominal compression and improves ventilation and venous return (Schonauer et al. 2004), and the horse shoe head-rest that allows ventilation without compromise of the intubation equipment. Theatre staff should be aware of parts of the body at risk from pressure effects. Excessive compression of the breast and male genitalia must be prevented by adequate padding.

2. Supine position: The patient is placed lying flat on their back, face up on the operating table with arms placed either on the side of the body or with the elbows flexed and palms on the chest. Transfer of the patient from the anesthetic table to the operating table is undertaken in a smooth coordinated manner. A minimum of four people including the anaesthetist are recommended (Charney 2003). Ulnar nerve injury resulting from pressure of the elbow at the edge of the operating table should be prevented by ensuring that the arm does not slip off the operating table and that there is soft padding around the elbow. Excessive external pressure on the humerus that could lead to radial nerve injury should also be avoided. Soft support on the lumbosacral area of the back will prevent backache. Soft padding over the sacrum and a

pillow under the occiput prevents the development of pressure sores. Intraoperatively, theatre staff should not 'prop themselves up' on the patient as this can lead to pressure sores, reduced ventilation and reduced venous return. Pressure on the calf muscle can increase the risk of DVT and should be reduced by wearing thrombo-embolic deterrent (TED) stockings and pneumatic compression devices.

3. Lithotomy position: The patient is laid supine and the distal end of the bed detached so that the legs can be elevated in stirrups. The medical history of the patient should be considered before placing the patient in the lithotomy position and any restrictions to hip, knee or ankle movements noted. It may be necessary to modify the lithotomy position taking these factors into account. Both legs should be moved slowly and simultaneously by two people when positioning the patient in and out of the stirrups to avoid excessive shear and torsional stresses at the hip joint and pelvis.

Nerve injuries following the lithotomy position are well documented. Concomitant hip flexion should be used when placing anesthetised patients in a lithotomy position where the lower limbs are abducted to greater than 30° to decrease the risk of obturator nerve injury (Litwiller et al. 2004). Stretching injures to the sciatic nerve should also be prevented by avoiding excessive external rotation of the hip with the knee in extension. Common peroneal nerve injuries resulting in foot drop and loss of sensation over the dorsum of the foot have been reported in literature (Warner et al. 1994) and should be avoided by correct placement of the legs in the stirrups.

Lower limb acute compartment syndrome after prolonged urological, colorectal, and gynaecological procedures are also well-documented. Simms & Terry (2005) estimate that 1 in 500 cystectomy procedures may result in a compartment syndrome. Theatre staff should communicate with ward staff postoperatively to ensure that a regular lower limb neurovascular assessments are made in patients placed in the lithotomy position for a prolonged period of time.

4. Lateral or decubitus position: The patient is positioned on their lateral side with their arms parallel to each other. The most important aspect is to maintain body alignment and stability. The neck is kept in a neutral position, and the body stabilised with positional devices to prevent the patient moving freely on the table. The patient is typically anaesthetised in the supine position, and then moved into the lateral position. Peroneal nerve injury may arise from pressure on the lateral aspect of the knee due to the weight of the other leg and could be reduced by appropriately placed padding under the lower knee. Padding between the knees should also be used to protect against pressure sores over medial condyles. Brachial plexus injuries are prevented by placing an axillary roll underneath the bottom arm. The general principles of avoiding skin necrosis and DVT apply.

How to Prevent Patient Mal-Positioning

Prior to the patient arriving in the anaesthetic room, theatre staff should ensure that the correct operating table and all necessary attachments are available and in good working condition. Sufficient personnel should be available to allow safe and controlled transfer of the patient. Following discussion with the anaesthetist and the medical or surgical practitioner, theatre staff should decide on the appropriate mode of patient transfer and positioning.

The patient must be free to move and all limbs controlled during transfer. Any attachments to the patient such as monitoring devices, catheters, intravenous access etc must be secured or temporarily removed. The patient should be transferred in a coordinated manner that is directed by the anaesthetist. Hyperextension of the extremities should be avoided at all costs (Edgecombe et al. 2008). Easyslide, Patslide, or Roll Boards may all be used in transferring the patient. Their basic principle involves gently rolling the patient slightly to one side and placing the device under them, then rolling the patient back to a supine position and sliding them onto the operating table. Finally the patient is gently rolled the other way and the device removed.

Once transferred and positioned the patient should be secured appropriately. Restraints must be secure but not excessively tight. Placing restraints over superficial nerves or bony prominences should be avoided. The position of the patient must not compromise the use and visualisation of monitoring equipment for the theatre staff as this could put the patient at risk.

Patient factors are also important in adverse outcomes in poorly positioned patients and must be addressed to minimise the risk of injury. Special care should be taken in obese individuals who face a greater likelihood of nerve and other pressure point injury (Meltzer 2001). The elderly population has also been observed to be more susceptible to pressure point injury due to their generally poorer peripheral circulation, friable skin and reduced capacity to tolerate circulatory compromise.

An algorithm to ensure correct patient positioning devised by the Association of Operating Room Nurses (2005) and is outlined below

- Plan for the procedure in advance.
- Identify the position that will be used and ensure that any equipment necessary for the safe transfer and positioning of the patient is available and in working order.
- A dedicated theatre member should coordinate the safe transfer and positioning of the patient.
- Ensure adequate theatre staff numbers and communicate the responsibility of each theatre member involved in the process of transfer and positioning.
- Consider repositioning the patient in long procedures to reduce the risk of pressure sores, DVT formation and compartment syndrome.
- Check the patient before and after the procedure for tell-tale signs of complications from the positioning. Ask the patient once awake if they have any unexpected pain or numbness.
- Consider preoperative and postoperative nerve conduction studies for patients at risk such as prolonged immobilisation in the prone position.

CONCLUSION

Every healthcare practitioner must ensure that patients are protected from harm where possible and correct patient positioning in theatre is crucial to avoid the preventable complications of pressure sores, nerve compressions, DVTs and compartment syndrome. It is important to plan for patient transfer and positioning in a safe and coordinated manner, and to use all aids and appliances available to prevent complications. It is also important to check the patient before and after the procedure for tell-tale signs of complications from the positioning.

REFERENCES

Association of Operating Room Nurses 2005 *Recommended practices for positioning the patient in the perioperative practice setting* In: *Standards, Recommended Practices, and Guidelines* Denver, *CO, AORN Journal.*

Carruthers I, Philip P 2006 *Safety first: a report for patients, clinicians and healthcare managers* London, UK, Department of Health Publications.

Charney W 2003 Preventing back injury to healthcare workers using lift teams: Data from 18 hospitals *Journal of Health and Safety* 1 21-29.

Donaldson J, Haddad B, Khan WS (2014). The Pathophysiology, Diagnosis and Current Management of Acute Compartment Syndrome. *The Open Orthop. J.* 8: 185-93.

Edgecombe H, Carter K, Yarrow S 2008 Anaesthesia in the prone position *British Journal of Anaesthesia* 100 165-183.

Kaffarnik M, Utzolino S 2009 Postoperative management of patients with BMI > 40 kg / m^2 *Zentralblatt für Chirurgie* 134 43-49.

Kamming D, Clarke S 2005 Postoperative visual loss following prone spinal surgery *British Journal of Anaesthesia* 95 257–260.

Lee LA 2003 Postoperative visual loss registry: preliminary analysis of factors associated with spine operations *American Society of Anaesthesiology Newsletter* 67 7–8.

Litwiller JP, Wells RE, Halliwill JR, Carmichael SW, Warner MA 2004 Effect of lithotomy positions on strain of the obturator and lateral femoral cutaneous nerves *Clinical Anatomy* 17 45-49.

Mabvuure NT, Malahias M, Hindocha S, Khan WS, Juma A (2012). Acute Compartment Syndrome of the Limbs: Current Concepts and Management. *Open Orthop. J.* 6: 535-43.

Makary MA, Sexton JB, Freischlag JA et al. 2006 Patient Safety in Surgery *Annals of Surgery* 243 628–635.

Malik AA, Khan WS, Chaudhry A, Ihsan M, Cullen NP 2009 Acute compartment syndrome-a life and limb threatening surgical emergency *Journal of Perioperative Practice* 19 137-142.

Meltzer B 2001 *A Guide to Patient Positioning* [Online] Available from: http://www.outpatientsurgery.net/2001/os04/f5.shtml [Accessed October 2009].

Millsaps CC 2006 Pay attention to patient positioning! *RN* 69 59-63.

National Institute for Health and Clinical Excellence 2007 *Venous thromboembolism* London, UK, Department of Health Publications.

Oragui E, Khan WS, Maruthainar N (2010). The Importance of Correct Patient Positioning in Theatres and Implications of Mal-positioning. *J. Perioper Pract.* 20(4): 143-7.

Parks BJ 1973 Postoperative peripheral neuropathies *Surgery* 74 348-357.

Pearse EO, Caldwell BF, Lockwood RJ, Hollard J 2007 Early mobilisation after conventional knee replacement may reduce the risk of postoperative venous thromboembolism *Journal of Bone & Joint Surgery* 89B 316-322.

Pronovost PJ, Weast B, Rosenstein B et al. 2005 Implementing and validating a comprehensive unit-based safety program *Journal of Patient Safety* 1 33-40.

Roher H, Onmann C, Beck L 2008 Acute compartment syndrome due to positioning during long-lasting gynecological operations in the lithotomy position. *Gynakologe* 41 1023-1026.

Rothrock J C 2003 *Alexander's care of the patient in surgery* (12th edition) St. Louis, MO, Mosby.

Schonauer C, Bocchetti A, Barbagallo G, Albanese V, Moraci A 2004 Positioning on surgical table. *European Spine Journal* 13 S50-S55.

Simms MS, Terry TR 2005 Well leg compartment syndrome after pelvic and perineal surgery in the lithotomy position. *Postgraduate Medical Journal* 81 534-536.

Stevens J, Nichelson E, Linehan W 2004 Risk factors for skin breakdown after renal and adrenal surgery. *Urology* 64 246-249.

Videman T, Rauhala H, Asp S et al. 1989 Patient-handling skill, back injuries, and back pain. An intervention study in nursing. *Spine* 14 148-156.

Warner M, Martin J, Schroeder D, Offord KP, Chute CG 1994 Lower-extremity motor neuropathy associated with surgery performed on patients in a lithotomy position. *Anesthesiology* 81 6-12.

Warner M 2004 *Patient positioning strategies* [Online] Available from: www. outpatientsurgery.net/2003/os08/patient_positioning_strategies.php [Accessed October 2009].

Winfree CJ, Kline DG 2005 Intraoperative positioning nerve injuries *Surgical Neurology* 63 5-18.

In: Perioperative Practice in Trauma and Orthopaedic Surgery ISBN: 978-1-63483-325-7
Editor: Wasim S. Khan

Chapter 10

THE USE OF IONISING RADIATION IN TRAUMA AND ORTHOPAEDIC THEATRES

Matthew S. Prime, Wasim S. Khan*, Sujay Dheerendra and Nimalan Maruthainar

Department of Trauma & Orthopaedics, Royal Free Hampstead NHS Trust, London, UK

ABSTRACT

Ionising radiation is used extensively in trauma and orthopaedic perioperative practice for operative planning and intraoperative decision making. Radiation poses risks to patients and theatre staff, and it is important to always justify, optimise and limit the exposure. This is facilitated by a thorough understanding and awareness of radiation, as well as a sound knowledge of the precautions required for using this technology to minimise the risks of radiation.

Keywords: Ionising radiation, trauma; orthopaedics, X-ray, risks, precautions

Ionising radiation is integral to trauma and orthopaedic perioperative practice, and is used extensively for operative planning and intraoperative decision making (Prime et al. 2010). It is important to consider the risks radiation poses to patients and theatre staff, and always justify, optimise and limit the exposure. There is a need for a thorough understanding and awareness of radiation, and sound knowledge of the precautions required for using this technology to minimise the risks. This chapter aims to cover these aspects of radiation.

X-rays were discovered by Rontgen in 1895 whilst experimenting with a cathode tube at Wuerzburg University in Germany (Van Tiggelen 2001). The invention of the high vacuum

* Corresponding Author: Mr W Khan, Clinical Lecturer, University College London Institute of Orthopaedic and Musculoskeletal Research, Royal National Orthopaedic Hospital, Stanmore, Middlesex, HA7 4LP, UK; Telephone number: +44 (0) 77791 025554; Fax number: +44 (0) 1707 655059; E-mail address: wasimkhan@doctors.org.uk.

X-ray tube by Coolidge in 1912 allowed X-rays of sufficient penetration to be generated that allowed Medicine to take advantage of the potential of radiation (Van Tiggelen 2001).

THE GENERATION OF X-RAYS

The X-ray emitting tube where X-rays are produced is a glass vacuum tube encased in lead that consists of a cathode and an anode (Armstrong & Wastie 2001). The cathode is a filament that is heated by the passage of electric current that allows electrons to leave the surface. A high potential of more than 50 kV between the cathode and anode accelerates these electrons towards the anode. On hitting the anode the electrons produce electromagnetic radiation or X-rays. The anodes are generally made of tungsten as this has a higher atomic number resulting in the production of more X-rays. The X-ray tube needs a cooling system as a large amount of heat is also produced. The X-rays are filtered as they leave the X-ray tube to remove low energy X-rays that do not contribute to image production. The X-rays then generally pass through some medium before reaching the image receptor. The image that they produce depends on the medium that they have travelled through. X-rays are high energy electromagnetic radiations that travel in straight lines at the speed of light and are not affected by electric or magnetic fields (Armstrong & Wastie 2001).

IMAGING PRINCIPLES IN CLINICAL PRACTICE

Radiology is the use of X-rays to cross materials to see inside them. When an exposure is taken X-rays are released from the X-ray tube as a primary beam. As the radiation passes through the body some of it is absorbed by a process known as attenuation. Anatomy that has increased density has a higher rate of attenuation, so bone has a higher attenuation rate than soft tissues. When the X-rays reach the image receptor the radiation that has passed through tissues with lower attenuation will receive more radiation and be processed as darker. This is why bone which is dense shows up as white and the lungs which are full of air show up as black. Because different materials have varying abilities to absorb the emitted radiation a two-dimensional image can be constructed from the absorption pattern on a detection film. This is known as a radiographic film.

Over the last century scientific advancement in radiology and the invention of the computer have allowed all modalities of imaging to be digitally represented. The introduction of the picture archiving and communication system (PACS) has dispensed with the need for hard copy radiographs, and allows images to be viewed in multiple locations simultaneously and on screens with all manner of enhancement tools (Kreel 1991). This includes the operating theatre where the recently introduced WHO surgical checklist has a special check-box for the availability of imaging (Haynes et al. 2009).

The Perioperative Uses of Radiation Imaging

The use of radiology in theatres can be divided into two broad categories. First, radiological investigations carried out prior to an operative procedure which aid preoperative planning and are available in theatre to assist in perioperative decision making; second, radiological investigations taken during a procedure, which again optimise and enhance surgery.

Most trauma and orthopaedic procedures require a plain film radiograph for operative planning that commonly includes templating fixation implants and prostheses. Trauma patients are managed according to Advanced Trauma Life Support (ATLS) guidelines and if appropriate undergo cervical spine, chest and pelvis X-ray after their initial assessment, as well as further imaging as indicated. Several specific fractures require more sensitive imaging modalities to fully assess the fracture configuration; computerised tomography (CT) scans are the gold standard in pelvic, tibial plateau and calcaneal fracture. Operative planning can be further enhanced by the use of three-dimensional reconstruction of the fracture pattern by a computer. Picture archiving and communication system (PACS) is a computer server dedicated to the storage, retrieval, distribution and presentation of images. This allows electronic images to be transmitted digitally and facilitates retrieval, distribution and display that are common problems with hard copy images. PACS now also has the provision of software programmes that allow templating for fixation implants and prostheses.

The use of X-rays in theatre has increased with the realisation that more accurate surgical reduction and stabilisation of fractures with X-rays results in better healing of the fracture. This also allows procedures to be performed through smaller incisions as full visual exposure is often not required. The image intensifier is a highly complex piece of equipment that uses X-rays to produce a continuous image feed which is displayed on a monitor (Kahler 2004). This is known as fluoroscopy and there are multiple examples of its use in trauma and orthopaedic theatres. A simple application is the insertion of dynamic hip screw for fixation of a fractured neck of femur. Fluoroscopy is used to achieve a good closed reduction of the fracture, then a guide wire followed by a screw are inserted into hip across the fracture under imaging and through a small incision. Fluoroscopy allows the angle and position of the screw within the bone to be checked in multiple views to confirm accurate reduction. Recent advances have seen work being done to replace the two-dimensional fluoroscopic image with intra-operative cone beam CT (Khoury et al. 2007).

How X-Rays Create a Radiation Hazard

X-rays are a form of ionising radiation that can in certain doses cause damage to living tissue, skin burns, radiation sickness and cancer, and in high enough doses, death. X-rays are harmful as they have the ability to ionise atoms and molecules, and potentially damage or kill living cells. X-rays interact with other atoms and molecules in two ways. Atoms consist of neutrons and protons in the nucleus and electrons in orbit around the nucleus. If an X-ray hits an inner orbit electron, the electron leaves the orbit and the X-ray is absorbed. This is called photoelectric absorption. If an X-ray hits an outer orbit electron, the electron leaves the orbit but the X-ray is not absorbed. Instead it is deflected but has a lower residual energy. This is called Compton scattering and results in a radiation field around the X-ray tube and poses a radiation hazard for those in the vicinity (Theodorakou & Farquharson 2008).

X-rays interact with atoms and molecules in living tissues in the same two ways described above. These interactions can have a direct and indirect effect. The direct effect on cells is by disruption of the molecular bonds of the structures within the cell including the DNA. This can result in apoptosis or cell death, or division of the cell to produce an abnormal mutated cell and carcinogenesis (Rothkamm & Lobrich 2003). The indirect effect of X-rays on cells is through the ionisation of water molecules that results in disruption of molecular bonds. The probability and the severity of the effect of radiation on living tissue increase with increasing radiation dose.

This principle is used to treat tumours with radiotherapy. Conventional radiotherapy machines create a targeted beam of ionising radiation, which penetrate tissues and cause the release of electrons which damage cells, mostly as a consequence of DNA damage. Since ionising radiation also damages normal tissue the challenge for the oncologist is to set a radiation dose that causes maximal damage to the cancer and minimal damage to the surrounding normal tissue (Vaidya et al. 2005).

Background Radiation

Radiation is the process by which energy is emitted by one body, travels through space or a material, and is absorbed by another body. It is called radiation because it radiates outwards from the source. Radiation is either non-ionising, such as thermal radiation or light, or ionising, such as alpha particles, beta particles and neutrons, which are the forms that are most dangerous but also have the most application for medical use.

Humans are constantly exposed to radiation in several different forms. Cosmic radiation comes from outside our solar system and is negligible in amount. Terrestrial radiation comes from sources like the chemical potassium found in buildings all around us. However, the biggest source of background radiation is from Radon-222 which is produced by decay from Radium-226. This is found wherever there is Uranium in the world and is released as a gas. Radiation exposure is measured in Sievert (Sv) where 1 Sv is equal to 1 J of energy absorbed per 1 kg of matter. The dose required for radiation poisoning is an acute dose of 5,000 mSv. The radiation from natural sources varies geographically between 2 mSv to 20 mSv per year (Dewey et al. 2005). Man-made sources of radiation are produced by medical procedures such as X-rays, nuclear medicine and radiation therapy. The typical radiation dose from a limb or joint X-ray is less than 0.01 mSv. The radiation dose for a pelvis X-ray is 0.7 mSv and increases to 10 mSv for a CT of the abdomen and pelvis. Man-made sources represent around 15% of the total average background radiation (Clark 1997).

Radiation Protection

All radiological procedures carry a risk. The International Commission on Radiological Protection (ICRP) has developed three important principles in radiological protections (ICRP 60 1991). These are 'justification, optimisation and limitation.'

Exposure to radiation should only be performed if it provides a net benefit. The risk incurred from undertaking the procedure must be balanced against the benefit for the patient from the information the imaging provides. All exposures should be kept as low as reasonably achievable. Individual exposure should be dose limited. The limits set for members of the public is 1 mSv and for occupationally exposed staff including theatre staff, 20 mSv. These limits do not include background radiation or radiation exposure for personal medical treatment.

Some human organs are more sensitive than others to the effects of radiation. The gonads are particularly vulnerable and are exposed in imaging of the lumbar spine and pelvis as well as in barium enemas. Precautions should therefore be taken to protect sensitive areas in patients with lead gowns. Finally, it should also be noted that irradiating the foetus *in utero* is especially hazardous because the rapidly dividing cells are very radiosensitive; the main risk is induction of childhood cancers. A risk benefit assessment should be made in any such cases and exposure to radiation in the first trimester should be avoided. This has implications not only the patient but also staff working in radiation-prone areas and local guidelines should be followed.

RISK TO THEATRE STAFF AND NECESSARY PRECAUTIONS

All staff in theatres or wards where radiological imaging techniques are being used are at risk from radiation exposure. For staff working regularly with radiation, the potential for harm comes from the cumulative effect of exposure over a length of time. There are many steps that can be taken to reduce this cumulative effect and these are summarised in Table 1.

Table 1. Necessary precautions for theatre staff exposed to radiation

Necessary precautions for theatre staff exposed to radiation
• The patient and the image intensifier should be placed at the optimum position.
• Image intensifier screening time and field size should be kept to a minimum.
• Theatre staff should stand as far away as is practical from the radiation source.
• All theatre staff should wear lead gowns, thyroid neck protectors and a personal radiation dosimeter under their protective gown.
• Lead gowns should be handled carefully to avoid cracking of the protective material.
• Ensure all equipment ranging from the image intensifier to the protective garments are regularly inspected by the radiology department.
• All staff should receive training and updates to make working with radiation as safe as possible for them and other members of the team.
• Team work and good communication.

In operating theatres, the patient and the image intensifier should be placed at the optimum position. Radiation exposure is greater at the image intensifier end with the X-ray tube and lower behind the image receptor. The image receptor should be placed as close as possible to the patient (Kahler 2004). Screening time should be kept to a minimum by reducing the number and duration of exposures. The field size should be kept to a minimum to reduce radiation. Most modern image intensifier machines have an image memory facility that should be used. Other methods and devices that reduce exposure include proper beam focusing and filtering as well safe housing of the radiation source (Herscovici & Sanders 2000). Theatre staff should stand as far away as is practical from the radiation source. X-rays obey the inverse square rule and the intensity of X-rays decreases as the square of the distance from the source increases. Moving away from one meter to two meters, reduces radiation exposure to a quarter; moving to three metres reduces exposure to a ninth. A study looking at the radiation dose operating staff receive during hip fracture surgery concluded that at a within a two-metre radius of the patient, gowns and thyroid neck protectors should be worn They also stated that at a distance of greater than two metres, theatre staff would not need to wear a lead gown because the very low dose of scattered radiation (Alonso et al. 2001). The authors however disagree with this and in a high-stress environment where the image intensifier may be changing positions it is difficult to fully adhere to the two-metre rule, and all theatre staff wearing lead gowns and thyroid neck protectors eliminates an additional potential hazard.

Lead gowns of 0.5-1.0mm should be worn to absorb the radiation and provide protection. These are available as one- and two-piece gowns. The gowns should be handled carefully to avoid cracking of the protective material. All staff exposed to radiation should wear a personal radiation dosimeter under their protective apron to record personal exposure. Additional protective garments include thyroid shields and lead acrylic glasses, or head shields with lead acrylic visors. Lead screens reduce exposure to X-ray radiation but are not commonly used in the UK trauma and orthopaedic theatre setting. They can be mounted on the operating table or the ceiling. All equipment ranging from the image intensifier to the protective garments should be regularly inspected by the radiology department (Herscovici & Sanders 2000). It is also important that all staff regularly exposed to radiation receive training and updates to make working with radiation as safe as possible for them and other members of the team.

The role of team work and good communication could not be over-emphasised. The radiographer has primary responsibility for screening and the operator has primary responsibility for the patient. Good communication between the radiographer and the operator is crucial to produce a satisfactory image and to reduce radiation exposure to patient and theatre staff. A lack of consistent names for various movements of the image intensifier and ambiguity in commands often leads to confusion between the radiographer and the operator. Knowledge of the movements of the image intensifier and consistent names for these various movements can improve the efficacy of communication between radiographers and operators, avoid confusion and improve theatre time utilisation (Chaganti et al. 2009).

CONCLUSION

X-rays have revolutionised the delivery of medicine and nowhere is this more evident than in the trauma and orthopaedic operating theatre. Despite the obvious integral role for X-rays it is important to bear in mind the risks it can pose to patients and theatre staff. This highlights the need for a thorough understanding and awareness of radiation, as well as a sound knowledge of the precautions required for using this technology.

REFERENCES

Alonso JA, Shaw DL, Maxwell A, McGill GP, Hart GC 2001 Scattered radiation during fixation of hip fractures, is distance alone enough protection? *Journal of Bone & Joint Surgery* 83B 815-818.

Armstrong P, Wastie ML 2001 *A Concise Textbook of Radiology* Arnold Publishing, Ontario, Canada.

Chaganti S, Kumar D, Patil S, Alderman P 2009 A language for effective communication between surgeons and radiographers in trauma theatre. *Annals of the Royal College of Surgeons of England* 91 509-512.

Clark RH 1997 Managing radiation risks *Journal of the Royal Society for Medicine* 90 88-92.

Dewey P, George S, Gray A 2005 Ionising radiation and orthopaedics *Current Orthopaedics* 19 1-12.

Haynes AB, Weiser TG, Berry WR et al. 2009 A surgical safety checklist to reduce morbidity and mortality in a global population *New England Journal of Medicine* 360 491-499.

Herscovici D Jr, Sanders RW 2000 The effects, risks, and guidelines for radiation use in orthopaedic surgery *Clinical Orthopaedics & Related Research* 375 126-132.

ICRP 60 1991 1990 Recommendations on the international commission on Radiological Protection *Annals of the ICRP* 21 1-3.

Kahler DM 2004 Image guidance: fluoroscopic navigation *Clinical Orthopaedics & Related Research* 421 70-76.

Khoury A, Siewerdsen JH, Whyne CM et al. 2007 Intraoperative cone-beam CT for image guided tibial plateau fracture reduction *Computer Aided Surgery* 12 195-207.

Kreel L 1991 Reviews in medicine, medical imaging *Postgraduate Medical Journal* 67 334-346.

Prime MS, Khan WS, Dheerendra S, Maruthainar N (2010). The Use of Ionising Radiation in Trauma and Orthopaedic Theatres. *J. Perioper. Pract.* 20(5): 165-8.

Rothkamm K, Lobrich M 2003 Evidence for a lack of DNA double strand break repair in human cells exposed to very low X-ray doses *Proceedings of the National Academy of Science USA* 100 5057-5062.

Theodorakou C, Farquharson MJ 2008 Human soft tissue analysis using x-ray or gamma-ray techniques *Physics in Medicine & Biology* 53 R111-R149.

Vaidya JS, Tobias JS, Baum M et al. 2005 TARGeted Intraoperative radiotherapy (TARGIT): an innovative approach to partial-breast irradiation *Seminars in Radiation Oncology* 15 84-91.

Van Tiggelen R 2001 Since 1895, orthopaedic surgery relies on x-ray imaging: a historical overview from discovery to computed tomography *Acta Orthopaedica Belgica* 67 317-329.

In: Perioperative Practice in Trauma and Orthopaedic Surgery ISBN: 978-1-63483-325-7
Editor: Wasim S. Khan

Chapter 11

THE CERVICAL SPINE RADIOGRAPH IN THE ADVANCED TRAUMA LIFE SUPPORT RADIOGRAPHIC TRAUMA SERIES

M. Chimutengwende-Gordon, J. Sidhu, W. Khan* and N. Maruthainar
Department of Trauma and Orthopaedics,
Royal Free Hampstead NHS Trust, London, UK

ABSTRACT

Plain cervical spine radiographs are the first line investigation in trauma patients to exclude cervical spine fractures and dislocations. Adequate views are essential to reduce the risk of missing diagnoses. Injuries may however not be visible on plain cervical spine radiographs despite adequate views. Additional imaging such as computer tomography scanning is indicated in the event of a normal plain radiograph if there is any clinical suspicion of injury.

Keywords: Trauma series, cervical spine radiograph, cervical spine trauma, advanced trauma life support

INTRODUCTION

In this chapter we review the cervical spine radiographs performed as part of the Advanced Trauma Life Support (ATLS) trauma series (Chimutengwende-Gordon et al. 2010a, 2010b, 2011). Cervical spine injury may lead to significant morbidity and mortality especially if diagnosis is delayed (Anderson et al. 2010). The clinical assessment of patients with potential cervical spine injuries includes a history of the injury mechanism and pain as well as a physical examination focusing on the presence of posterior midline tenderness and

* Tel.: +44 (0) 7791 025554; E-mail: wasimkhan@doctors.org.uk.

any neurological deficits (Graber and Kathol 1999). If radiological assessment of the cervical spine is considered necessary, plain radiography is often the first examination employed. It is a readily available, inexpensive, quick screening test for detection of cervical spine injury and is part of the radiographic trauma series in cases of major trauma (ATLS 2004, Anderson et al. 2010). The main limitation of plain cervical spine radiographs is that its sensitivity is low. If the cervical spine cannot be cleared on the basis of the clinical assessment, further imaging with a computer tomography (CT) scan is indicated even in the presence of a normal cervical spine radiograph (Anderson et al. 2010, Bhamra et al. 2012, Holmes and Akkinepalli 2005).

Anatomy of the Cervical Spine

The cervical spine protects the spinal cord and provides support for the head. Figures 1-3 illustrate the normal anatomical structures visualised on the cervical spine radiographs.

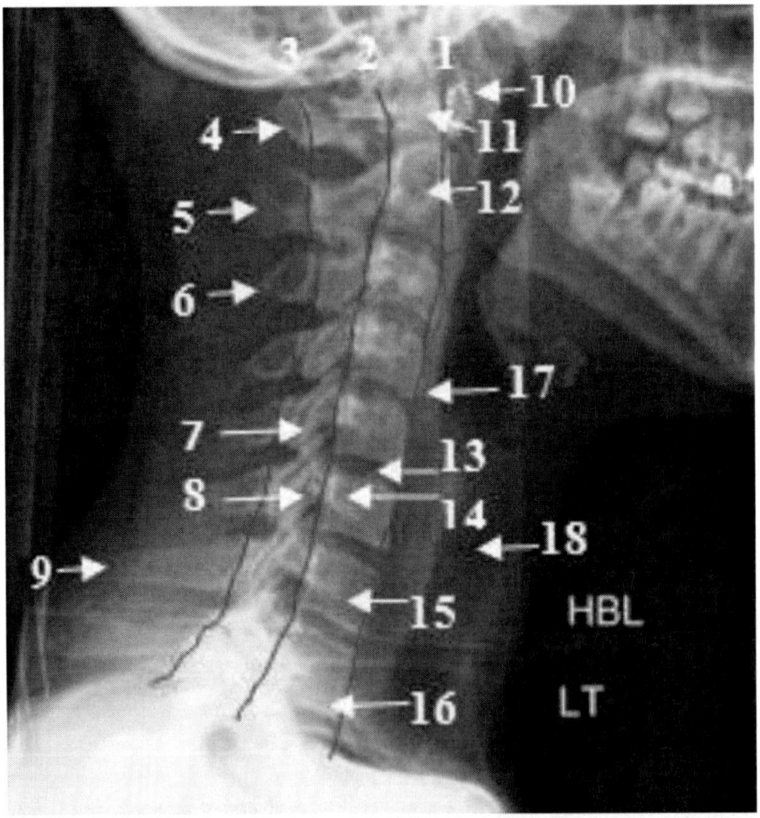

Figure 1. Adequate lateral cervical spine radiograph showing all seven cervical vertebrae and the cervicothoracic junction. The anterior vertebral line (1), posterior vertebral line (2), spinolaminar line (3), posterior arch of atlas (4), spinous process of axis (5), spinous process of C3 (6), C5 lamina (7), C6 pedicle (8), C7 spinous process (vertebra prominens) (9), anterior arch of atlas (10), odontoid process (11), body of axis (12), C5/C6 intervertebral disc space (13), C6 transverse process (14), body of C7 (15), body of T1 (16), prevertebral soft tissues (17), trachea (18) are illustrated.

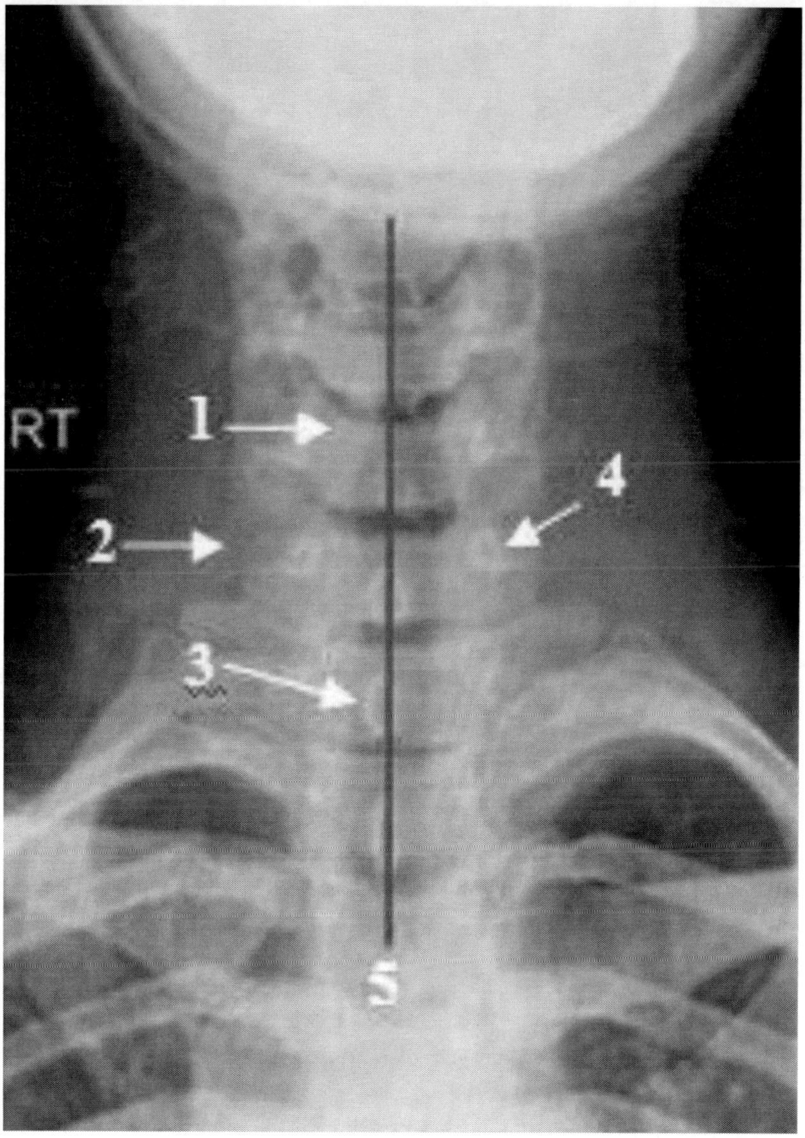

Figure 2. Normal anteroposterior cervical spine radiograph illustrating the vertebral body (1), transverse process (2), spinous process (3), pedicle (4) and the line showing alignment of spinal processes (5).

The seven cervical vertebrae (C1-C7) form the skeleton of the neck. The cervical vertebrae are smaller than the thoracic, lumbar and sacral vertebrae inferior to them and bear less weight. Anatomical features which distinguish the cervical vertebrae from other vertebrae are the presence of the small foramina of the transverse processes and the large vertebral foramen. The two most superior cervical vertebrae are termed atypical cervical vertebrae. The C1 vertebrae or 'atlas' is a ring shaped bone which does not contain a vertebral body or a spinous process. It is the widest of the cervical vertebrae and consists of anterior and posterior arches. It has two concave superior articular surfaces which articulate with the occipital condyles on the inferior aspect of the skull forming the atlanto-occipital joints (Moore and Dalley 1999).

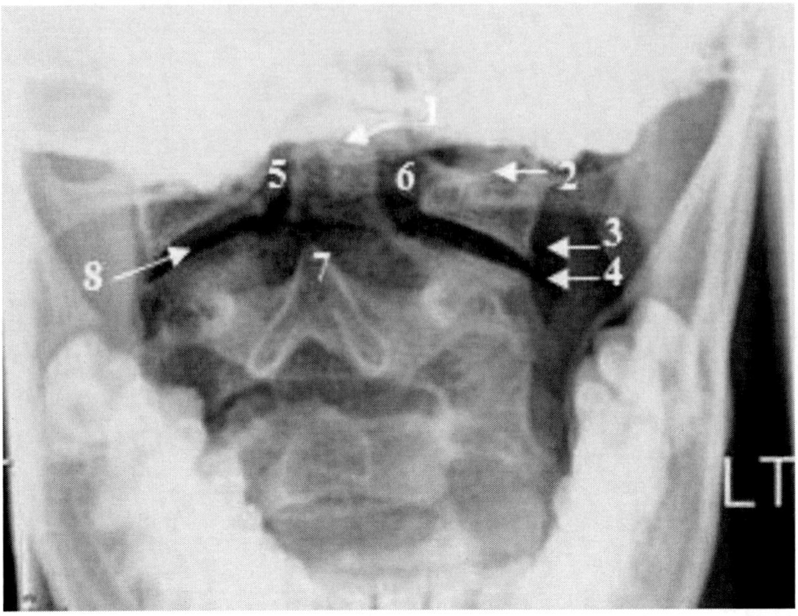

Figures 3. Normal 'open-mouth' odontoid view illustrating the odontoid process (1), lateral mas of atlas (2), and the lateral margin of atlas (3) aligning with lateral margin of axis (4). The space between odontoid process and lateral mass of the atlas on right (5) is smaller than the space between the lateral mass of the atlas on the left (6). This due to rotation as 3 and 4 are aligned. The body of the axis (7) and the atlantoaxial joint (8) are also illustrated.

The C2 vertebrae or 'atlas' which carries the skull rotates around the axis when a person turns their head to one side. The axis has large oval facets and pedicles which articulate with the inferior facets of the atlas. The distinguishing feature of the axis is the odontoid process, also known as the dens or the odontoid peg, which a tooth-like process which projects superiorly from the body of the axis and is held in place by the transverse ligament of the atlas (Moore and Dalley 1999). The vertebrae from C3-C7 are termed typical cervical vertebrae (Moore and Dalley 1999).

These vertebrae have a large triangular vertebral foramen which allows for the cervical enlargement of the spinal cord. The vertebral bodies are smaller and wider from side to side than from anteroposteriorly with a concave superior surface and a convex inferior surface. The vertebral bodies get progressively larger and bear more weight inferiorly. The cervical vertebrae have two transverse processes each containing a small foramen which transmits the vertebral arteries. These foramina are small or absent in C7. Each vertebra has a single spinous process which is short and often bifid. C7 is the exception as it has a long spinous process and is therefore known as the 'vertebra prominens.' In addition to this, typical cervical vertebrae contain two pedicles, two laminae and two superior articular surfaces (Moore and Dalley 1999).

The intervertebral discs are interposed between adjacent vertebral bodies (Moore and Dalley 1999). Several ligaments contribute to the stability of the cervical spine. The anterior and posterior longitudinal ligaments are closely applied to the anterior and posterior aspects of the vertebral bodies and intervertebral discs respectively. The ligamentum flavum connects the laminae of the vertebrae. The interspinous ligaments connect the spinous processes. The supraspinous ligaments are attached to the tips of the spinous processes and overlie the interspinous ligaments (Moore and Dalley 1999).

Indications for Cervical Spine Radiography

Trauma patients requiring cervical spine imaging are those who report neck pain, have posterior midline neck tenderness on examination or have signs of a neurological deficit associated with the cervical spine. Trauma patients who cannot be assessed due to altered consciousness level, intoxication, distracting injuries such as extremity fractures, and age also require cervical spine imaging (Daffner and Hackney 2007, Graber and Kathol 1999). Adult patients who are asymptomatic, fully conscious and have no distracting injuries are unlikely to have a cervical spine injury and therefore do not require imaging of their cervical spine (Anderson et al. 2010, Daffner and Hackney 2007).

There should be a high index of suspicion for vertebral or spinal cord injury. The patient's neck should remain immobilised supine supported on a spine board with a cervical collar and immobilisation apparatus such as sandbags and tape until an adequate full cervical spine series can be obtained in the radiology department (ATLS 2004). The cervical collar should be radiolucent so that radiographs may be taken with the patient fully immobile (Graber and Kathol 1999).

The Standard Plain Radiographic Views

The three standard radiographic views required following acute trauma are the true lateral radiograph (Figure 1), an anteroposterior (AP) view (Figure 2) and an 'open-mouth' odontoid view (Figure 3) (Raby et al. 2005). The single portable cross-table lateral radiograph which may be obtained in the resuscitation is insufficient to exclude a cervical spine fracture (Spain et al. 1990). The lateral cervical spine view should be taken in the radiology department with the X-ray beam horizontal to the long axis of the patient (Nicholas 2006). The lateral and AP views should include all seven cervical vertebrae and the first thoracic vertebra. The standard AP view is performed with the patient on a spine board support and the mid-sagittal plane aligned. The central ray is angled 15 to 20 degrees cephalic. The first three vertebrae are often difficult to image on the AP view because of the mandible and the base of the skull (Nicholas 2006, Raby et al. 2005). The odontoid view is taken with the mouth open. The central ray is angled up to 25 degrees caudally so it passes through the upper incisors and the base of the skull. This view is only possible when the patient is alert and cooperative. A CT scan is performed if there is any altered consciousness (Nicholas 2006, Raby et al. 2005).

Additional views not part of the standard cervical spine trauma radiographic series include the lateral oblique views and flexion-extension views. The lateral oblique views may be considered if there is a question of fracture on the other three films or if an adequate lateral view cannot be obtained (Graber and Kathol 1999). Flexion-extension views are appropriate for alert patients with negative cervical spine radiographs who have persistent symptoms, provided that the entire cervical spine can be visualised on standard views. They are often used to identify unstable cervical spine injuries which may have been missed on the standard cervical spine series or to determine the stability of a known fracture. Flexion-extension views add little to the acute evaluation of patients with blunt trauma and their use is debatable (Pollack et al. 2001, Freedman et al. 2005).

Approach to Interpretation of Cervical Spine Radiographs

A systematic approach is essential when reviewing cervical spine radiographs. The first step is to assess the adequacy of the film. Failure to adequately visualise the region of the injury is the commonest cause of missed cervical spine injuries (McCormick 2002). An adequate lateral view must include all seven cervical vertebrae and the cervicothoracic junction including the junction between the seventh cervical vertebra and the first thoracic vertebra as illustrated in Figure 1. If the view is inadequate (Figure 4), traction on the arms may be applied provided there is no upper limb injury. A 'swimmer's view' may also allow visualisation of the whole cervical spine and is performed with one arm extended over the head (Nicholas 2006, Raby et al. 2005). The alignment of the vertebrae on the lateral film is assessed. Three contour lines may be traced as illustrated in Figure 1. These lines should be smooth curves with no steps. The anterior vertebral line joins the anterior margins of the vertebral bodies.

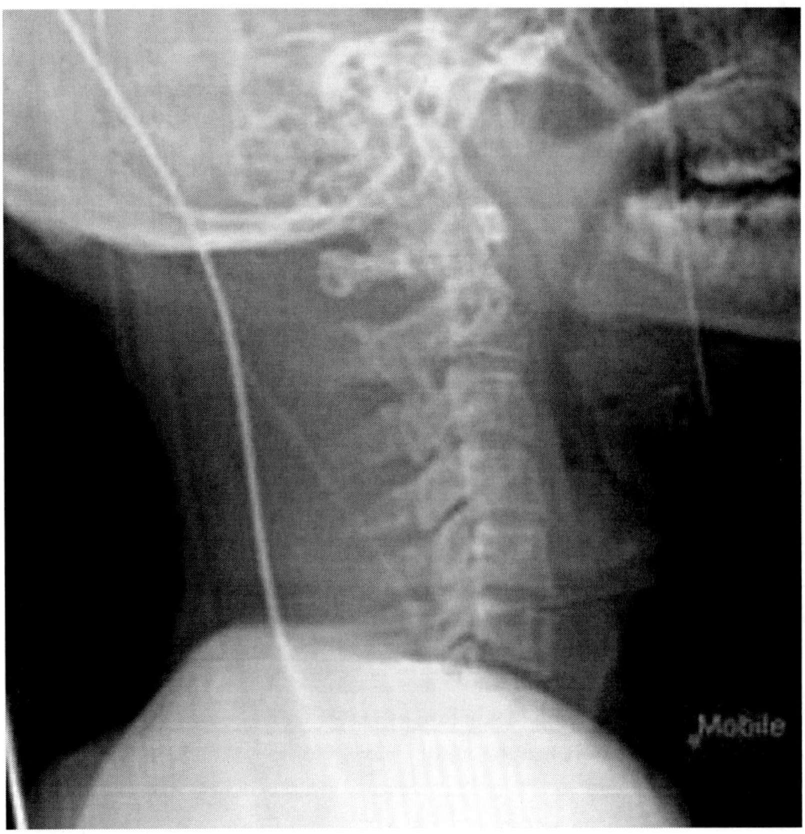

Figure 4. Inadequate lateral cervical spine radiograph that fails to demonstrate the C7-T1 junction.

When this line is continued superiorly it merges with the anterior aspect of the odontoid process. The posterior vertebral line joins the posterior margins of the vertebral bodies and when continued superiorly merges with the posterior aspect of the odontoid process. The spinolaminar line joins the bases of the spinous processes. The spinolaminar line may show a step at the level of the axis. This malalignment is more common in children. A step of up to 2 mm between the spinous process of the axis and the smooth curve between atlas and C3 is accepted as normal (Raby et al. 2005).

The predental space is the space between the odontoid process and the anterior arch of atlas (Figure 5). This space should be less than 3 mm in adults and less than 5 mm in children. An increase in this space suggests a fracture of the atlas, the odontoid process or a ligamentous injury. Harris' ring is seen as a white ring projected over the base of the odontoid process and over part of the body of the axis (Figure 5). The most inferior aspect of Harris' ring may be incomplete. If any other part of the ring appears disrupted, it may indicate a fracture of the odontoid process (Raby et al. 2005).

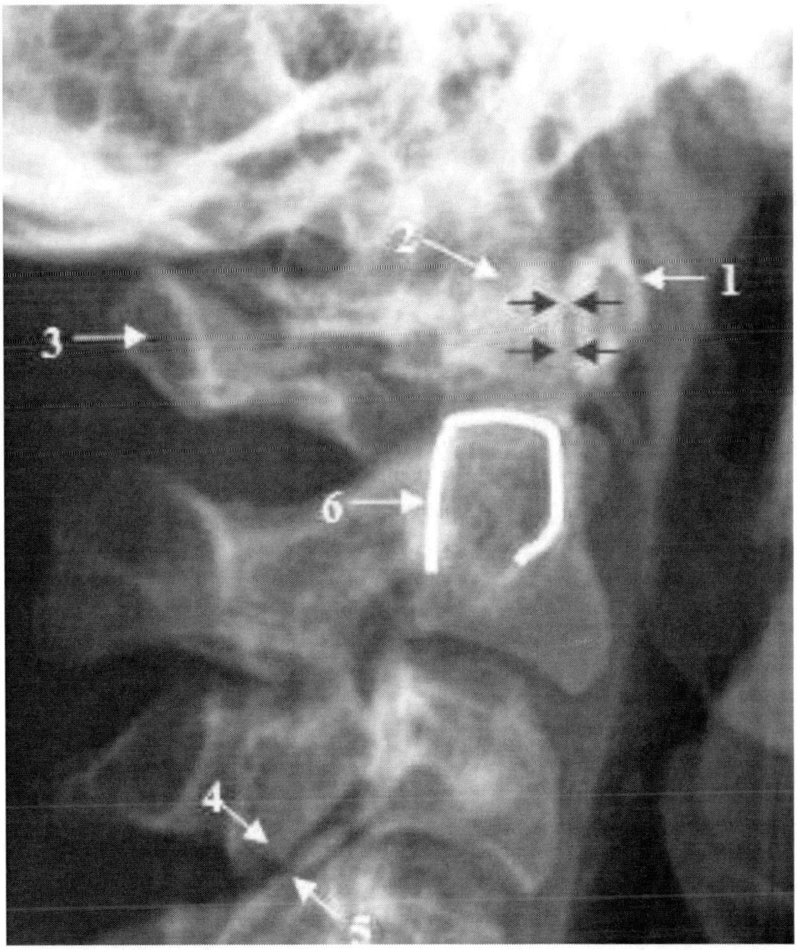

Figure 5. Lateral view of the upper cervical vertebrae illustrating the anterior arch of atlas (1), odontoid process (2), posterior arch of atlas (3), inferior articulating facet of C3 (4), superior articulating facet of C4 (5), Harris' ring (6) and the predental space (red arrows).

Each vertebral body and spinous process should be examined. The anterior and posterior heights of the vertebral bodies should be equal. The spaces between the spinous processes are assessed. Widening of this space may indicate a ligamentous injury or a fracture. The intervertebral disc spaces should also be examined. The disc spaces should be of uniform height. Finally, the prevertebral soft tissues are examined (Figure 1). Soft tissue swelling of more than 7 mm at the level of the axis or more than 22 mm at C6 is abnormal (Raby et al. 2005).

On the AP view, the spinous processes should be seen to be in alignment and in the midline as illustrated in Figure 2. The distance between the spinous processes should be approximately equal. No single space should be 50 percent wider than the one above or below unless the neck is flexed due to muscle spasm. The bones are then systematically examined for the presence of any fractures (Raby et al. 2005).

The odontoid process is examined for fractures on the odontoid view. Overlying teeth may obscure the odontoid process. A repeat view to try to get the teeth out of the field or a CT may be needed to overcome this and achieve an adequate view. The lateral margins of the atlas should be aligned with the lateral margins of the axis. The distance between each side of the odontoid process and the lateral margins of the atlas should be equal. Slight rotation of the neck may cause these spaces to appear unequal. If the lateral margins of the atlas and the axis remain normally aligned, the asymmetry can be attributed to rotation (Figure 3) (Raby et al. 2005).

Cervical Spine Injuries

Cervical spine injuries detected on plain radiography should be assumed to be unstable and investigated further, except spinous process fractures. Patients should be referred to the orthopaedic or neurosurgical team and remain immobilised until definitive treatment is instituted.

1. Fractures and Dislocations of the Atlas

Fractures of the atlas account for approximately 5 percent of cervical spine fractures. Approximately 40 percent of atlas fractures are associated with fractures of the axis. The Jefferson fracture is the commonest fracture of the atlas (see Case study 1). It is a burst fracture which is usually the result of axial loading or vertebral compression, for example when a load falls vertically onto the head. The odontoid view shows displacement of the lateral aspects of the atlas and a widened predental space of more than 3 mm (ATLS 2004).

Atlanto-occipital dislocation is an uncommon, highly unstable injury that results from severe traumatic flexion and distraction. It is fatal in many cases, causing death by brainstem destruction and apnoea. Survivors are often left with severe neurological deficits. Radiological diagnosis using plain radiographs is challenging as landmarks may be indistinct and during patient positioning, the landmarks may sometimes align and conceal disruption of the joint. Several methods exist to diagnose atlanto-occipital dislocation on lateral cervical spine radiographs.

Case study 1.

> Mr FC, a 27 year old rugby player was brought to hospital by ambulance after an attempted head-on tackle on the rugby field with a lowered head. The patient suffered from a momentary loss of consciousness before coming round. He complained of neck pain and stiffness but did not have any neurological symptoms.
> The patient was managed in accordance with the ATLS guidelines. In the AandE department, he was alert and orientated. He was tender in the midline of his cervical spine but there were no palpable abnormalities, and he had a normal neurologic examination. Any other significant chest, abdominal, pelvis or limb injury was not evident during the primary survey.
> Trauma series radiographs of the cervical spine were performed and showed a burst fracture of Cl. He then went on to have a CT scan of his head and neck that failed to show any significant head injury. He was treated in a halo-vest for eight weeks and a rigid cervical collar for a further eight weeks. Physiotherapy was then started and normal cervical range of motion and strength were restored after a further six weeks.

For example, the basion-dens interval is measured as the distance between the basion (the midpoint on the anterior margin of the foramen magnum on the occipital bone) and the odontoid process.

A basion-dens interval of more than 10 mm is considered abnormal. If there is a clinical suspicion of atlanto occipital dislocation and plain radiographs are non-diagnostic or show the presence of upper cervical prevertebral soft tissue swelling, additional imaging should be obtained without delay (ATLS 2004, Garrett et al. 2010).

Atlanto-axial rotary subluxation is due to loss of ligamentous stability between the atlas and the axis and is most common in children and adolescents. It may occur spontaneously or following trauma. It is also associated with Down's syndrome, rheumatoid arthritis and pharyngeal infections in children (Grisel's syndrome). This highly unstable injury may appear on an odontoid view as the spaces between the odontoid process and the two lateral masses of the atlas being unequal and an increased predental space (ATLS 2004, Karkos et al. 2007).

2. Fractures of the Axis

Acute fractures of the axis account for approximately 18 percent of all cervical spine injuries. Odontoid fractures may be identified by a lateral or odontoid view. Type I fractures involve the tip of the odontoid process and are rare. Type II fractures are the most common odontoid fracture. They occur through the base of the odontoid process. Type III fractures occur through the base and extend obliquely into the body of the axis (Figure 6). Odontoid fractures may be difficult to see on plain radiographs and CT scans are generally used to delineate the injury further (Pryputniewicz and Hadley 2010).

Hangman's fracture is an unstable fracture through the pars interarticularis (the posterior elements of the axis). The mechanism of injury is sudden deceleration such as during hanging or hyperextension, for example in motor vehicle accidents. Variations of the hangman's fracture seen on plain radiographs include bilateral pedicle or lateral mass fracture of the axis, with or without anterior subluxation (ATLS 2004).

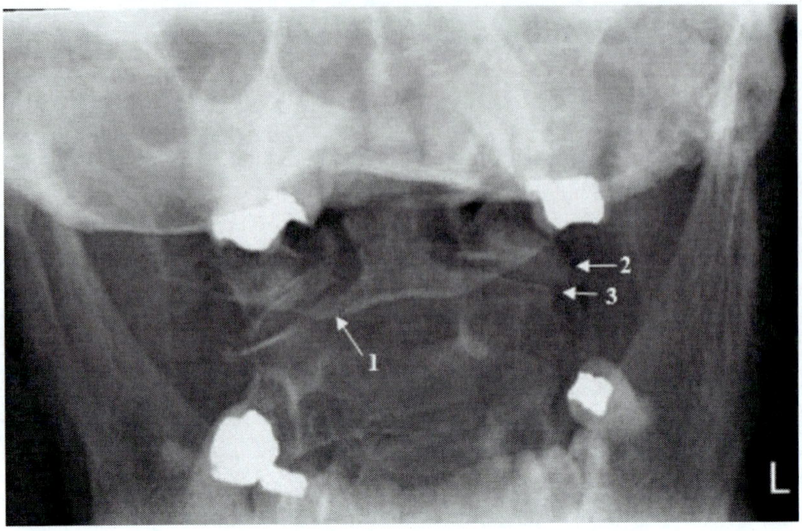

Figure 6. An odontoid process fracture (1) with loss of alignment between the lateral margins of the atlas (2) and the axis (3) on an odontoid view.

3. Fractures and Dislocations of C3-C7 Vertebrae

Wedge compression fractures occur due to flexion. The anterior vertebral body bears most of the force. The lateral view shows the anterior vertebral column loses height, whereas the posterior column remains intact as seen in Figure 7 (Davenport 2009). The usual mechanism of burst fractures is axial loading. Radiographs show a comminuted vertical fracture through the vertebral body and posterior elements. There may be retropulsed fragments which result in varying degrees of narrowing of the canal (Wheeless 2008).

The teardrop fracture is a fracture of the anteroinferior aspect of the vertebral body. Flexion teardrop fractures occur due to compression of the anterior vertebral aspect due to sudden and forceful hyperflexion.

This is a highly unstable injury and is associated with significant ligamentous disruption. The plain radiograph shows a large wedge at the anterior aspect of the vertebrae. There may be malalignment due to the ligamentous instability (Wheeless 2008, Davenport 2009). The extension teardrop fracture shows similar radiological features but the injury occurs due to sudden hyperextension resulting in the anterior longitudinal ligament pulling the fracture away from the inferior aspect of the vertebrae. This avulsion fracture is stable in flexion, but highly unstable in extension (Davenport 2009).

Figure 8 shows an old teardrop fracture that fails to show any evidence of instability on flexion-extension views.

Anterior subluxation occurs when the posterior ligamentous complexes rupture, but the anterior longitudinal ligament remains intact. Radiographs show widening of the interspinous space.

The anterior and posterior vertebral lines illustrated in Figure 1 are disrupted in flexion views. This injury is usually stable and rarely associated with neurological deficits (Graber and Kathol 1999).

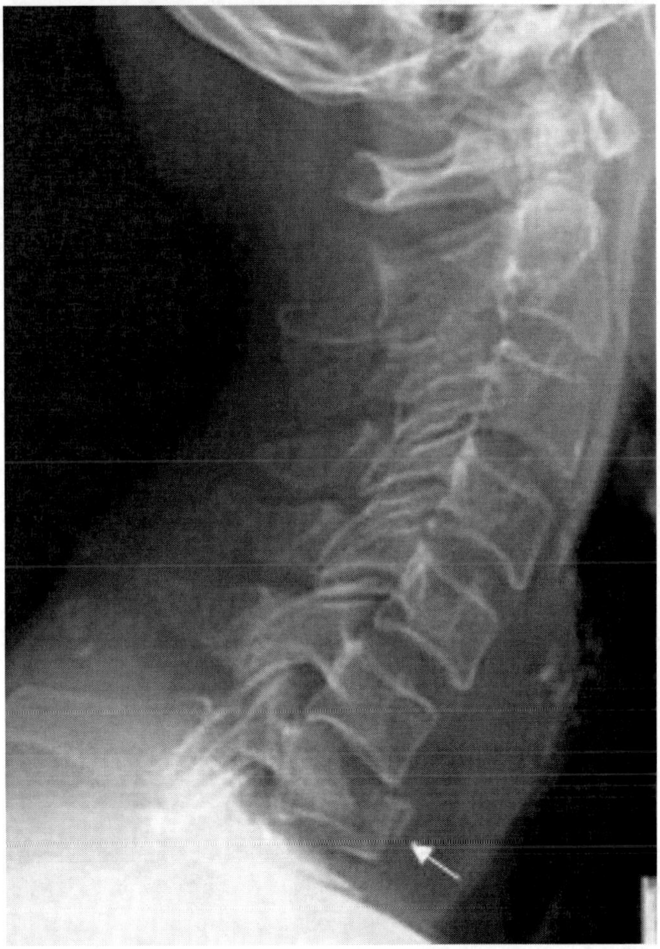

Figure 7. A lateral cervical spine radiograph illustrating a C7 wedge compression fracture.

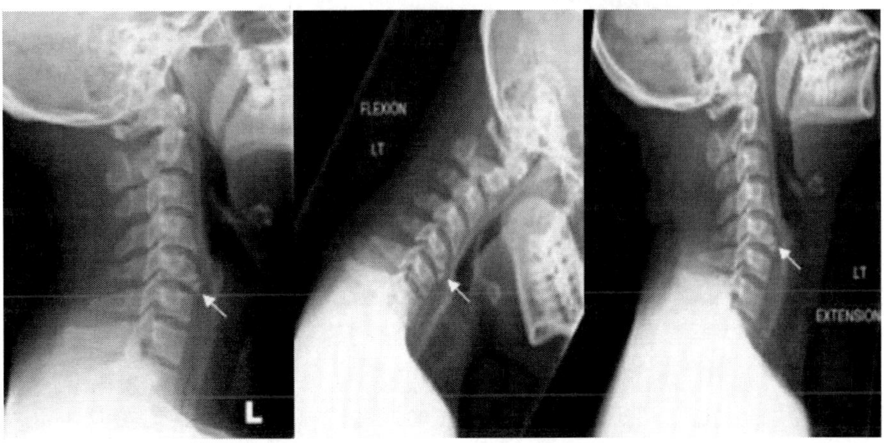

Figure 8. A stable old C5 teardrop fracture on a lateral radiograph with no significant disruption evident on flexion-extension views.

Unilateral facet dislocation occurs when flexion combined with rotation forces one inferior articular facet of a vertebra to pass superiorly and anteriorly to the superior facet of the vertebra below (Figure 9). This occurs due to disruption of the posterior longitudinal ligament. The vertebrae are locked in place, thus making this a stable injury.

Radiographs show an anterior displacement of the spine at the involved level of less than one half of the diameter of the vertebral body. The AP radiograph shows malalignment of the spinous processes at the level of the dislocation (Figure 10) (Graber and Kathol 1999, Davenport 2009).

Bilateral facet dislocation involves the posterior ligamentous complex, the anterior longitudinal ligament as well as the annulus fibrosus (see Case study 2). At the level of the injury, the inferior articulating facets of the upper vertebra pass superiorly and anteriorly to the superior articulating facets of the lower involved vertebra.

The mechanism of injury is extreme flexion. Bilateral facet dislocation is seen as displacement of more than half the anteroposterior diameter of the vertebral body seen on the lateral view.

This injury is highly unstable and is associated with a high prevalence of spinal cord injuries (Graber and Kathol 1999, Davenport 2009).

Clay-Shoveler fracture is a very stable injury and often an incidental finding. The mechanism is flexion. Radiographically, it is seen as an avulsion of the posterior aspect of the spinous process (Figure 11) (Graber and Kathol 2009).

FURTHER IMAGING

If an abnormality is seen or suspected on the plain cervical spine series, a CT scan is recommended to confirm the diagnosis and delineate the injury in more detail. Cervical spine radiographs have a low sensitivity and approximately 15 percent of fractures are missed (Anderson et al. 2010, Mower et al. 2001).

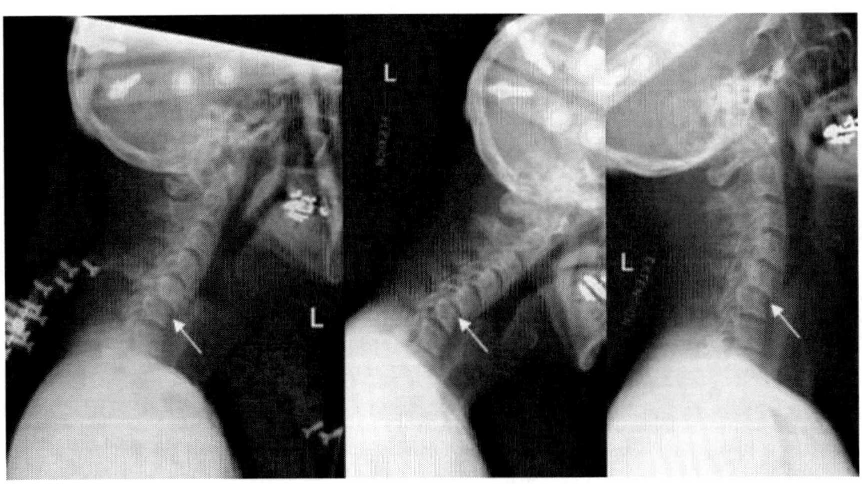

Figure 9. A lateral cervical spine radiograph and flexion-extension views illustrating a C5/C6 unilateral facet dislocation.

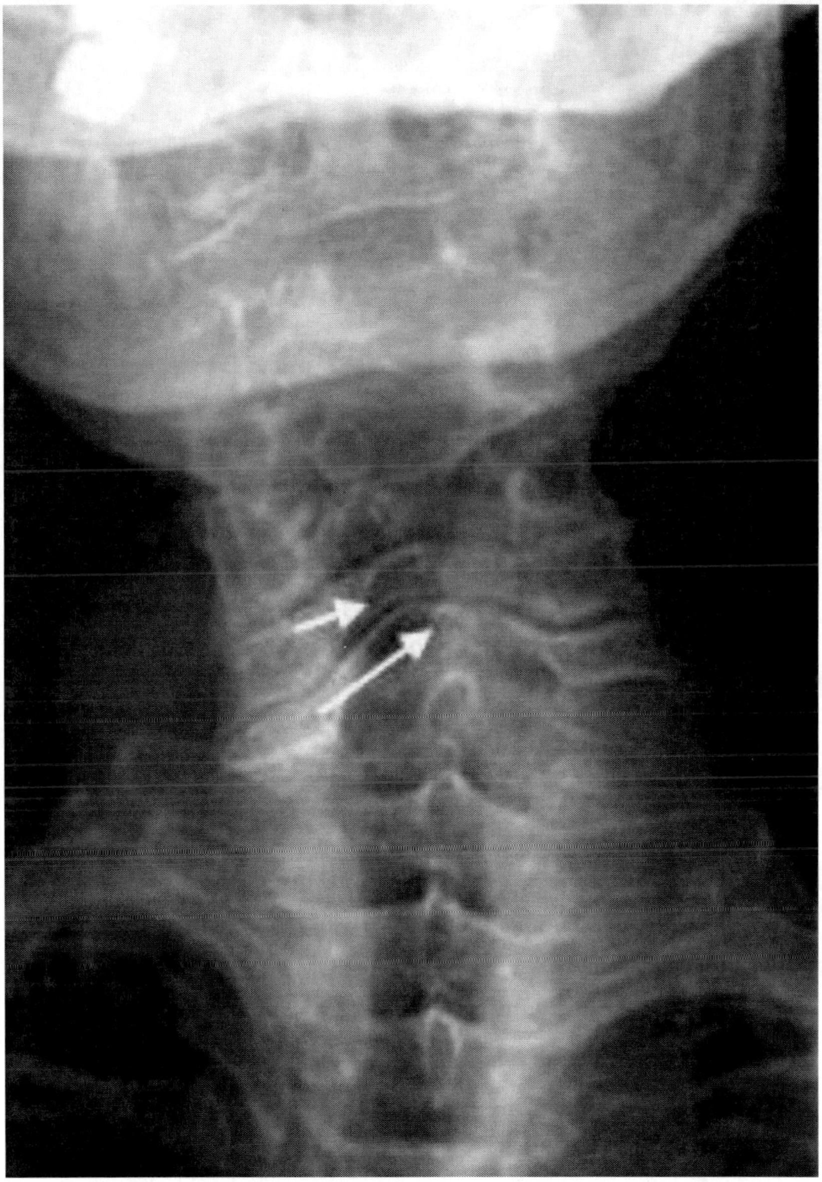

Figure 10. An anteroposterior view of the unilateral facet dislocation with arrows pointing out loss of alignment between spinous processes.

A CT scan is also recommended if adequate plain views are not obtainable despite appropriate manoeuvres described above, or if the patient has persistent symptoms despite normal plain radiographs and a significant mechanism of injury (Anderson et al. 2010).

A CT or Magnetic Resonance Imaging (MRI) scan is recommended in unconscious patients, whose cervical spines cannot be cleared on the basis of clinical examination (Rabb et al. 2007, Sliker et al. 2005). CT scanning is highly sensitive for detecting bony injuries, and MRI scan is better at identifying spinal cord injury or ligamentous injuries (Daffner and Hackney 2007).

Case study 2.

Mr KJ, a 34 year old lawyer was brought to hospital by ambulance after the car he was driving lost control and rolled. The fire brigade helped extricate him from the car. He did not lose consciousness and was complaining of isolated neck pain but no neurological symptoms.

The patient was managed in accordance with the ATLS guidelines. In the AandE department, he was found to be alert and orientated. Cervical spine examination revealed bruising and midline tenderness over the lower cervical region in addition to a palpable step deformity. On neurological examination, the patient was noted to have Medical Research Council (MRC) grade 3 power in the intrinsic muscles of both hands suggesting T1 nerve root compression. Power in other muscle groups as well as tone, reflexes and sensation were normal. Anal tone and perianal sensation were also normal. No other significant chest, abdominal, pelvis or limb injury was evident during the primary survey.

Cervical spine radiographs revealed complete bilateral fracture dislocation of C6 on C7. He then went on to have a CT scan and MRI scan of the cervical spine. The patient went to theatre for reduction of the dislocation and posterior cervical spine stabilisation with sublaminar wires and bone grafting. He was then placed in a halo-vest for twelve weeks before commencing physiotherapy.

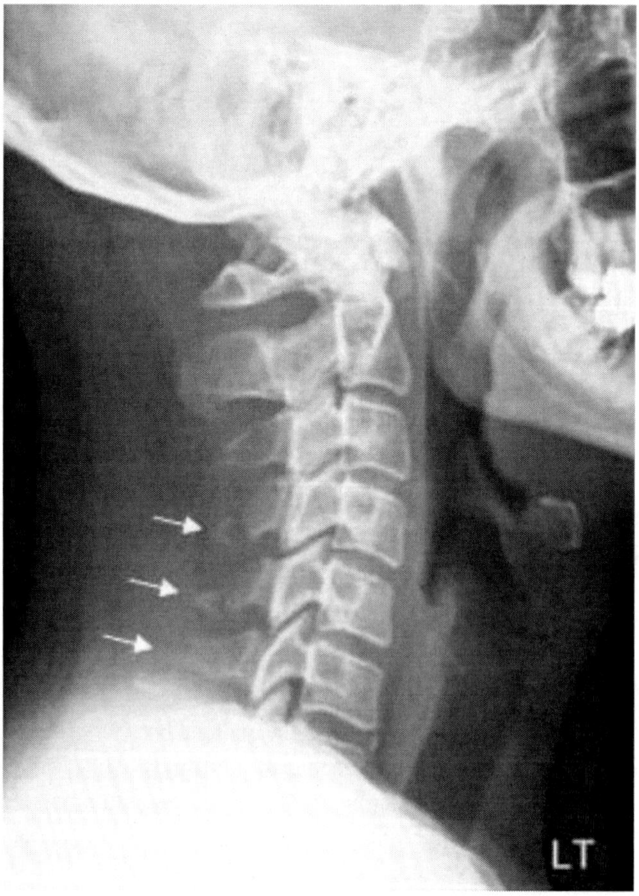

Figure 11. A lateral cervical spine radiograph illustrating spinous process fractures of C4-C6. Note that the radiograph is inadequate as it does not demonstrate the C7-T1 junction.

CONCLUSION

Interpretation of cervical spine radiographs may be challenging and significant injuries may not always be apparent on plain radiographs. The history and clinical examination dictate the need for plain radiographs and further imaging. Patients who are alert, do not have distracting injuries and are asymptomatic are unlikely to have significant cervical spine injuries. Symptomatic patients should be immobilised until imaging has defined the diagnosis and appropriate treatment by an orthopaedic or neurosurgeon has been instituted. The key to interpretation of cervical spine radiographs is to ensure films adequately visualise the entire cervical spine and to take a systematic approach.

REFERENCES

Advanced Trauma Life Support (ATLS) Student Course Manual Seventh Edition, 2004 178-189.

Anderson P. A., Gugala Z., Lindsey R., Schoenfels A. J., Harris M. B. 2010 Clearing the Cervical Spine in the Blunt Trauma Patient. *Journal of the American Academy of Orthopaedic Surgeons,* 18 149-159.

Anderson P. A., Muchow R. D., Munoz A., Tontz W. L., Resnick D. K. 2010 Clearance of the asymptomatic cervical spine: a meta-analysis. *Journal of Orthopaedic Trauma*, 24 100-106.

Bhamra J. S., Morar Y., Khan W. S., Deep K., Hammer A. (2012). Cervical Spine Immobilization in Sports Related Injuries: Review of Current Guidelines and a Case Study of an Injured Athlete. *Open Orthop. J.*, 6: 548-52.

Chimutengwende-Gordon M., Sidhu J., Khan W. S., Maruthainar N. (2010a). Advanced trauma life support radiographic trauma series: Part 1- The cervical spine radiograph. *J. Perioper. Pract.,* 20(9): 322-8.

Chimutengwende-Gordon M., Khan W. S., Sidhu J., Longo U. G., Maruthainar N. (2010b). Advanced trauma life support radiographic trauma series: Part 2- The chest radiograph. *J. Perioper. Pract.*, 20(12): 430-5.

Chimutengwende-Gordon M., Khan W. S., Sidhu J., Maruthainar N. (2011). Advanced trauma life support radiographic trauma series: Part 3- The pelvic radiograph. *J. Perioper. Pract.*, 21(1): 16-21.

Daffner R. H., Hackney D. B. 2007 ACR Appropriateness Criteria on suspected spine trauma. *Journal of the American College of Radiology,* 4, 762-765.

Davenport M. 2009 Fracture, Cervical Spine EMedicine.

Freedman I., van Gelderen D., Cooper D. J. 2005 Cervical Spine Assessment in the Unconscious Trauma Patient: A Major Trauma Service's Experience with Passive Flexion-Extension Radiography. *Journal of Trauma*, 58 1183-1188.

Garrett M., Consiglieri G., Kakarla U. K., Chang S. W., Dickman C. A. 2010 Occipitoatlantal Dislocation. *Neurosurgery,* 66, A48-A55.

Graber M. A., Kathol M. 1999 Cervical Spine Radiographs in the Trauma Patient. *American Family Physician*, 59, 331-342.

Holmes J. F., Akkinepalli R. 2005 Computer tomography versus plain radiography to screen for cervical spine injury: A meta-analysis. *Journal of Trauma,* 58, 902-905.

Karkos P. D., Benton J., Leong S. C. et al., 2007 Grisel's syndrome in otolaryngology: a systematic review. *International Journal of Paediatric Otorhinolaryngology*, 71, 1823-1827.

McCormick P. C. 2002 Radiographic Assessment of the Cervical Spine in Symptomatic Trauma Patients. *Neurosurgery,* 50, S36-S43.

Moore K. L., Dalley A. F. 1999 Back Clinically Oriented Anatomy Fourth Edition Lippincott Williams & Wilkins, 432-467.

Mower W. R., Hoffman J. R., Pollack C. V. Jr. et al. 2001, Use of plain radiography to screen for cervical spine injuries. *Annals of Emergency Medicine,* 38 1-7.

Nicholas J. 2006 Trauma Radiography Series CEEssentials, LLC.

Pollack C. V. Jr., Hendey G. W., Martin D. R. et al. 2001 Use of flexion-extension radiographs of the cervical spine in blunt trauma. *Annals of Emergency Medicine,* 38 8-11.

Pryputniewicz D. M., Hadley M. N. 2010, *Axis Fractures Neurosurgery,* 66 A68-A82.

Rabb C., Johnson J., VanSickle D. et al. 2007, Are upright lateral cervical radiographs in the obtunded trauma patient useful? A retrospective study. *World Journal of Emergency Surgery*, 2.

Raby N., Berman L., de Lacy G. 2005 Cervical Spine Accident and Emergency. *Radiology Elsevier Saunders*, 144-169.

Sliker C. W., Mirvis S. E., Shanmuganathan K. 2005 Assessing Cervical Spine Stability in Obtunded Blunt Trauma Patients: *A Review of Medical Literature Radiology*, 234 733-739.

Spain D. A., Trooskin S. Z., Flancbaum L., Boyarsky A. H., Nosher J. L. 1990 The adequacy and cost effectiveness of routine resuscitation-area cervical spine radiographs. *Annals of Emergency Medicine*, 19 276-278.

Wheeless C. R. 2008 Cervical Spine Wheeless' Textbook of Orthopaedics online.

In: Perioperative Practice in Trauma and Orthopaedic Surgery ISBN: 978-1-63483-325-7
Editor: Wasim S. Khan

Chapter 12

THE CHEST RADIOGRAPH IN THE ADVANCED TRAUMA LIFE SUPPORT RADIOGRAPHIC TRAUMA SERIES

M. Chimutengwende-Gordon, W. S. Khan*, J. Sidhu, and N. Maruthainar
Department of Trauma and Orthopaedics,
Royal Free Hampstead NHS Trust, London, UK

ABSTRACT

The chest radiograph is used as a screening test to exclude significant thoracic injuries in cases of major trauma. A systematic approach to reviewing chest radiographs is necessary for accurate interpretation. Radiographic findings should be considered in conjunction with clinical assessment.

Keywords: Trauma series, chest radiograph, thoracic trauma, advanced trauma life support

INTRODUCTION

In this chapter we are reviewing the chest radiographs performed as part of the Advanced Trauma Life Support (ATLS) trauma series (Chimutengwende-Gordon et al. 2010a, 2010b, 2011). Thoracic trauma is a significant cause of morbidity and mortality (Peters 2010, Gavelli 2002). A portable chest radiograph may be carried out in the resuscitation room and is the first-line radiological investigation used to diagnose thoracic injuries.

Chest radiography is indicated for all major trauma patients as part of the ATLS protocol. It is a useful screening test that facilitates prompt detection of potentially life-threatening injuries that may require rapid intervention. In the case of critically ill patients, the chest

* Tel.: +44 (0) 7791 025554; E-mail: wasimkhan@doctors.org.uk.

radiograph may be the only investigation that may be performed without the risk of further decompensation (Ho 2009).

The review of the chest radiograph should be guided by the findings from the clinical examination. In turn, the radiographic findings may then be used to focus further clinical examination and to direct decisions regarding the need for further investigations such as thoracic computed tomography (CT), arteriography or echocardiography. Clinical re-evaluation and repeat chest radiographs may be required if the patient's clinical status changes (ATLS 2004).

Mechanisms of Thoracic Injury

The majority of thoracic injuries may be classified as blunt or penetrating injuries. Blunt trauma refers to a closed injury which may be due to direct impact from moving solid objects, sudden deceleration, compressive or shear forces.

Most blunt thoracic injuries in the developed world are caused by road traffic accidents (Mayberry 2000, Zinck 2000). Falls, physical attacks and crush injuries are other causes of blunt trauma. Penetrating injuries occur when the skin and tissues are pierced by items such as knives, glass, bullets etc. These items enter the body and may damage organs and vascular structures. Less common mechanisms include burns, radiation and blast injuries (Ho 2009, Ursic 2010).

Thoracic Anatomy

A clear understanding of the normal anatomy of the thoracic cavity is essential for accurate interpretation of the chest radiograph. Figure 1 shows a normal chest radiograph with the main anatomical features labelled. The thoracic cavity is the superior part of the trunk between the neck and the abdomen. It extends from the supraclavicular fossae to the diaphragm. It contains several vital organs and structures. The thoracic wall surrounds the cavity and consists of skin, fasciae, nerves, muscles and bone. The skeleton of the thoracic wall includes twelve thoracic vertebrae and intervertebral discs, twelve pairs of ribs and costal cartilages and the sternum. This osteocartilaginous cage protects the heart and lungs as well as some abdominal organs such as the liver (Moore 1999).

The thoracic cavity is divided into two compartments that contain the lungs. The right lung is divided into three lobes by horizontal and oblique fissures. The left lung has two lobes separated by an oblique fissure (Moore 1999).

The bronchi and vessels enter and leave the lung at the hilum (Raby 2005). Each lung is surrounded by a pleural sac that consists of two serous membranes called the pleurae. The parietal pleura lines the thoracic wall and the visceral pleura lines the surfaces of the lungs. The pleural cavities are potential spaces between the layers of pleura which only become visible on a chest radiograph when abnormal e.g. when fluid, blood or air collects within the pleural cavity.

The mediastinum is a central compartment within the thoracic cavity located between the two pleural sacs.

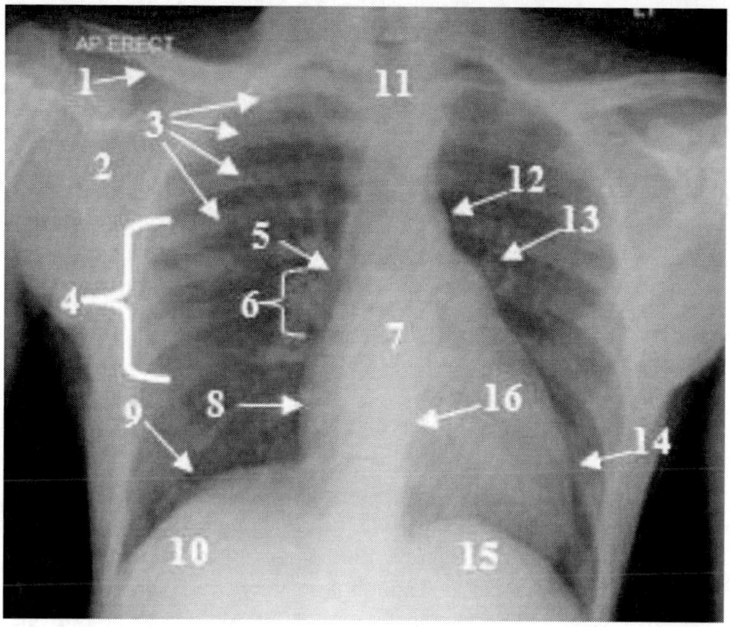

Figure 1. A normal chest radiograph illustrating the clavicle (1), scapula (2), ribs (3), lung field (4), superior vena cava (5), pulmonary artery (6), heart (7), right atrium of heart (8), diaphragm (9), liver (10), trachea (11), arch of the aorta (12), pulmonary artery (13), left ventricle of heart (14), stomach (15) and thoracic vertebrae (16).

It contains the heart which is enclosed by the pericardial sac, great vessels related to the heart such as the aorta, the vena cava and the azygous venous system. The distal part of the trachea and the oesophagus are also located within the mediastinum (Moore 1999).

Interpretation of the Chest Radiograph for Identification of Thoracic Injuries

It is important to have a structured, consistent approach for interpretation of chest radiographs. A useful mnemomic for reviewing a chest radiograph is 'ABCDEF' (Medicalmnemonics.com). A useful approach for the preliminary assessment of the chest radiograph and the systematic assessment of the main regions of the chest are summarised in Table 1 and Table 2 respectively.

Thoracic Injuries and Associated Radiological Findings

1. Chest Wall

Subcutaneous emphysema is the presence of air within the subcutaneous soft tissues (Figures 2-4). It may result from airway injury, lung injury or chest wall infection. The air appears on the chest radiograph as radiolucencies within the subcutaneous tissues.

Table 1. Preliminary assessment of the chest radiograph

Preliminary Assessment of the Chest Radiograph		
A	Antero-posterior (AP) or a postero-anterior (PA) film	Most chest radiographs in trauma patients will be AP films. On an AP chest radiograph, the heart will appear slightly larger than on a PA film.
B	Body position	It should be noted whether the patient is supine or upright. In trauma patients who are critically ill or when unstable spinal fractures have not been excluded an upright chest radiograph may not be possible (Gavelli 2002). Erect chest radiographs increase the sensitivity for detecting small haemothoraces, pneumothoraces and diaphragmatic injuries. Blunt upper abdominal injury is an indication for an erect chest radiograph. In the absence of any rotation of the film, the medial ends of each clavicle are equidistant to the spinous process of the vertebra at that level.
C	Confirm the patient details	It is important to confirm that the film being viewed is that of the correct patient.
D	Date	The date that the film was taken on should be checked.
E	Exposure	The thoracic intervertebral disc spaces are barely visible behind the heart on an adequately penetrated chest radiograph. Slightly overpenetrated films allow better visualisation of the thoracic spine, paraspinal lines and aortic outline.
F	Films for comparison	Reviewing old films on the same patient may be helpful.

This may be seen as the 'gingko leaf' sign which is the presence of radiolucent striations outlining the fibres of the pectoralis major muscles. Subcutaneous emphysema is usually self-limiting, but the underlying injury must be addressed (Ho 2009, ATLS 2004).

A subcutaneous haematoma is the collection of blood within the soft tissues. They may develop due to damage to the thoracic vessels, muscles or ribs.

Haematomas appear on chest radiographs as radiodense opacities overlying the chest wall. A lateral radiograph or a CT scan is useful to localise the presence of the haematoma to the chest wall. Subcutaneous haematomas usually resolve spontaneously (Collins 2000).

Thoracic trauma may lead to a variety of skeletal injuries. The ribs are commonly injured and may have significant consequences.

Table 2. Systematic assessment of the main regions of the chest. ABCDEF is a pneumonic to remember a systematic way of going through chest radiographs. A stands for airway that includes the trachea and main bronchi, B for bones of the chest, C for cardiac shadow, D for diaphragm, E for edges of the lung fields, and F for fields of the lung. This pneumonic only applies to radiographs and should not be confused with the ABCDE (Airway, Breathing, Circulation, Disability, Exposure) that is used in the primary survey of a trauma patient

Systematic Assessment of the Main Regions of the Chest		
A	Airways	The radiograph should be assessed for the presence of interstitial or pleural air that may indicate a large airway injury. Tracheal lacerations that may present as pneumomediastinum, pneumothorax, and subcutaneous emphysema of the neck should be looked for (ATLS 2004).
B	Bones	Fractures of the ribs, sternum, clavicle or scapula may accompany major thoracic injuries. The soft tissues should also be assessed, for example the presence of subcutaneous air or foreign bodies should be identified.
C	Cardiac	An enlarged cardiac silhouette occurs when there is air or blood within the pericardium. A widened mediastinum suggests aortic rupture.
D	Diaphragm	The radiograph should be carefully evaluated for evidence of diaphragmatic irregularity or obliteration. The right hemidiaphragm is usually slightly higher than the left. Excessive diaphragmatic elevation indicates diaphragmatic injury. The presence of stomach, bowel gas or a nasogastric tube above the diaphragm indicates rupture (Zinck 2000, ATLS 2004).
E	Edges	The apices should be assessed in particular for the presence of a pneumothorax. Abnormal fluid collections in the pleural space may represent a haemothorax.
F	Fields	The lung fields are assessed for infiltrates that may suggest pulmonary contusion, haematoma, aspiration etc. Pulmonary contusions appear as air space consolidation that can be irregular and patchy, homogenous, diffuse or extensive. The lung parenchyma should be assessed for evidence of laceration. Lacerations appear as a haematoma and areas of consolidation.

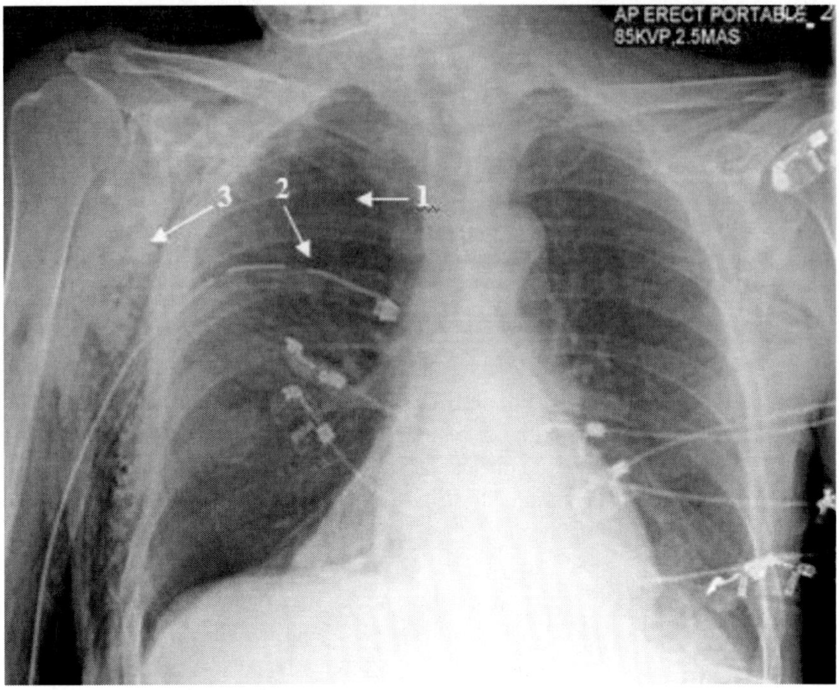

Figure 2. A chest radiograph showing a pneumothorax (1) managed with a chest drain (2). There is also subcutaneous emphysema (3) accompanying the pneumothorax.

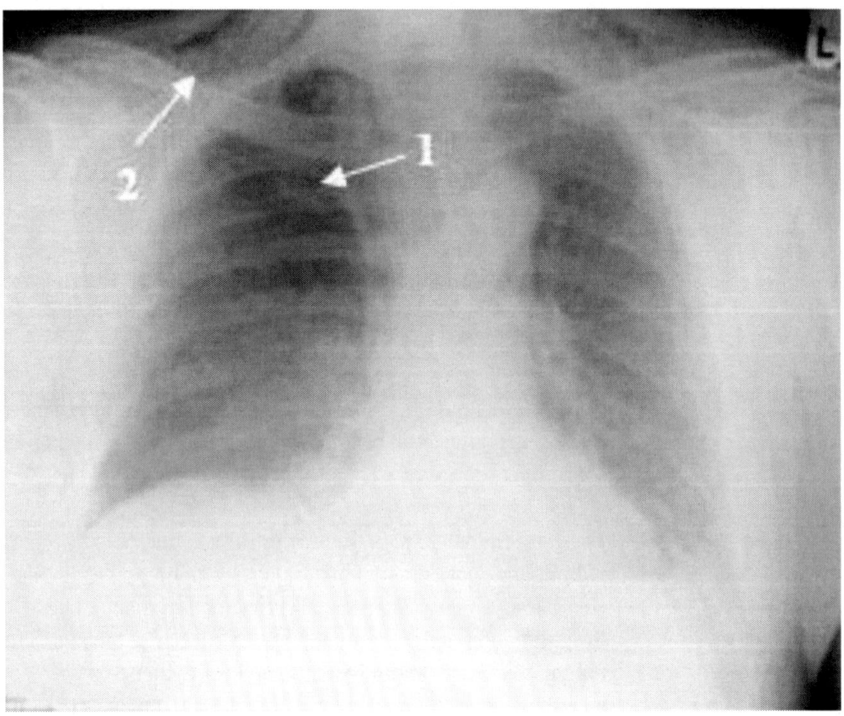

Figure 3. A chest radiograph showing a pneumothorax (1) and subcutaneous emphysema (2).

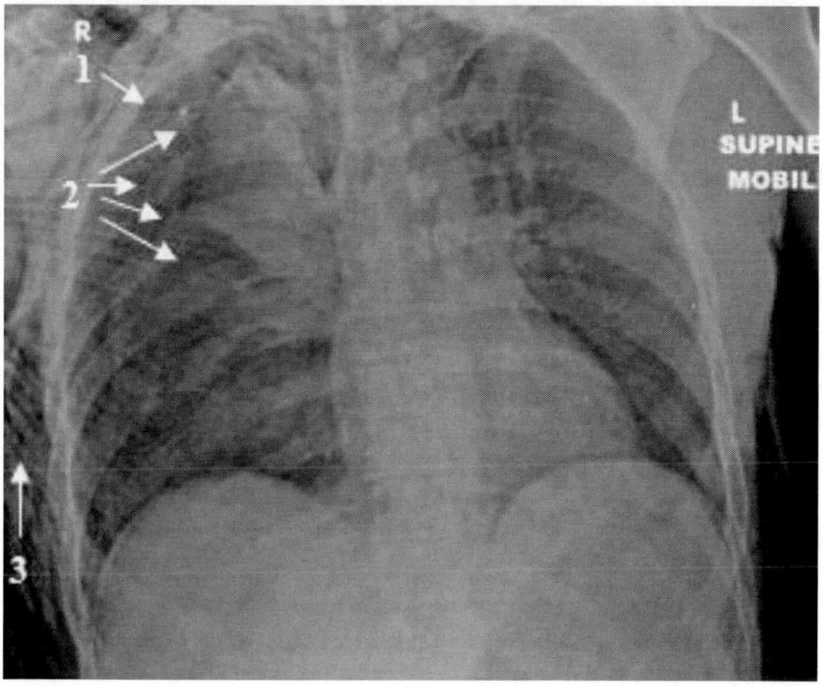

Figure 4. A chest radiograph showing a tension pneumothorax (1) and multiple rib fractures (2). There is also subcutaneous emphysema (3) accompanying the tension pneumothorax (3).

Multiple rib fractures are seen in Figure 4 and Figure 5. Pain results in splinting of the thorax reducing the effectiveness of ventilation, oxygenation and effective coughing. These factors increase the risk of atelactasis (collapse of part or the entire lung) and pneumonia, especially if there is pre-existing lung disease. Fractures to the upper ribs (1-3) are uncommon as they are protected by the shoulder girdles and musculature (Collins 2000). Fractures of these ribs indicate significant energy transfer and may be associated with injuries to the great vessels, brachial plexus, lungs, head and neck.

Fractures to the middle ribs (4-9) often occur due to antero-posterior compression of the thoracic cavity and may be associated with intrathoracic injuries such as pneumothorax. Young patients have more flexible chest walls and multiple rib fractures indicate high forces being applied to the chest.

Lower rib fractures (10-12) may be associated with injuries to the upper abdominal organs such as the liver, spleen and kidneys (ATLS 2004). A flail chest occurs when three or more adjacent segmental rib fractures or five or more contiguous single fractures are present. It results in paradoxical motion of the chest wall during inspiration or expiration and may lead to underlying lung injuries with pulmonary contusions. Treatment consists of adequate ventilation and fluid resuscitation (Ho 2009).

Fractures of the sternum and scapula may be identified on chest radiographs, although CT scans, and sternal or scapular radiographs are more sensitive in diagnosing these injuries (Collins 2000, Ho 2009). Clavicle fractures are common injuries easily identified on chest radiographs (Figure 6 and Figure 7).These injuries require significant application of force to the thoracic cavity. Sternal fractures may be associated with blunt cardiac injury and lung injuries.

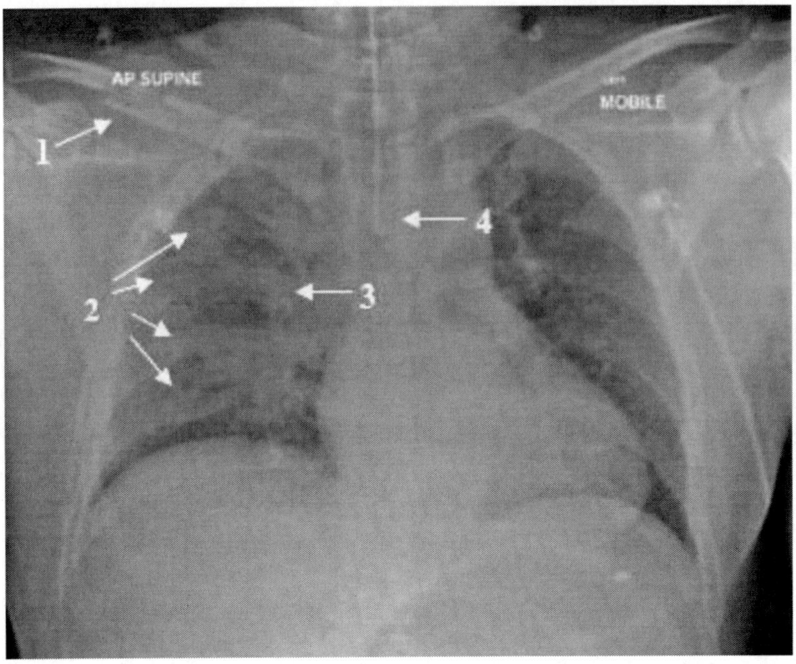

Figure 5. A chest radiograph showing a right clavicle fracture (1) and multiple rib fractures (2). There is also air space shadowing within right lung consistent with pulmonary contusion (3) and an endotracheal tube at the level of T3 (4).

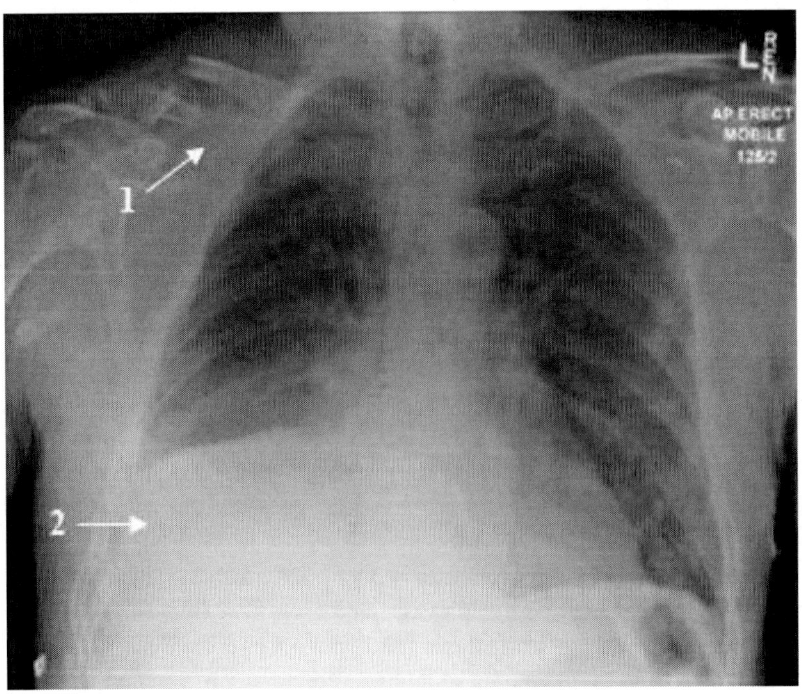

Figure 6. A chest radiograph showing a comminuted displaced right clavicle fracture (1) and a right-sided haemothorax (2).

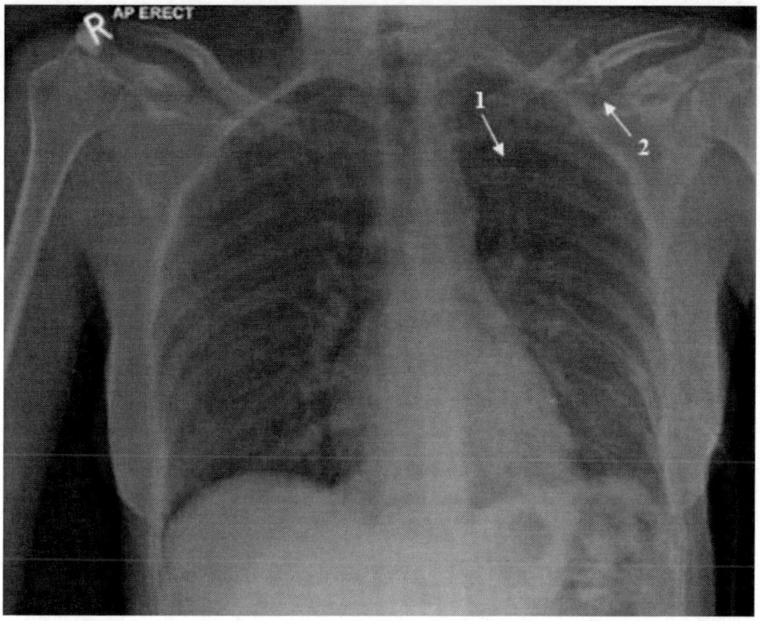

Figure 7. A chest radiograph showing a chest drain with tip lying against the left hilum which is draining left pneumothorax (1). There is also a left clavicle fracture (2).

2. Pleura

A pneumothorax occurs when air enters the potential space between the visceral and parietal pleura. This may occur as a result of blunt or penetrating trauma. This appears as an apical lucent area without bronchial or vascular markings on a chest radiograph (Figures 2, 3, 7 and 8). A pneumothorax is generally treated with a chest drain placed in the fourth or fifth intercostal space, just anterior to the midaxillary line (ATLS 2004).

A tension pneumothorax (see Case study 1) occurs when air is forced into the thoracic cavity but cannot escape due to the development of a 'one-way-valve' air leak from the lung or through the chest wall. As the air collects, the affected lung collapses completely. The mediastinum is displaced to the opposite side, which decreases the venous return and compresses the opposite lung (ATLS 2004). Chest radiographic signs include a unilateral hyperlucent lung field with collapse of the lung, tracheal deviation and mediastinal displacement (Figure 4) (Ho 2009).

As tension pneumothorax is a life-threatening emergency, time should not be wasted obtaining a chest radiograph. The diagnosis should be made on the basis of clinical findings of chest pain, respiratory distress, tachycardia, hypotension, tracheal deviation, unilateral absence of breath sounds and neck vein distension.

Immediate treatment consists of insertion of a large-calibre needle into the second intercostal space in the mid-clavicular line in order to convert it to a simple pneumothorax. Chest drain insertion is the definitive treatment (ATLS 2004).

A haemothorax (see Case study 2) can result from lung laceration or vascular injury. The chest radiograph appearance of a small haemothorax consists of layering of fluid and blunting of the costophrenic angles.

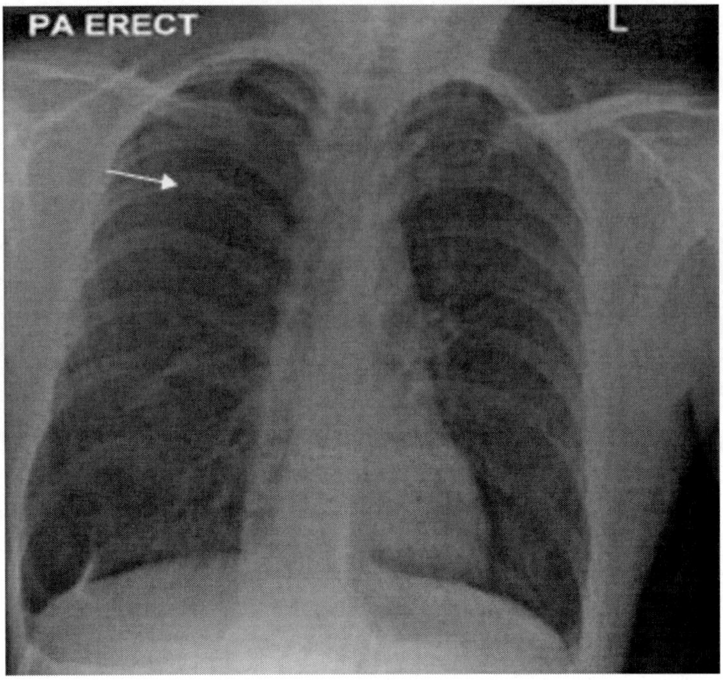

Figure 8a. A chest radiograph showing a small to moderate sized right sided pneumothorax (arrow).

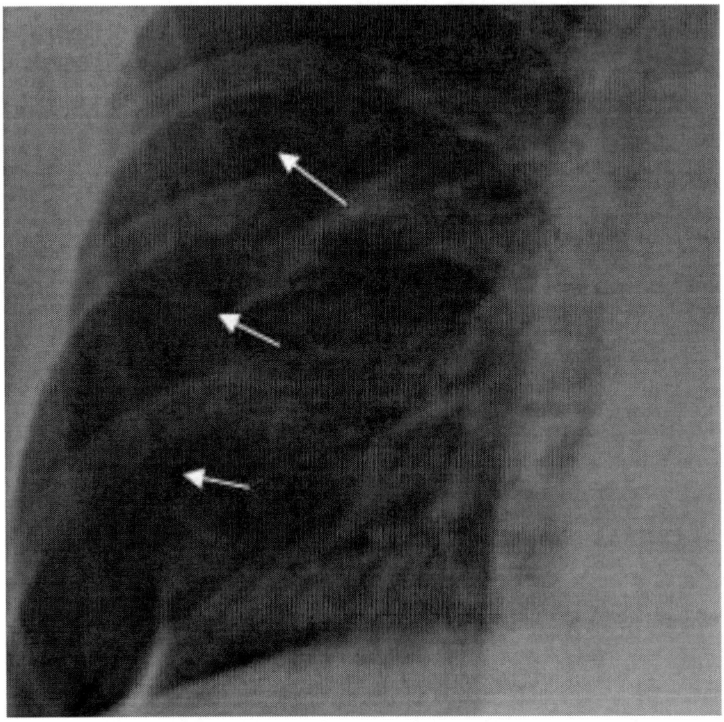

Figure 8b. A magnified version of the pneumothorax illustrated in Figure 8a showing the junction between lung markings and pneumothorax.

Case study 1.

Mrs RC, a 47 year old journalist was brought to hospital by ambulance after being crushed on her bicycle between a reversing bus and a wall. She was complaining of right sided chest and right wrist pain. She was noted to have bruising over her right chest wall and a deformed right wrist.

The patient was managed in accordance with the ATLS guidelines. In the A&E department, the patient was found to be dyspnoeic, disorientated and agitated. Although her blood pressure was normal she was tachycardic and tachypnoeac. Her oxygen saturation was only 68% despite being on high flow oxygen via a rebreather mask. On examination her trachea was deviated away from the right side, she had hyperresonance of the right chest wall on percussion and decreased breath sounds.

A clinical diagnosis of tension pneumothorax was made and it was decompressed with a needle in the right second anterior rib space. This was followed by a chest drain inserted into the fifth mid-axillary rib space.

The patient then had a chest radiograph confirming the pneumothorax and correct placement of the chest drain. It also showed the presence of associated rib fractures. A right sided distal radius fracture was identified and stabilised in the secondary survey. The chest drain was removed on day 4 after the patient had her distal radius fracture operation, and once the pneumothorax had resolved.

Case study 2.

Mr AP, a 20 year old student was brought to hospital by ambulance after the car he was driving was hit from the right side by another car at a junction. He was unconscious and noted to have bruising over his right chest wall and a deformed right thigh.

The patient was managed in accordance with the ATLS guidelines and had been intubated and ventilated at the scene. In the A&E department, the patient was noted to be hypotensive and tachycardic but was responding to fluid resuscitation. On examination the trachea was in the midline but the right chest wall was dull to percussion and had decreased breath sounds. The deformed thigh was aligned and stabilised in a splint.

The patient then had a chest radiograph confirming a right sided haemothorax. A chest drain was inserted in the fifth mid-axillary rib space to drain the haemothorax. After an initial drainage of 700 ml of blood, the drainage stopped. A mid-shaft femoral fracture was identified in the secondary survey. The chest drain was removed on day 6 after the patient had intra-medullary nailing of his femoral fracture, and after the haemothorax had resolved.

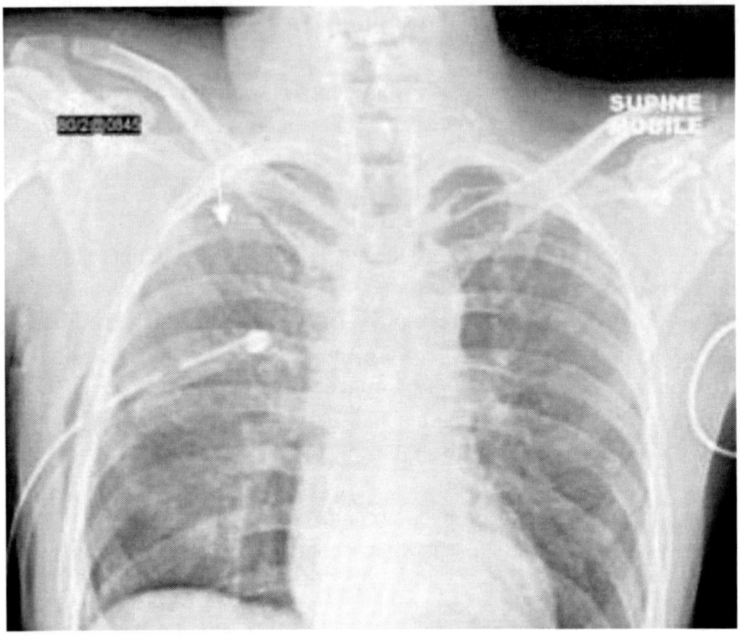

Figure 9. A chest radiograph showing a right sided haemopneumothorax with a chest drain *in situ* (arrow).

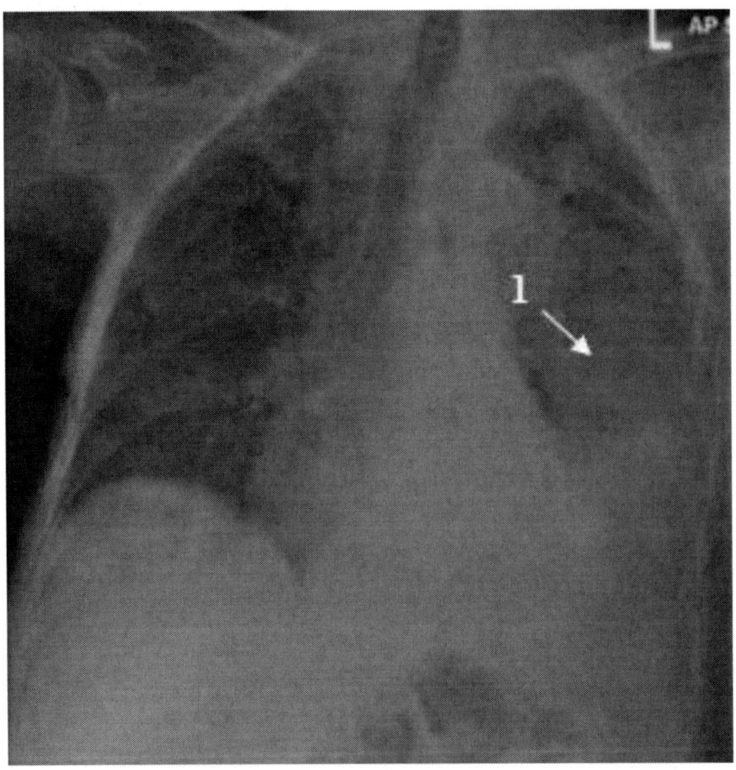

Figure 10. A chest radiograph showing a large left sided haemothorax (arrow).

Figure 6 shows the appearance of a haemothorax on an erect chest radiograph. Figure 9 and Figure 10 show the appearance of haemothoraces in supine patients. Small haemothoraces resolve spontaneously. A large haemothorax may appear radiographically as complete opacification of the hemithorax. Large haemothoraces are treated with chest drainage and fluid resuscitation or blood transfusion in hypovolaemic patients (Ho 2009). If 1,500 ml of blood is immediately evacuated on insertion of the chest drain, or if haemorrhage continues at a rate of 100-200 ml per hour for more than two hours, thoracotomy by a suitably trained surgeon is indicated (ATLS 2004).

3. Lungs

Pulmonary contusions occur when lung injuries result in leakage of blood and oedema into the interstitial and alveolar spaces. Areas of air-space shadowing are seen within the lung fields (Figure 5). Contusions are usually evident within six hours after trauma and usually resolve within a week (Ho 2009).

4. Mediastinum

Pneumomediastinum is the presence of air within the mediastinal structures. It may be due to tracheobronchial, pharyngeal or oesophageal rupture. Chest radiographs show air outlining the mediastinal soft tissue structures and the parietal pleura (Zinck 2000).

Mediastinal widening and irregularity are signs of aortic injury (Figure 11). This is often difficult to identify and chest radiographs may be normal. Clinical suspicion of aortic dissection is more important than chest radiograph appearances (Raby 2005).

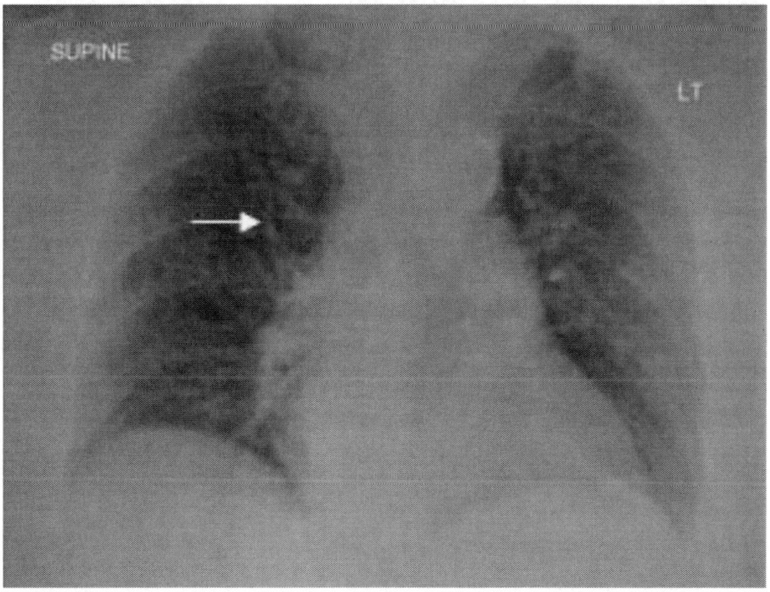

Figure 11. A chest radiograph showing a widened mediastinum (arrow) in aortic dissection.

Traumatic aortic dissection may show non-specific signs on radiographs such as an irregular aortic silhouette, discontinuous calcification of the arch of the aorta or intraluminal displacement of a calcified aortic intima (Ho 2009). CT or arteriography is required for further investigation of aortic injury (Fishman 2000).

Oesophageal rupture and foreign body injury may lead to mediastinitis (mediastinal infection). Chest radiographs may show oedema, haemorrhage and gas production in the mediastinum. Pleural effusions and lower lobe consolidation may also occur (Ho 2009).

Cardiac tamponade occurs when the pericardium fills with blood from the heart, great vessels or pericardial vessels. A relatively small amount of blood may impair cardiac filling and result in venous pressure elevation, decline in arterial pressure and muffled heart sounds on auscultation (Beck's triad) (ATLS 2004).

Chest radiography may occasionally show a global enlargement of the cardiac silhouette (Ho 2009). Echocardiography is the usual method of making the diagnosis. Prompt removal of small amounts of fluid by needle periocardiocentesis may result in immediate haemodynamic improvement (ATLS 2004).

5. Diaphragm

Diaphragmatic rupture may be identified on chest radiographs as hemidiaphragmatic elevation, irregular diaphragmatic contours and the presence of upper abdominal organs within the thoracic cavity. A CT scan has a considerably greater sensitivity and is usually required to make the diagnosis. The treatment for diaphragmatic rupture is surgical repair (Shanmuganathan 2000).

Alternative Radiological Tests for the Initial Investigation of Thoracic Trauma

CT scanning of the chest is more sensitive and specific for the detection of lung lesions than plain chest radiographs (De Wever 2000, Traub 2007). It has been suggested that CT scanning could be used as a routine screening test for patients presenting with chest trauma. However, as CT scanning cannot be performed in the resuscitation room and takes longer to perform, its use as an initial screening test would only be appropriate in selected clinically stable patients who are alert and do not have evidence of chest wall tenderness, reduced air-entry or abnormal respiratory effort (Traub 2007). Ultrasound scanning has also been found to be more sensitive than supine plain chest radiography and as sensitive as CT for the detection of traumatic pneumothoraces (Rowan 2002). Focused assessment sonography in trauma (FAST) may be performed rapidly at the patient's bedside to detect other traumatic thoracic lesions such as haemothoraces, pericardial effusions, pulmonary contusions and rib fractures (Rowan 2002, Chan 2003, Chan 2009). It has the added advantage of enabling immediate ultrasound guided pericardiocentesis in the presence of cardiac tamponade (ATLS 2004) or chest drainage for pneumothoraces or haemothoraces (Laws 2003). This is only possible if the facilities are available in the Emergency Department and the operator has appropriate expertise.

Conclusion

Thoracic trauma is common and may lead to life-threatening complications. Diagnosis of thoracic injuries should be prompt to allow early intervention and prevent unnecessary deaths. Clinical assessment and accurate interpretation of plain chest radiographs is the basis of diagnosis. Some thoracic injuries may produce subtle clinical signs which may be missed in the emergency department but usually recognised on chest radiographs. Other thoracic injuries result in classical dramatic clinical signs and lead to rapid deterioration. Tension pneumothoraces, for example, should be diagnosed clinically and treated immediately without the delay of obtaining a chest radiograph. Some injuries may be underestimated or not easily diagnosed on plain chest radiography and require further investigations such as CT scans (Miller 2006).

References

Advanced Trauma Life Support (ATLS) Student Course Manual Seventh Edition, 2004 103-130.

Chan S. S. 2003 Emergency bedside ultrasound to detect pneumothorax *Academic Emergency Medicine*, 10(1) 91-94.

Chan S. S. 2009 Emergency bedside ultrasound for the diagnosis of rib fractures. *American Journal of Emergency Medicine*, 27(5) 617-620.

Chest X-ray interpretation Medicalmnemonics.com.

Chimutengwende-Gordon M., Sidhu J., Khan W. S., Maruthainar N. (2010a). Advanced trauma life support radiographic trauma series: Part 1- The cervical spine radiograph. *J. Perioper. Pract.*, 20(9): 322-8.

Chimutengwende-Gordon M., Khan W. S., Sidhu J., Longo U. G., Maruthainar N. (2010b). Advanced trauma life support radiographic trauma series: Part 2- The chest radiograph. *J. Perioper. Pract.*, 20(12): 430-5.

Chimutengwende-Gordon M., Khan W. S., Sidhu J., Maruthainar N. (2011). Advanced trauma life support radiographic trauma series: Part 3- The pelvic radiograph. *J. Perioper. Pract.*, 21(1): 16-21.

Collins J. 2000 Chest Wall Trauma. *Journal of Thoracic Imaging*, 15(2) 112-119.

De Wever W., Bogaert J., Verschakelen J. 2000, Radiology of lung trauma. *JBR-BTR*, 83(4):167-73.

Fishman J. E. 2000 Imaging of Blunt Aortic and Great Vessel Trauma, *Journal of Thoracic Imaging,* 15(2) 97-103.

Gavelli G., Canini R., Bertaccini P. et al. 2002 Traumatic injuries: imaging of thoracic injuries. *European Radiology*, 12(6) 1273-1294.

Ho M., Gutierrez F. 2009 Chest Radiography in Thoracic Polytrauma. *American Journal of Roentgenology*, 192 599-612.

Laws D., Neville E., Duffy J.; Pleural Diseases Group, Standards of Care Committee, British Thoracic Society, 2003 BTS guidelines for the insertion of a chest drain. *Thorax,* 2003 58 (Suppl. 2)ii53-ii59.

Leblang S. D., Dolich M. O. 2000 Imaging of Penetrating Thoracic Trauma. *Journal of Thoracic Imaging*, 15(2) 128-135.

Mayberry J. C. 2000 Imaging in Thoracic Trauma: The Trauma Surgeon's Perspective. *Journal of Thoracic Imaging*, 15(2) 76-86.

Miller L. A. 2006 Chest wall, lung and pleural space trauma. *Radiologic Clinics of North America,* 44(2) 213-224.

Moore K. L., Dalley A. F. 1999 Thorax Clinically Oriented Anatomy Fourth Edition Lippincott Williams & Wilkins, 60-172.

Peters S., Nicholas V., Heyer C. M. 2010 Multidetector computer tomography-spectrum of blunt chest wall and lung injuries in polytraumatized patients. *Clinical Radiology*, 65(4) 333-338.

Raby N., Berman L., de Lacy G. 2005 Chest Accident and Emergency. *Radiology Elsevier Saunders*, 256-269.

Rowan K. R., Kirkpatrick A. W., Liu D. 2002 Traumatic pneumothorax detection with thoracic US: correlation with chest radiography and CT – initial experience. *Radiology*, 225(1) 210-214.

Shanmuganathan K., Killeen K., Mirvis S. E., White C. S. 2000, Imaging of Diaphragmatic Injuries. *Journal of Thoracic Imaging*, 15(2) 104-111.

Traub M., Stevenson M., McEvoy S., et al. 2007 The use of chest computed tomography versus chest X-ray in patients with major blunt trauma. *Injury,* 38(1) 43-47.

Ursic C., Curtis K. 2010 Thoracic and neck trauma. *International Emergency Nursing,* 18 47-53.

Zinck S. E., Primack S. L. 2000 Radiographic and CT Findings in Blunt Chest Trauma. *Journal of Thoracic Imaging*, 15(2) 87-96.

In: Perioperative Practice in Trauma and Orthopaedic Surgery ISBN: 978-1-63483-325-7
Editor: Wasim S. Khan

Chapter 13

THE PELVIC RADIOGRAPH IN THE ADVANCED TRAUMA LIFE SUPPORT RADIOGRAPHIC TRAUMA SERIES

Mukai Chimutengwende-Gordon, Wasim S. Khan*, Jasmeet Sidhu and Nimalan Maruthainar
[1]Department of Trauma and Orthopaedics,
Royal Free Hampstead NHS Trust, London, UK

ABSTRACT

Pelvic fractures are often high energy injuries and are associated with a high morbidity and mortality. The plain antero-posterior pelvis radiograph is part of the Advanced Trauma Life Support radiographic trauma series and is used as a screening test. As the main limitation of plain antero-posterior pelvic radiographs is the difficulty in identification of some fractures, in particular posterior fractures, radiographic findings should be considered in conjunction with clinical assessment.

Keywords: Trauma series, antero-posterior pelvis radiograph, pelvic trauma, pelvic fracture, advanced trauma life support

INTRODUCTION

In this chapter we review pelvic radiographs performed as part of the Advanced Trauma Life Support (ATLS) trauma series (Chimutengwende-Gordon et al., 2010a, 2010b, 2011).

Pelvic injuries often occur due to high velocity injuries such as road traffic accidents, and may be associated with polytrauma (i.e. multiple injuries) (See Case Study 1 and Case study 2). Low velocity pelvic injuries such as falls usually occur in the elderly but may occur in young athletic patients due to sudden muscular contraction leading to avulsion injuries (Koval

* Tel.: +44 (0) 7791 025554; E-mail: wasimkhan@doctors.org.uk.

2006). Pelvic ring fractures account for 1.5% of all joint fractures and have a high morbidity and mortality (Theumann 2002, Sathy 2009). Life-threatening major haemorrhage is the leading cause of death in patients with a pelvic fracture and may occur if the pelvic vessels are injured. It may also be due to accompanying extrapelvic injuries (ATLS 2004, Balogh 2007). Methods of immediate haemorrhage control include wrapping a pelvic binder around the pelvis and external fixation (Koval 2006). The use of pelvic angiography with embolization may improve patient outcomes if haemorrhage continues despite these measures (Wiss 2001).

Structures such as the bladder, urethra, rectum and uterus are at risk due to sharp bone edges of the fracture lacerating adjacent organs. The elastic recoil of the tissues may result in the bone fragments returning to a near-normal position. As a result, even minimally displaced pelvic fractures may be associated with significant organ damage (Case Study 2). Therefore, injury severity cannot be predicted according to the degree of displacement seen radiographically (Raby 2005, Gardner 2010).

There should be a high index for suspicion for pelvic fractures to enable rapid identification in order to reduce the risk of fatality (Raby 2005). It is important to recognise when interpreting these films that some fractures such as posterior fractures involving the sacrum and sacro-iliac joints are not always visible (Lunsjo 2007).

ANATOMY

The pelvic cavity contains organs such as the urinary bladder, the rectum, the inferior parts of the ureters and the reproductive system, as well as blood vessels, lymphatics and nerves.

Case Study 1.

A 59 year old woman was driving a car with a seatbelt and headrest when she had a high-velocity impact to the front of her vehicle. She was extracted from the vehicle by an ambulance crew and had a pelvic binder applied. She was taken to A&E where she had a Glasgow Coma Scale (GCS) score of 14, pulse rate of 120 beats/min, respiration rate of 24/min, and blood pressure of 104/68 mm Hg. Following primary survey she had radiographs of her pelvis showing pelvic ring disruption with bilateral sacroiliac disruption and left superior and inferior pubic rami fractures. Initial hemoglobin level was 6.6 g/dL and the patient received 2 units of blood but remained haemodynamically unstable. Because of the fracture pattern and likelihood of ongoing pelvic hemorrhage, pelvic angiography was performed. Pelvic angiography revealed substantial bleeding from the left internal pudendal artery. The feeding vessel was selectively cannulated and embolised successfully. Four days later, the patient had open reduction and internal fixation of the pelvis, and was subsequently discharged on day 16.

Case Study 2.

> A 39 year old construction site worker got caught between two trucks for almost one minute. When the ambulance crew arrived, he was unable to stand and complained of pain over the left sacroiliac joint and abdomen. He was brought to A&E and following the primary survey, had pelvic radiographs revealing an 'open book' type of pelvic fracture with left and right sacroiliac joint disruption. An ultrasonogram of the abdomen revealed free fluid. Initial resuscitation efforts failed to provide haemodynamic stability and the patient was taken to theatre. After application of the external fixator, a midline laparotomy was performed. A liver laceration was identified and repaired. The patient remained haemodynamically stable and six days later underwent open reduction and internal fixation of the pelvis following a CT scan.

The bony pelvis is a ring of bone formed by the two innominate bones anteromedially, the sacrum posteriorly and the coccyx which is inferior to the sacrum. The innominate bones consist of three parts, namely the ilium, ischium and pubis (Moore 1999). The pelvis has several joints. The lumbosacral joints are articulations formed by the intervertebral disc between the fifth lumbar vertebral body and the first sacral vertebral body. The sacrococcygeal joint unites the sacrum and the coccyx. The sacroiliac joints are strong articulations between the sacrum and the ilium. The pubic symphysis is where the innominate bones join anteriorly in the midline. There are anatomical differences between the male and female pelves. The female pelvis is broader and wider as an adaptation for childbearing (Moore 1999). Figure 1 illustrates the main anatomical features of the bony pelvis.

The pelvis is described as having three bony rings which are shown in Figure 2. The main pelvic ring contains the pubic symphysis and the sacroiliac bones. The two smaller rings, which are known as the obturator foramina, are formed by the pubic and ischial bones (Raby 2005). The pelvis is divided into the 'true' (lesser) pelvis and the 'false' (greater) pelvis by the pelvic brim. The pelvic brim is formed by arcuate lines passing from the sacral promontory to the superior border of the pubis anteriorly. The 'true' pelvis is below the pelvic brim and contains the pelvic viscera. The 'false' pelvis is above the pelvic brim and contains some of the abdominal viscera (Koval 2006).

The bony pelvis is stabilised by several strong ligaments. The long and short posterior sacroiliac ligaments, the interosseous ligaments within the sacroiliac joints and the sacrotuberous ligaments resist forces leading to vertical translation between the ilia and the sacrum. The anterior sacroiliac, symphyseal and sacrospinous ligaments are arranged transversely and resist forces that lead to rotation of the pelvis (Theumann 2002).

Plain Pelvic Radiographic Views

A portable pelvis radiograph taken in the resuscitation room is usually the first line investigation performed to diagnose pelvic fractures in patients with major trauma. It is used as a screening test as part of the ATLS trauma series following the primary survey (i.e. the initial clinical assessment) to identify pelvic fractures that may need further investigation.

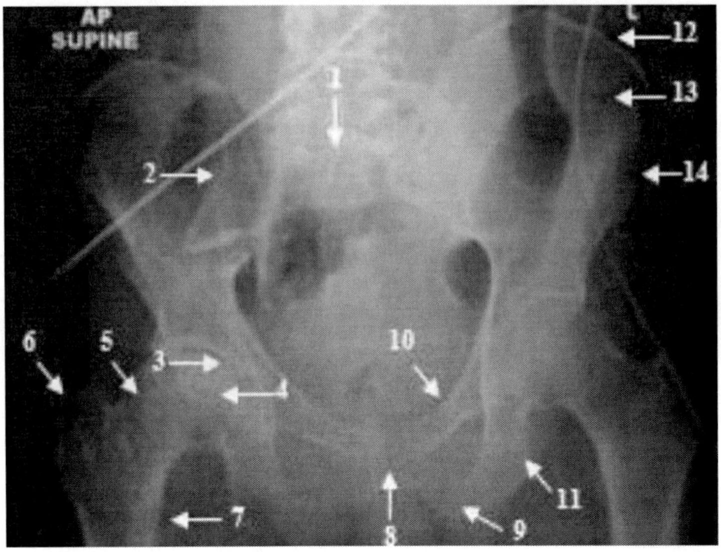

Figure 1. A normal plain antero-posterior pelvic radiograph illustrating the bony anatomy: sacrum (1), sacroiliac joint (2), acetabulum (3), femoral head (4), femoral neck (5), greater trochanter (6), lesser trochanter (7), pubic symphysis (8), ischium (9), superior pubic ramus (10), inferior pubic ramus (11), iliac crest (12), iliac wing (13), anterior superior iliac spine (14).

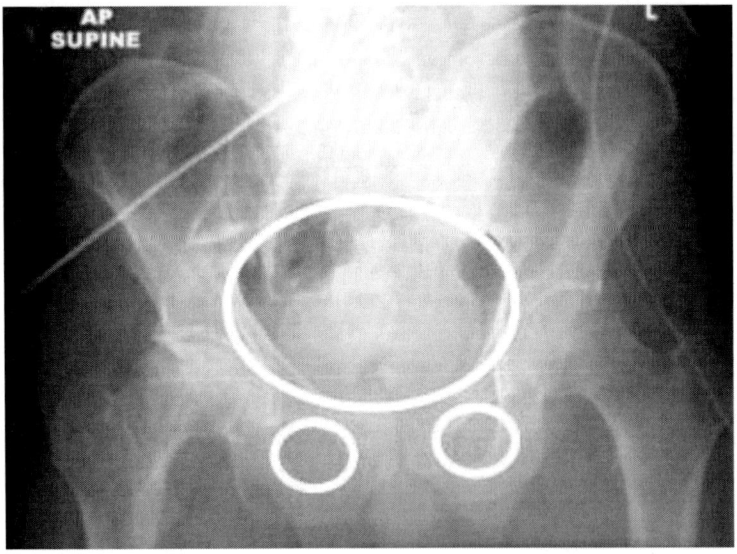

Figure 2. A normal plain antero-posterior pelvic radiograph highlighting the three bony rings.

This view is taken with the patient supine and the feet approximately 15 degrees internally rotated. The central beam is directed vertically towards the mid-portion of the pelvis. The Antero-Posterior (AP) pelvis radiograph should demonstrate the iliac bone, sacrum, pubis, ischium, proximal femur, greater trochanter and lesser trochanters (Nicholas 2006). Additional views include the pelvic inlet and outlet views, and Judet views. The pelvic inlet (superior pelvic aperture) is the opening into the 'true' pelvis which contains the urinary bladder and rectum as well as the uterus in females.

This view is taken with the patient supine and the X-ray tube angled 45 degrees inferiorly and perpendicular to pelvic brim. This view is useful for diagnosing and assessing the degree of displacement of the sacroiliac joint, sacrum or iliac wing. Additionally, it may be useful to diagnose internal or external rotation of the hemipelvis, pubic diastasis (separation) or overlap and the presence of subtle sacral fractures or sacral impaction (Koval 2006, Nicholas 2006). The pelvic outlet view may demonstrate the magnitude of vertical hemipelvis displacement. Sacral foramina as well as some sacral/pubic rami fractures may be visualized better on the outlet view than the AP. The outlet view is obtained with the patient supine and the X-ray tube angled 45 degrees superiorly and perpendicular to the pelvic brim (Koval 2006, Nicholas 2006). Oblique Judet views are 45 degree internal and external rotation views. They are useful for visualization of suspected acetabular fractures (Theumann 2002).

Approach to Interpretation of the Plain AP Pelvic Radiographs

An adequate AP pelvis view will include the anatomy from the top of both iliac crest superiorly through to the iliac tuberosities and will include the lesser trochanters of the femur as shown in Figure 1. The lateral margins of the film should include the anterior portions of the iliac wings. The radiographic exposure technique should demonstrate good bone detail.

A systematic inspection of the radiograph should be made. Firstly, the main pelvic ring and the two small rings should be examined for continuity. Following this, the sacroiliac joints should be inspected. They should have equal widths. The pubic symphysis is examined. The width of the joint should not be more than 5mm. Additionally, the superior surfaces of the pubic bones should align. The sacral foramina are then assessed for any evidence of disruption of the smooth arcuate lines which would indicate a fracture (see Figure 3). Both sides should be compared (Raby 2005). Finally, the acetabula should be examined. The continuity of the four lines shown in Figure 4 should be assessed. These lines are the iliopectineal line which is formed by the anterior column of the acetabulum, the ilioischial line which is formed by the posterior column of the acetabulum, the anterior and posterior lips of the acetabulum (Solomon 2001, Wheeless 2008).

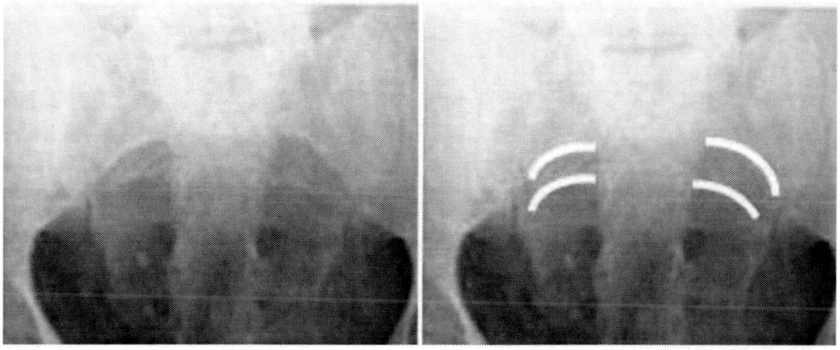

Figure 3. The normal smooth curves of the arcuate lines forming the margins of the sacral foramina.

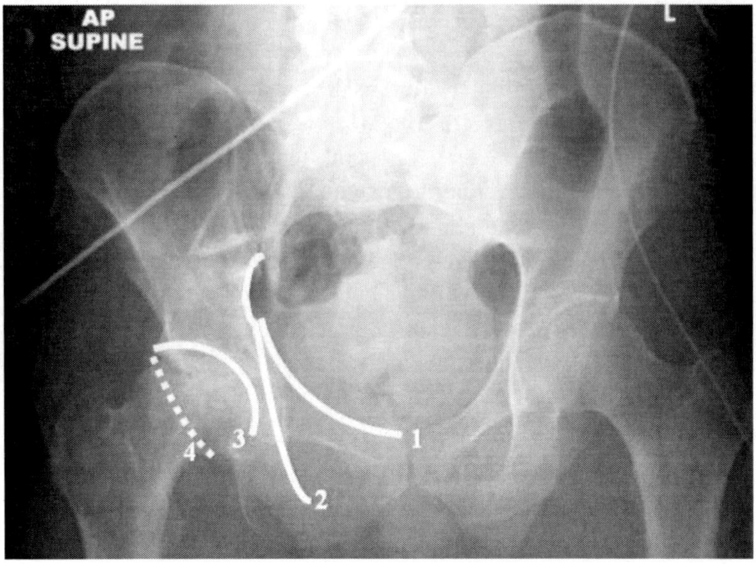

Figure 4. Four pelvic lines: iliopectineal line (1), ilioischial line (2), anterior lip (3), posterior lip (4) on a antero-posterior pelvic radiograph.

Patterns of Pelvic Injury

The Young and Burgess classification system may be used to describe patterns of pelvic injury and categorises injuries according to four mechanisms (Koval 2006):

1. Lateral Compression

This occurs due to a laterally applied force and may result in transverse or oblique fractures of the pubic rami which may be either ipsilateral or contralateral to a posterior injury.

Type I - Sacral compression on the side of impact associated with coronal pubic rami fractures

Type II - Posterior iliac wing fracture or sacroiliac joint disruption on the side of impact

Type III - An external rotation injury due to force being transmitted to the contralateral hemipelvis resulting in disruption of the sacroiliac, sacrotuberous and sacrospinous ligaments (Koval 2006, Slater 2010).

2. AP Compression

These injuries include external rotation injuries, diastasis of the pubic symphysis or longitudinal fractures of the pubic rami. This occurs due to direct application of force to the pubis or the posterior pelvis or indirect application of force transferred via the lower limbs (Theumann 2002, Koval 2006).

Type I - Diastasis of the pubic symphysis of less than 2.5cm or anterior sacroiliac joint disruption. There may be longitudinal fractures of the pubic rami. The sacrotuberous, sacrospinous and posterior sacroiliac ligaments remain intact.

Type II - Diastasis of the pubic symphysis of more than 2.5cm, widening of the anterior sacroiliac joint caused by disruption of the anterior sacroiliac, sacrotuberous and sacrospinous ligaments. The posterior sacroiliac ligaments remain intact.

Type III (open book fracture) - There is complete disruption of the pubic symphysis and the sacroiliac joint. This leads to extreme rotational instability and lateral displacement. The anterior and posterior sacroiliac, sacrotuberous and sacrospinous ligaments are disrupted. This injury is associated with a high risk of vascular injuries and haemorrhage (Koval 2006, Slater 2010).

3. Vertical Shear

This is due to longitudinally applied forces and may result in diastasis of the pubic symphysis and complete disruption of the sacrotuberous, sacrospinous and sacroiliac ligaments. These injuries are highly unstable (Koval 2006, Slater 2010).

4. Combined Mechanical Injuries

These injuries involve a combination of patterns and are often due to crush injury. Lateral compression with vertical shear is the most common combination (Koval 2006). The main limitation of this and other classifications of pelvic fracture patterns is that there is a degree of inter- and intraobserver variability among orthopaedic surgeons when applying it. However, this degree of variability is less when the classification systems are applied by specialists in pelvic surgery (Koo 2008, Furey 2009).

Pelvic Fractures

1. Disruption of the Main Pelvic Ring

A fracture at one site is very likely to be associated with disruption of the ring at a second site. Disruption of the ring is not necessarily a fracture of a bone. For example, the ring may be broken by diastasis of the pubic symphysis or the sacroiliac joint due to ligamentous disruption as shown in Figure 5 (Solomon 2001, Raby 2005).

2. Acetbular Fractures

Acetabular fractures most commonly involve disruption of the acetabular socket when the hip is driven backwards during a road traffic accident. Acetabular fractures are frequently comminuted and osteoarthritic degeneration is a potential long-term consequence.

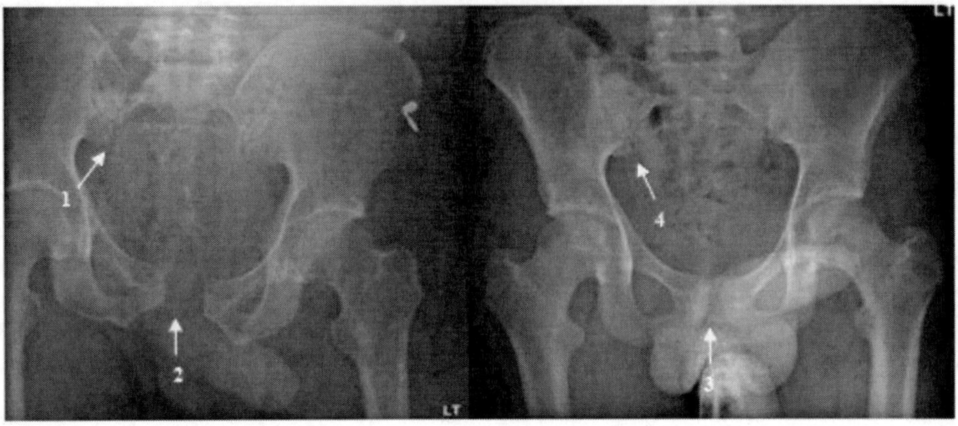

Figure 5. Antero-posterior pelvic radiograph demonstrating a cortical discrepancy along the sacral body adjacent to the sacroiliac joint consistent with a longitudinal fracture (1), wide diastasis of the pubic symphysis (2), diastasis of the pubic symphysis (3), irregularity of the sacroiliac joint (4).

Judet views and computer tomography (CT) scanning are needed to classify the type of acetabular fracture and to guide treatment (Dandy 2004). Examples of acetabular fractures are shown in Figure 6.

3. Sacral Fractures

Sacral fractures are often difficult to detect on the AP radiograph leading to missed or delayed diagnosis commonly. Up to a quarter of sacral fractures are associated with neurological injury (Mehta 2006, Slater 2010).

Impacted vertical fractures of the sacrum and nondisplaced fractures of the posterior sacroiliac complex are stable. Fractures may appear as asymmetry of the sacral arcuate lines. Diastasis of the fracture of more than 5mm and ligamentous disruption are features of unstable sacral fractures (Wheeless 2008).

4. Coccygeal Fractures

Fractures of the coccyx result from a direct impact such as a fall onto the buttocks. The diagnosis is made clinically and radiography is unnecessary as findings do not change the management (Dandy 2004, Raby 2005).

5. Iliac Wing Fractures

Fractures of the iliac wing occur due to a direct impact or crush injury. An isolated fracture of the iliac wing with an intact pelvic ring is a stable injury and may be treated non-operatively provided that it is not associated with significant complications such as haemorrhage or visceral injury (see Figure 7) (Dandy 2004, Abrassart 2009).

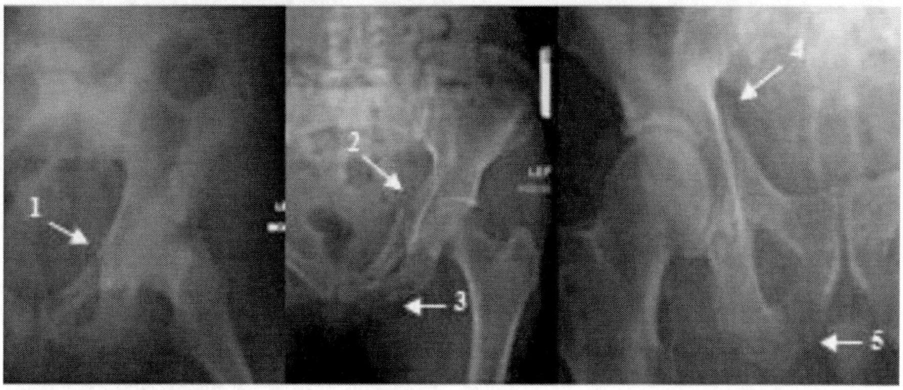

Figure 6. Antero-posterior pelvic radiograph demonstrating a fracture through the acetabulum affecting the superior pubic ramus (1), displaced fracture of the superior (2) and inferior (3) pubic rami extending into the acetabulum, and fracture through the acetabulum (4) associated with fracture of the inferior pubic ramus (5).

6. Pubic Ramus Fractures

Pubic rami fractures are common in the elderly patients with osteoporosis following falls. They may be associated with posterior ring injuries (Solomon 2001, Cosker 2005). Figure 8 shows several examples of pubic rami fractures.

7. Avulsion of an Apophysis

These fractures usually result from repeated or sudden violent muscle contraction in young athletic patients (Solomon 2001, Raby 2005). For example, Figure 9 shows avulsion fractures of the anterior superior iliac spine. The anterior superior iliac spine is the attachment of the sartorius and the tensor fascia lata.

Further Radiological Investigations

Fractures identified on plain radiography may be further investigated to delineate the fracture pattern by CT scanning. CT is very useful for the assessment of the posterior aspect of the pelvis, including the sacrum and the sacroiliac joint. Magnetic Resonance Imaging (MRI) is more accurate than CT for imaging of the genitourinary and pelvic vascular structures, however, is usually not practical as it limits access to the injured patient, takes longer to perform than other imaging modalities and is not immediately available in some settings (Koval 2006).

There are several interventional radiological techniques to investigate and treat significant soft tissue injuries. Pelvic angiography and embolization to control haemorrhage due to damage to pelvic vessels has reduced the mortality associated with pelvic fractures (Case study 1).

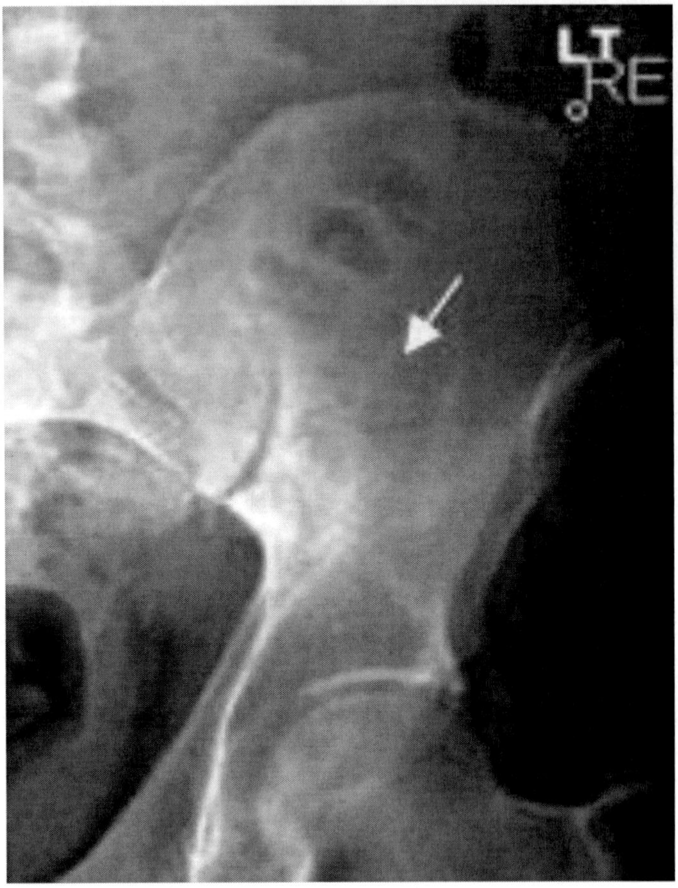

Figure 7. Iliac wing fracture (arrow).

Investigations for bladder and urethral injury include intravenous cystourethrograms (intravenous contrast material is used to visualize the bladder and ureters on plain radiographs) or retrograde cystourethrograms (the contrast material is injected into the urethra and flows into the bladder).

Several studies have shown that the sensitivity of the AP pelvis is low and have claimed that there is a diminishing role for routine AP pelvis radiographs in trauma (Berg 1996, Guillamondegui 2002, Their 2004).

A study of the radiological findings of 1386 patients who had undergone multidetector CT in serious blunt trauma revealed that only 55% of pelvic fractures were detected by plain pelvic radiography. The sensitivity of pelvic radiography varied depending on the anatomical region. For example, the sensitivity was better antero-inferiorly (i.e. pubic symphysis, pubic ramus and proximal femur). The sensitivity was poor posteriorly (i.e. sacroiliac joint and sacrum) (Their 2004). It has been suggested that routine AP pelvis radiography often adds little to the management of the trauma patient and that haemodynamically stable patients who undergo an abdominopelvic CT during their immediate management do not require an AP pelvis radiograph (Berg 1996, Guillamondegui 2002, Vo 2004, Kessel 2007).

This view is controversial. Some have argued that the role of the AP pelvis radiograph is broader than to simply diagnose pelvic fractures.

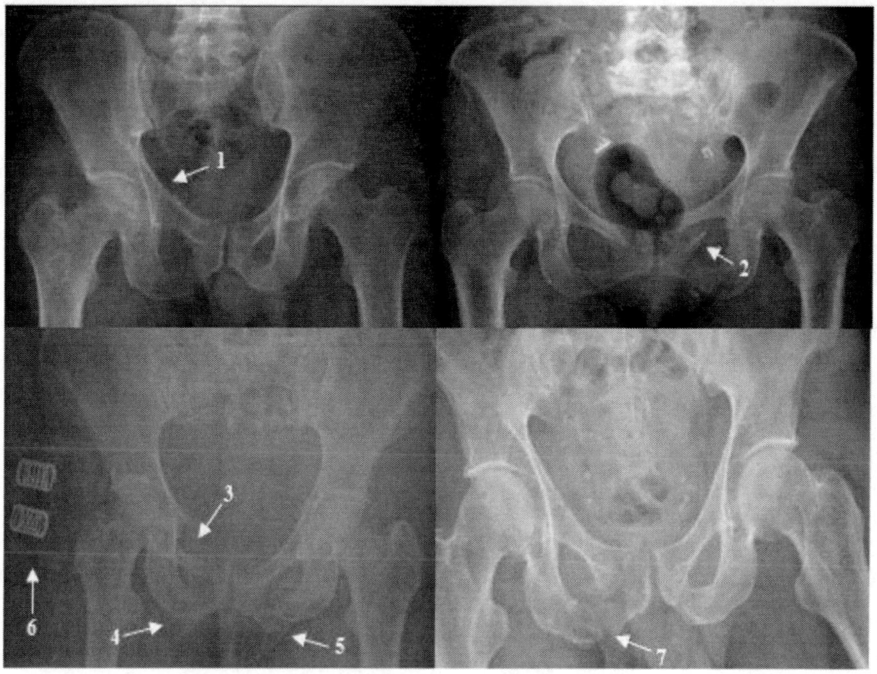

Figure 8. Antero-posterior pelvic radiograph demonstrating superior pubic rami fractures (1-3), inferior pubic rami fractures (4, 5), pelvic binder (6), and comminuted inferior pubic ramus fracture (7).

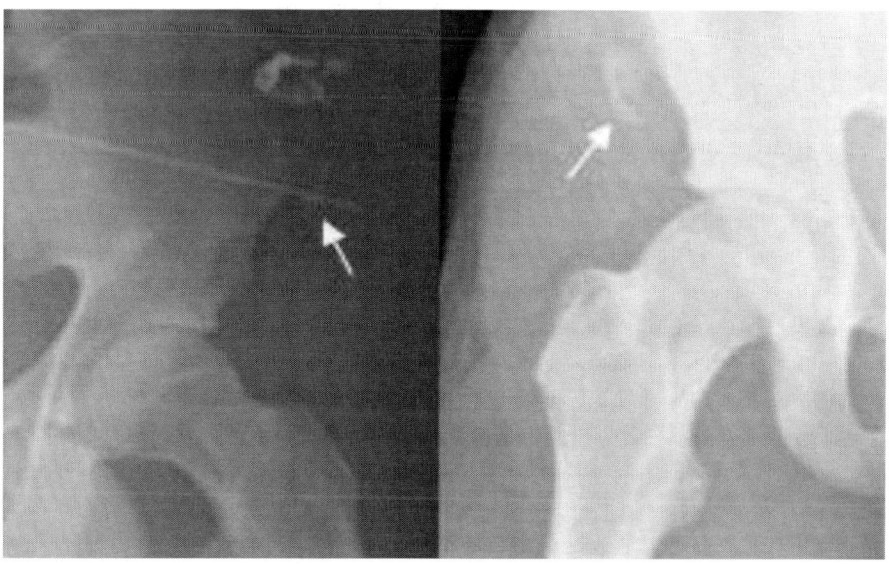

Figure 9. Avulsion of the anterior superior iliac spine (arrows).

It may be considered as having a role as an adjunct to the ATLS secondary survey by guiding the process of diagnosis and planning during the ATLS assessment. Omission of this rapid screening test could potentially cause delays in the full appreciation of the extent of injury (Flint 2002).

CONCLUSION

It is essential that pelvic fractures are identified rapidly in cases of major trauma due to the risk of life-threatening haemorrhage. Although a systematic approach to interpretation of the AP pelvis radiograph increases the identification of injuries, it may not be possible to visualise all fractures. Additional plain radiographic views such as pelvic inlet, outlet and oblique Judet views may facilitate diagnosis. Other imaging modalities such as CT are useful to provide more detailed information in haemodynamically stable patients.

REFERENCES

Abrassart S., Stern R., Peter R. 2009 Morbidity associated with iliac wing fractures. *Journal of Trauma*, 66 (1) 200-203.

Advanced Trauma Life Support (ATLS) Student Course Manual Seventh Edition. 2004, 141 – 142.

Berg E., Chebuhar C., Bell R. 1996 Pelvic Trauma Imaging: A Blinded Comparison of Computed Tomography and Roentgenograms. *Journal of Trauma,* 41 (6) 994-998.

Balogh Z., King K. L., Mackay P. et al. 2007 The Epidemiology of Pelvic Ring Fractures: A Population-Based Study. *Journal of Trauma*, 63 (5) 1066-1073.

Chimutengwende-Gordon M., Sidhu J., Khan W. S., Maruthainar N. (2010a). Advanced trauma life support radiographic trauma series: Part 1- The cervical spine radiograph. *J. Perioper. Pract.*, 20(9): 322-8.

Chimutengwende-Gordon M., Khan W. S., Sidhu J., Longo U. G., Maruthainar N. (2010b). Advanced trauma life support radiographic trauma series: Part 2- The chest radiograph. *J. Perioper. Pract.*, 20(12): 430-5.

Chimutengwende-Gordon M., Khan W. S., Sidhu J., Maruthainar N. (2011). Advanced trauma life support radiographic trauma series: Part 3- The pelvic radiograph. *J. Perioper. Pract.*, 21(1): 16-21.

Cosker T. D. A., Ghandour A., Gupta S. K., Tayton K. J. J. 2005 Pelvic ramus fractures in the elderly: 50 patients studied with MRI. *Acta Orthopaedica,* 76 (4) 513-516.

Dandy D. J., Edwards D. J. 2004 Injuries to the Trunk. Essential Orthopaedics and Trauma Fourth Edition, Churchill Livingstone, 161-177.

Flint L. 2002 Editorial Comment, Pelvic Radiography in Blunt Trauma Resuscitation: A Diminishing Role. *Journal of Trauma*, 53 (6) 1047.

Furey A., O'Toole R., Nascone J. et al., 2009 Classification of pelvic fractures: analysis of inter- and intraobserver variability using the Young-Burgess and Tile classification systems. *Orthopaedics*, 32 (6) 401.

Gardner M., Krieg J., Simpson T., Bottlang M. 2010 Displacement After Simulated Pelvic Ring Injuries: A Cadaveric Model of Recoil. *Journal of Trauma,* 68 (1) 159-165.

Guillamondegui O., Pryor J., Gracias V. et al. 2002 Pelvic Radiography in Blunt Trauma Resuscitation: A Diminishing Role. *Journal of Trauma,* 53 (6) 1043-1047.

Kessel B., Sevi R., Jeroukhimov I. et al. 2007 Is routine portable pelvic X-ray in stable multiple trauma patients always justified in a high technology era? *Journal of Trauma*, 38 (5) 559-563.

Koo H., Leveridge M., Thompson C. et al. 2008 Interobserver Reliability of the Young-Burgess and Tile Classification Systems for Fractures of the Pelvic Ring. *Journal of Orthopaedic Trauma*, 22 (6) 379-384.

Koval K., Zuckerman J. 2006. Handbook of Fractures:Third Edition, Lipincott Williams and Wilkins 275-301.

Lunsjo K., Tadros A. M. A., Hauggaard A. et al. 2007 Acute plain anterioposterior radiograph of the pelvis is not useful in detecting fractures of iliac wing and os sacrum: A prospective study of 73 patients using CT as gold standard. *Australasian Radiology*, 51 (2) 147-149.

Mehta S., Auerbach J., Born C., Chin K. 2006 Sacral Fractures. *Journal of the American Academy of Orthopaedic Surgeons,* 14 (12) 656-665.

Moore K. L., Dalley A. F. 1999 Pelvis and Perineum. Clinically Oriented Anatomy Fourth Edition, Lippincott Williams and Wilkins 337-340.

Nicholas J. 2006 Trauma Imaging of the Pelvis CEEssentials, LLC.

Raby N., Berman L., de Lacy G. 2005 Chest. Accident and Emergency Radiology, *Elsevier Saunders*, 180-189.

Sathy A. K., Starr A. J., Smith W. R. et al. 2009 The Effect of Pelvic Fracture on Mortality After Trauma: An Analysis of 63,000 Trauma Patients. *Journal of Bone and Joint Surgery –American*, 91(12) 2803-2810.

Slater S. J., Barron D. A. 2010, Pelvic fractures – A guide to classification and management. *European Journal of Radiology*, 74 (1) 16-23.

Solomon L., Warwick D., Nayagam S. 2001 Injuries of the Pelvis. Apley's System of Orthopaedics and Fractures, Eighth Edition, Arnold 667-679.

Their M., Bensch F., Koskinen S., Handolin L., Kiuru M. 2005 Diagnostic value of pelvic radiography in the initial trauma series in blunt trauma. *European Radiology*, 15 (8) 1533-1537.

Theumann N., Verdon J., Mouhsine E. et al. 2002 Traumatic Injuries: Imaging of pelvic fractures. *Emergency Radiology*, 12 1312-1330.

Vo N. J., Gash J., Browning J., Hutson R. K. 2004, Pelvic imaging in the stable trauma patient: is the AP pelvic radiograph necessary when abdominopelvic CT shows no acute injury? *Emergency Radiology*, 10 (5) 246-249.

Wheeless C. R. 2008, AP view of Pelvis. Wheeless' Textbook of Orthopaedics online.

Wiss D. 2001, What's New in Orthopaedic Surgery. *Journal of Bone and Joint Surgery – American,* 83-A (11) 1762-1772.

In: Perioperative Practice in Trauma and Orthopaedic Surgery ISBN: 978-1-63483-325-7
Editor: Wasim S. Khan

Chapter 14

THE USE OF BONE CEMENT IN TRAUMA AND ORTHOPAEDICS

C. J. O'Dowd-Booth, J. J. E. White, P. Smitham, W. Khan* and D. R. Marsh

University College London Institute of Orthopaedic and Musculoskeletal Sciences, Royal National Orthopaedic Hospital, Stanmore, Middlesex, UK

ABSTRACT

Bone cement has been increasingly used in orthopaedic surgery over the last 50 years. Since Sir John Charnley pioneered the use of polymethylmethacrylate cement in total hip replacements, there have been developments in cementing techniques and an expansion in the number of orthopaedic procedures that use cement. This chapter covers the perioperative issues surrounding bone cement including storage, cementing techniques and complications. It also discusses specific orthopaedic applications of bone cement and future developments.

Keywords: Bone cement, polymethylmethacrylate, complications, orthopaedics, developments

INTRODUCTION

This chapter discusses perioperative issues, orthopaedic applications and future developments in bone cement (O'Dowd-Booth et al. 2011). Bone cement was originally developed in1943 for use in the field of dentistry (Kühn 2005).

There are now a number of different types of bone cement and these vary in their biomechanical properties. The first and most commonly used bone cement is Polymethylmethacrylate (PMMA) acrylic cement.

* Tel.: +44 (0) 7791 025554; E-mail: wasimkhan@doctors.org.uk.

In 1958, Sir John Charnley first used PMMA cement in orthopaedics to create a more secure fixation of the femoral and acetabular components in a total hip replacement (Charnley 1960 and 1970). The interface between the stiff metal implant and the more elastic bone was referred to as the weak link due to the difference in mechanical properties, resulting in loosening over time (Gupta et al. 2006). PMMA cement has an elasticity value between that of implant and bone, allowing for additional shock absorption and a more even distribution of contact forces between the two materials (Webb and Spencer 2007). Figure 1 shows the radiograph of a cemented total hip replacement. Bone cement acts more like a grouting agent than an adhesive 'cement' (Gupta et al. 2006).

PMMA has proved to be one of the most versatile and lasting biomaterials in orthopaedics having an important role in joint replacement (Dheerendra et al. 2010, Khan et al. 2011) as well as spinal and tumour surgery (Webb and Spencer 2007). It is by far the most common choice of bone cement due to its workability and is widely used in orthopaedic theatres (Wang and Dunne 2008). The addition of Chlorophyllin gives bone cement a distinctive green colour, aiding visualisation and correct placement, and allowing for a better distinction between the cement and surrounding bone (Hendriks et al. 2004). Barium sulphate is also added to allow visualisation on postoperative radiographs and assess the quality of the cement mantle (Figure 1).

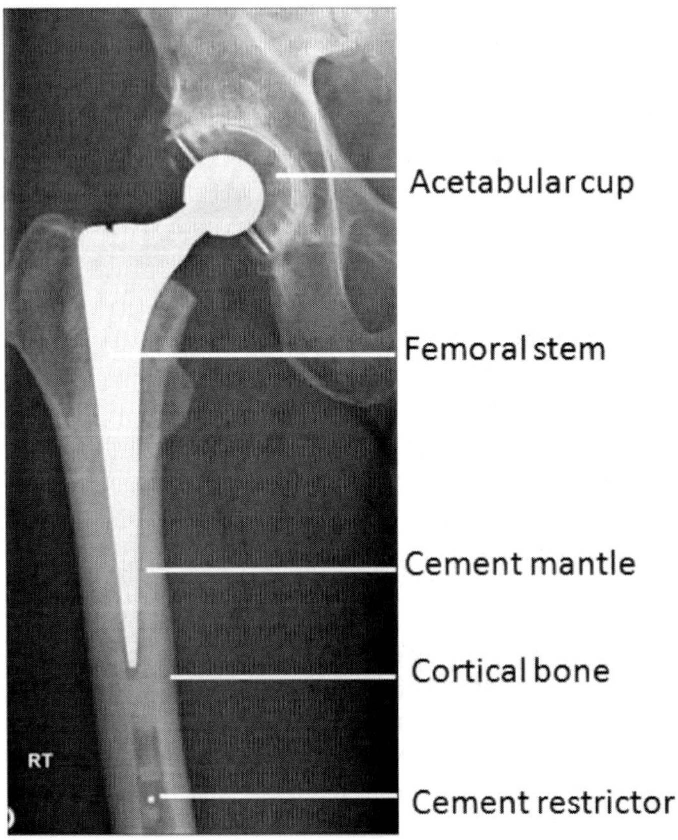

Figure 1. Anterioposterior radiograph of a cemented total hip replacement showing the cemented femoral and acetabular components, cement mantle, cortical bone and cement restrictor.

PERIOPERATIVE ISSUES SURROUNDING BONE CEMENT

1. Storage

PMMA cement is packaged in the form of a liquid monomer and a powder copolymer constituent. These are mixed together at the time of use and undergo polymerisation to form a viscous material which can be moulded and inserted into the required location (Chatterjee and Blunn 2007).

It is vital that the cement curing time is known so that it can be manipulated and inserted before the cement becomes unusable. From the initial mixing of the monomer and activator the time should be monitored.

The transition from a liquid to a useable paste is quick with the change to a solid and hence setting to be around nine minutes after mixing (Turner et al. 1981). International Standard Organization (ISO) standard 5833 set a limit of 3 to 15 minutes for the working time of bone cement. The storage conditions of these constituents affects the structural properties of the cement, and it is important to ensure storage at an ambient temperature of around 21°C (Lewis and Son 2008). Cement constituents stored at warmer temperatures set quickly and can cause procedural difficulties.

When the powder copolymer has been sterilised with ethylene oxide gas, it is thermally stable and available for use immediately. Gamma-irradiated powders however should be stored for a period of at least three weeks in an ambient environment to allow the development of increased stability post-sterilisation (Lewis and Son 2008).

2. Cementing Technique

A satisfactory interface between bone and cement is vital to prevent aseptic loosening, and cementing technique can directly influence the outcome (Ota et al. 2005). The process for cement preparation in hip replacement surgery has undergone several generations of development.

First generation cementating technique in which the cement was finger-packed, lead to radiographic evidence of aseptic loosening in 19-40% of cases (Ota et al. 2005). Results improved with the development of second generation techniques during the 1970s. These included intramedullary canal preparation with pulsatile lavage, use of a cement restrictor, and the introduction of a cement gun to allow a more even distribution of cement, greater pressurisation and better penetration into bone interstices (Ota et al. 2005). This promoted a strong bone-cement interface with good stability and greater fixation strength (Jaeblon 2010). Third generation techniques that are currently employed involve the vacuum mixing of cement to minimise any air inclusion and intramedullary pressurisation of cement with a proximal femoral seal (Ota et al. 2005).

This achieves an adequate level of cement penetration and reduces the degree of cement porosity that may compromise the cement mantle. These techniques have also benefitted the fixation of acetabular components in hip replacement surgery although the use of cemented sockets remains a controversial point and current trends favour an uncemented approach (Corten et al. 2009).

3. Complications

Bone cement implantation syndrome (BCIS) poses a significant risk of morbidity and mortality during cemented procedures. It is usually associated with total hip arthroplasty although it is not restricted to this procedure. The clinical features may include hypoxia, hypotension, cardiac arrhythmias and cardiovascular collapse. There is a wide spectrum of activity that ranges from a non-fulminant reaction characterised by a significant, momentary drop in arterial oxygen saturation and systemic blood pressure, to a profound intraoperative compromise in cardiovascular function and potential arrhythmias, shock and cardiac arrest (Donaldson et al. 2009). Problems typically occur shortly after cement insertion; hypotension is common, independent of the anaesthetic technique used and worsened if there is any degree of hypovolaemia present. The aetiology and pathophysiology of BCIS is poorly understood. Initial theories purposed direct toxicity of the MMA cement monomer on the cardiovascular system. Current thinking suggests that the changes observed in BCIS are secondary to the release of micro-emboli into the systemic circulation secondary to cement pressurisation. These emboli have been shown to include molecules of fat, marrow, cement, air and bone (Donaldson et al. 2009). Due to the serious nature of BCIS, the anaesthetic team should be informed prior to cement insertion to ensure frequent and diligent monitoring of blood pressure and cardiorespiratory function. The postoperative team should also be aware of the potential for persistent hypotension, pulmonary emboli, pulmonary hypertension and anaphylactoid reactions (Memtsoudis et al. 2007). Thermal injury poses a risk to both the patient and theatre staff. The polymerisation reaction generated during cement formation is exothermic and temperatures can reach as high as 110°C (Meyer et al. 1973). This can result in tremendous heat transfer to the surrounding tissues with the potential to cause thermal damage to skin, bone and surrounding neurovascular structures (Mjoberg et al. 1984). Should the patient or member of the surgical team be exposed such temperatures, thermal damage can result, with less than one second needed to cause transdermal necrosis when exposed to surface temperatures exceeding 70°C (Dunn and Orr 2007). PMMA cement is used extensively in orthopaedics, particulary joint arthroplasties, and therefore all members of the surgical team will have a level of occupational exposure to its component monomer methyl methacrylate (MMA) (Leggat et al. 2009). Combined inhalational and contact exposure can lead to problems with hypersensitivity, asthmatic reactions, local neurological symptoms, and localised irritation/dermatological reactions. The compound is not currently thought to pose a carcinogenic risk under conditions of normal use. To reduce these potential risks, room ventilation and airflow should be optimised, direct contact should be avoided and latex gloves should be inspected for possible compromise as a result of cement contact (Leggat et al. 2009).

Orthopaedic Applications of Bone Cement

1. Joint Reconstruction

Joint reconstruction is the most common orthopaedic application of bone cement. A wide range of procedures utilise cement including hip, knee and shoulder arthroplasties (Schlegel et al. 2010). Bone cement is used because of its ability to augment the interface between bone and implant and facilitate the transfer of forces. This accounts for the excellent long-term survival of cemented prostheses (Wang and Dunne 2008). Clinical studies and joint registries data strongly support the continued use of cemented prostheses in total hip and knee replacements (Webb and Spencer 2007). According to the National Joint Registry, cemented prostheses comprise 36% of total hip replacements and 83% of total knee replacements respectively in the United Kingdom (Hooper et al. 2009, Ellams et al. 2010). There has been a recent trend towards uncemented techniques for total hip arthroplasty, for which the reasons are not fully understood (Dunbar 2009). There is evidence that cemented techniques are associated with reduced pain postoperatively and improved mobility with no significant difference in perioperative complications (Parker et al. 2010). The use of bone cement is likely to continue to play an integral role in primary arthroplasty for the foreseeable future (Dheerendra et al. 2010).

It is inevitable that joint arthroplasties will eventually require revision and the use of bone cement adds an extra dimension to the complexity of this procedure. This difficult and time-consuming process requires optimal visualisation of the prosthesis and bone-cement interface (Takaqui et al. 2009). Cement removal usually involves curettage through the use of flexible and narrow osteotomes, chisels, high-speed burs and reamers. Ultrasonic extraction systems (e.g. OSCAR, Orthosonics) and Laser techniques have also been developed to improve cement removal (Birnbaum and Gutknecht 2010). Should these techniques fail or be unavailable, an osteotomy may be needed. In these rare situations that this is required there are associated complications of bone loss, cortical perforation and further fracture (Goldberg et al. 2007). The addition of chlorophyllin or methylene blue to the PMMA cement improves visualisation and facilitates cement removal (Graves and Sands 2007).

PMMA cement is also used in two-stage revisions for infected hip and knee arthroplasties. In these cases antibiotic-loaded cement spacers are used. These spacers can either be static or mobile, the former being the traditionally preferred option but mobile, articulating spacers are increasingly used due to there ability to allow limited weight bearing and hence facilitate mobility and reduce bone loss (Jacobs et al. 2009). The use of these spacers allows local antibiotic delivery though impregnated PMMA cement. Broad-spectrum antibiotics such as vancomycin and tobramycin are commonly used however this can potentiate the development of antibiotic resistance and continued infection (Fink 2009). It is therefore advisable to obtain antibiotic sensitivities prior to spacer insertion (Fink 2009).

2. Spinal Surgery

Vertebral crush fractures are one of the most common fractures associated with osteoporosis affecting 20% of those aged over 70 years. Bone cement has been used in the treatment of these fractures (Ghofrani et al. 2010).

Percutaneous vertebroplasty and kyphoplasty both aim to stabilise the vertebral body and achieve pain reduction (Dionyssiotis 2010). Percutaneous vertebroplasty is a procedure that involves the injection of PMMA cement into the vertebral body (Hu et al. 2006). Kyphoplasty differs in that before the PMMA cement is injected, a balloon is inserted and inflated inside the vertebral body. The aim is to attempt to decompress any existing bone so as to create a larger cavity to inject the cement (Dionyssiotis 2010). This leads to some correction of the deformity and fracture stabilisation (Hu et al. 2006). These procedures are performed under radiological control and the cement contains additional opacifiers such as tungsten or barium sulphate, added to aid with radiological monitoring (Prime et al. 2010).

Lowering the temperature of the cement prior to insertion has been shown to lead to a significant increase in working time. Cooling the cement-filled syringes to 12°C increases the working time by more than 30 minutes (James and Connell 2006). Chavali et al. (2003) found that cooling the cement to around 0.5ºC can extend its injectability to over two hours. This does however reduce cement viscosity and increases the chance of cement leakage. It is therefore advisable to wait for a sufficient period of time until a suitable viscosity is achieved (James and Connell 2006).

There are a number of disadvantages to using PMMA cement to correct and stabilise vertebral crush fractures. The rigidity caused by the cement can lead to further fractures in the adjacent vertebral bodies due to a difference in biomechanical properties between adjacent bodies (Berlemann et al. 2002). There is also a risk of thermal damage to surrounding neurovascular structures as the cement undergoes polymerisation (Ghofrani et al. 2010).

3. Oncology

Bone cement has a significant role in the management of tumours affecting the bone. It is used in massive prostheses that are employed in wide excision, requiring a large portion of bone and joint to be removed. Bone cement also plays a vital role in the treatment of giant cell tumours of bone where it has been used since 1969 as a packing material after a curettage procedure (Remedios et al. 1997). The PMMA cement polymerisation process is exothermic and leads to the destruction of any remaining tumour cells in the cavity. The cement also provides stability to the bone by filling the cavity. It has been shown that the use of cement gives greater mechanical properties than a bone graft in the early stages (Remedios et al 1997).

The principles behind the technique of vertebroplasty or kyphoplasty can also be applied for the treatment of pathological fracture of the vertebral body (Chi and Gokaslan 2008).

4. Additional Applications

Antibiotics were incorporated into PMMA as early as 1970 by Buchholz and Engelbrecht, who used gentamycin to aid in the management of infected arthroplasty (Webb and Spencer 2007). Antibiotic-impregnated bone cements are now commonly used for the prophylaxis and management of infected prostheses, osteomyelitis and infected non-union in conjunction with systemic antibiotics (McKee et al. 2010). In total hip replacements, gentamicin-loaded PMMA cement has been shown to reduce deep infection (Josefsson et al. 1990). In two-stage hip revision procedures for infection, antibiotic-loaded cement insertion after the first stage results in a 40% reduction in infection (Parvizi et al. 2008). Antibiotic-loaded cement beads have also been used in the management of chronic non-haematogenous osteomyelitis to provide localised therapy (McKee et al. 2010).

Bone cements are also used in situations where there is a decrease in bone quality, such as in osteoporosis. Augmentation of cancellous bone screws would be one such application, due to the stresses present at the screw-bone interface. Cement is used to increase stability and improve fixation (Al-Rasid et al. 2010).

FUTURE DEVELOPMENTS

Cement contracts as it cools at the end of polymerisation, potentially leading to compromise of the bone-cement interface and aseptic loosening (Webb and Spencer 2007). These factors have generated interest in alternative options. Glass ionomer cements have been used in dental surgery since the 1970s and undergo non-exothermic reactions during curing (Hatton et al. 2008). This avoids the risks of cement contracture (Wood and Hill 1991). Unlike PMMA cement, they are adhesive to both bone and metal surfaces resulting in enhanced mechanical interlocking with bone and metal (Hatton et al. 2008). Their mechanical properties however are not as ideal as PMMA cement, and they release ions into the biological environment (Hatton et al. 2008).

Calcium phosphate cements are also available and have attracted a great deal of attention due to their bioactivity and ability to self-set *in vivo* (Ginebra et al. 2006). Calcium phosphate has a number of advantages over PMMA in terms of biocompatibility and osteoconductivity, and its biomechanical properties are continuing to be improved (Stadelmann et al. 2010). Its clinical use so far has been limited to revision operations where a graft layer with bioresorbable cement is desired (Speirs et al. 2005).

There remains potential for expansion in the use of cement as a delivery medium for potential therapeutics, including antibiotics (Webb and Spencer 2007). Through the use of calcium phosphate cements it may be possible to impregnate anti-inflamatory drugs, anti-cancer agents, and hormones such as bone morphogenic proteins or transforming growth factors (Ginebra et al. 2006). The development of a system that would allow the selection of single or combined drug options at the time of cement implantation would improve the versatility of bone cement, however the effects of these additions on the physical properties of the cement needs greater research (Ginebra et al. 2006).

With continued study and developments in different biomaterials, particularly bioactive materials, we may see the function of PMMA and other bone cements change as we develop our understanding of their mechanical behaviour (Jaeblon 2010). The applications of cement will no doubt increase and provide a continued support in a large number of orthopaedic procedures.

REFERENCES

Al-Rashid M., Khan W. S., Vermulapali K. 2010 Principles of fracture fixation in orthopaedic trauma surgery. *Journal of Perioperative Practice,* 20 113-117.

Berlemann U., Ferguson S. J., Nolte L. P., Heini P. F. 2002 Adjacent vertebral failure after vertebroplasty: A biomechanical investigation. *Journal of Bone and Joint Surgery*, 84B 748-752.

Birnbaum K., Gutknecht N. 2010 Scanning electron microscopy investigation of PMMA removal by laser irradiation (Er:YAG) in comparison with an ultrasonic system and curettage in hip joint revision arthroplasty. *Lasers in Medical Science*, 25 (4) 595-603.

Charnley J. 1960 Anchorage of the femoral head prosthesis to the shaft of the femur. *Journal of Bone and Joint Surgery*, 42B 28-30.

Charnley J. 1970 Acrylic cement in orthopaedic surgery, Williams and Wilkins.

Chatterjee S., Blunn G. 2007 Biomaterials, in Basic orthopaedic sciences: The Stanmore guide, Ramachandran M. ed. Hodder Arnold 154-164.

Chavali R., Resijek R., Knight S. K., Choi I. S. 2003 Extending polymerization time of polymethylmethacrylate cement in percutaneous vertebroplasty with ice bath cooling. *American Journal of Neuroradiology*, 24 545-546.

Chi J. H., Gokaslan Z. L. 2008 Vertebroplasty and kyphoplasty for spinal metastases. *Current Opinions in Supportive Palliative Care,* 2 9-13.

Corten K., Au K., Bourne R. B. 2009 Acetabular options: notes from the other side. *Orthopedics*, 32 (9) 664.

Coultrup O. J., Hunt C., Wroblewski B. M., Taylor M. 2010 Computational assessment of the effect of polyethylene wear rate, mantle thickness, and porosity on the mechanical failure of the acetabular cement mantle. *Journal of Orthopaedic Research*, 28 565-570.

Dheerendra S., Khan W. S., Saeed M. Z., Goddard N. J. 2010 Recent developments in total hip replacements: cementation, articulation, minimal-invasion and navigation. *Journal of Perioperative Practice*, 20 133-138.

Dionyssiotis Y. 2010 Management of osteoporotic vertebral fractures. *International Journal of General Medicine*, 3 167-171.

Donaldson A. J., Thomson H. E., Harper N. J., Kenny N. W. 2009 Bone cement implantation syndrome. *British Journal of Anaesthesia*, 102 (1) 12-22.

Dunbar M. J. 2009 Cemented femoral fixation: the North Atlantic divide. *Orthopedics,* 32 (9) 662.

Dunne N. J., Orr J. F. 2007 Curing characteristics of acrylic bone cement Journal of Materials Science. *Materials in Medicine*, 13 (1) 17-22.

Ellams D., Forsyth O., Mistry A. et al. 2010 National Joint Registry For England and Wales 7th Annual Report.

Fink B. 2009 Revision of late periprosthetic infections of total hip endoprostheses: pros and cons of different concepts. *International Journal of Medical Sciences,* 6 (5) 287-295.

Ghofrani H., Nunn T., Robertson C. et al. 2010 An evaluation of fracture stabilization comparing kyphoplasty and titanium mesh repair techniques for vertebral compression fractures: is bone cement necessary? *Spine*, 35 E768-E773.

Ginebra M. P., Traykova T., Planell J. A. 2006 Calcium phosphate cements as bone drug delivery systems: a review. *Journal of Controlled Release,* 113 102-110.

Goldberg S. H., Studders E. M., Cohen M. S. 2007 Ultrasonic cement removal in revision arthroplasty. *Orthopedics,* 30 632-635.

Graves R. M., Sands K. C. 2007 Making a cost-effective contrast bone cement with or without antibiotics, using aqueous methylene blue for easy cement removal in revision and primary total joint arthroplasty. *Orthopedics,* 30 825-827.

Gupta R., Caiozzo V. J., Skinner H. B. 2006 Basic science in orthopaedics, in Current diagnosis and treatment: Orthopaedics, 4th edn. Skinner HB ed. Lange /McGraw-Hill 1-64.

Hatton P. V., Kearns V. R., Brook I. M. 2008 Bone-cement fixation: glass-ionomer cements, in Joint replacement technology, Revell PA ed. Woodhead Publishing Limited. 252-263.

Hendriks J. G., van Horn J. R., van der Mei H. C., Busscher H. J. 2004 Backgrounds of antibiotic-loaded bone cement and prosthesis-related infection. *Biomaterials,* 25 545-556.

Hooper G. J., Rothwell A. G., Stringer M., Frampton C. 2009 Revision following cemented and uncemented primary total hip replacement: a seven-year analysis from the New Zealand Joint Registry. *Journal of Bone and Joint Surgery*, 91B 451-458.

Hu S. S., Tribus C. B., Tay B. K. B., Bhatia N. N. 2006 Disorders, diseases and injuries of the spine, in Current diagnosis and treatment: Orthopaedics, 4th edn. Skinner HB ed. Lange/McGraw-Hill 221-298.

ISO 5833 2002 Implants for Surgery-Acrylic Resin Cements.

Jacobs C., Christensen C. P., Berend M. E. 2009 Static and mobile antibiotic-impregnated cement spacers for the managment of prosthetic joint infection. *The Journal of the American Academy of Orthopaedic Surgeons,* 17 (6) 356-368.

Jaeblon T. 2010 Polymethylmethacrylate: properties and contemporary uses in orthopaedics. *Journal of American Academy of Orthopedic Surgeons,* 18 297-305.

James S. L., Connell D. A. 2006 The effect of temperature reduction on cement working time in percutaneous vertebroplasty. *Clinical Radiology*, 61 797-799.

Josefsson G., Gudmundsson G., Kolmert L., Wijkstrom S. 1990 Prophylaxis with systemic antibiotics versus gentamicin bone cement in total hip arthroplasty. A five-year survey of 1688 hips. *Clinical Orthopaedcs and Related Research,* 253 173-178.

Khan W. S., Oragui E., Longo U. G. Recent Developments in Total Hip Arthroplasty-Cementation, Articulation, Minimal-Invasion and Navigation. pp 211-24. In Advances in Medicine and Biology, Volume 27, Editor Berhardt LV, 2011, Nova Science Publishers, New York.

Kühn K. D. 2005 Properties of bone cement: what is bone cement, in The well cemented hip arthroplasty: Theory and practice, Steffen H. M. and Breusch J. ed. 52-60.

Leggat P. A., Smith D. R., Kedjarune U. 2009 Surgical applications of methyl methacrylate: a review of toxicity. *Archives of Environmental and Occupational Health,* 64 (3) 207-212.

Lewis G., Son Y. 2008 Thermal stability of acrylic bone cement powder under shelf storage conditions: an isothermal microcalorimetric study. *Biomedical Materials in Engineering*, 18 83-90.

McKee M. D., Li-Bland E. A., Wild L. M., Schemitsch E. H. 2010 A prospective, randomized clinical trial comparing an antibiotic-impregnated bioabsorbable bone substitute with standard antibiotic-impregnated cement beads in the treatment of chronic osteomyelitis and infected non-union. *Journal of Orthopaedic Trauma*, 24 483-490.

Memtsoudis S. G., Rosenberger P., Walz J. M. 2007 Critical care issues in the patient after major joint replacement. *Journal of Intensive Care Medicine,* 22 (2) 92-104.

Meyer P. R. Jr., Lautenschlager E. P., Moore B. K. 1973 On the setting properties of acrylic bone cement. *Journal of Bone and Joint Surgery,* American Volume, 55 (1) 149-156.

Mjoberg B., Pettersson H., Rosenqvist R., Rydholm A. 1984 Bone cement, thermal injury and the radiolucent zone. *Acta Orthopaedica Scandinavia,* 55 597-600.

Ota J., Cook J. L., Lewis D. D. et al. 2005 Short-term aseptic loosening of the femoral component in canine total hip replacement: effects of cementing technique on cement mantle grade. *Veterinary Surgery*, 34 345-352.

Parker M. J., Gurusamy K. S., Azegami S. 2010 Arthroplasties (with and without bone cement) for proximal femoral fractures in adults. *Cochrane Database Systematic Reviews,* 6 CD001706.

Parvizi J., Saleh K. J., Ragland P. S., Pour A. E., Mont M. A. 2008 Efficacy of antibiotic-impregnated cement in total hip replacement. *Acta Orthopaedica,* 79 335-341.

Prime M. S., Khan W. S., Dheerendra S., Maruthainar N. 2010 The use of ionising radiation in trauma and orthopaedic theatres. *Journal of Perioperative Practice,* 20 165-168.

Remedios D., Saifuddin A., Pringle J. 1997 Radiological and clinical recurrence of giant-cell tumour of bone after the use of cement. *Journal of Bone and Joint Surgery,* 79B 26-30.

Sauri Arce J. C., Cardenas R. G. 2009 Hemodynamic complications of cemented hip arthroplasty. *Acta Ortopaedica Mexica*, 23 277-280.

Schlegel U. J., Knifka J., Rollinghoff M. et al. 2010 Effects of impaction on cement mantle and trabecular bone in hip resurfacing. *Archives of Orthopaedics and Trauma Surgery*, [Epub ahead of print].

Speirs A. D., Oxland T. R., Masri B. A., Poursartip A., Duncan C. P. 2005 Calcium phosphate cement composites in revision hip arthroplasty. *Biomaterials*, 26 7310-7318.

Stadelmann V. A., Bretton E., Terrier A., Procter P., Pioletti D. P. 2010 Calcium phosphate cement augmentation of cancellous bone screws can compensate for the absence of cortical fixation. *Journal of Biomechanics,* [Epub ahead of print].

Takaqui M., Tamaki Y., Kabayashi S., Sasaki K., TakakuboY., Ishii M. 2009 Cement removal and bone bed preparation of the femoral medullary canal assisted by flexible endoscope in total hip revision arthroplasty. *Journal of Orthopaedic Science*, 14 (6) 719-726.

Turner R. C., Atkins P. E., Ackley M. A., PArk J. B. 1981 Molecular and macroscopic properties of PMMA bone cement: free-radical generation and temperature change versus mixing ratio. *Journal of Biomedical Materials Research,* 15 (3) 425-435.

Wang J. S., Dunne N. 2008 Bone cement fixation: acrylic cements, in Joint replacement technology, Revell PA ed. Woodhead Publishing Limited, 212-251.

Webb J. C., Spencer R. F. 2007 The role of polymethylmethacrylate bone cement in modern orthopaedic surgery. *Journal of Bone and Joint Surgery*, 89B 851-857.

Wood D., Hill R. 1991 Glass ceramic approach to controlling the properties of a glass-ionomer bone cement. *Biomaterials,* 12 164-170.

In: Perioperative Practice in Trauma and Orthopaedic Surgery ISBN: 978-1-63483-325-7
Editor: Wasim S. Khan

Chapter 15

PRINCIPLES OF FRACTURE FIXATION IN ORTHOPAEDIC TRAUMA SURGERY

Wasim Khan[1,*], Mamun Al-Rashid[2] and Kishan Vemulapalli[2]

[1]University College London Institute of Orthopaedic and Musculoskeletal Sciences, Royal National Orthopaedic Hospital, Stanmore, Middlesex, UK
[2]Barking, Havering and Redbridge NHS Trust, Queen's Hospital, Rom Valley Way, Romford, Essex, UK

ABSTRACT

Fractures are common injuries, and their management has evolved over the last 30 years with a greater propensity to treat fractures surgically. There have also been accompanying advances with a better understanding of the principles of bone healing and their implications on implant choice. The purpose of this chapter is to highlight the various surgical fixation devices available for the management of fractures and their underlying principles.

Keywords: Fracture, healing, fixation, devices

INTRODUCTION

This chapter deals with the principles of fracture fixation in trauma and orthopaedics (Al-Rashid et al. 2010). Fractures are common injuries with an incidence of 3.6 fractures per 100 people per year. The lifetime fracture prevalence exceeds 50% in middle-aged men, and 40% in women over the age of 75 years (Donaldson et al. 2008). The management of fractures

* Corresponding Author: Mr W Khan, Clinical Lecturer, University College London Institute of Orthopaedic and Musculoskeletal Research, Royal National Orthopaedic Hospital, Stanmore, Middlesex, HA7 4LP, UK, Telephone number: +44 (0) 7791 025554, Fax number: +44 (0) 1707 655059, E-mail address: wasimkhan@doctors.org.uk.

takes up the more time and resources in emergency theatres than any other type of injury (Tambe et al. 2005). This chapter aims to describe the principles of successful fracture management and how fractures heal. This is followed by a description of commonly used implants used for fracture repair and the biomechanical principles that guide their use.

SUCCESSFUL FRACTURE MANAGEMENT

Successful fracture management aims to achieve early fracture union without significant complications. It is important to restore patients to a pre-fracture level of function. Fractures need to be reduced to a satisfactory position if they are displaced significantly. Following this the fractures need to be held or stabilised in a satisfactory position to allow fracture healing. In most cases, fracture stabilisation could be achieved using non-operative measures e.g. plaster casts, slings or straps. In some cases however surgical fixation or prolonged periods of traction is needed to stabilise a fracture till union is achieved.

Surgical fixation of fracture fragments can give sufficient stability permitting immediate joint movement, earlier weight-bearing, shorter hospital stay and early return to work and other activities. Early active pain-free mobilisation enhances articular cartilage nutrition by the synovial fluid. It also allows a rapid return of normal blood supply to bone and soft tissues. Early weight-bearing decreases post-traumatic osteoporosis by restoring the equilibrium between bone resorption and bone formation. Surgical fixation prevents many of the disastrous sequelea associated with non-operative management of fractures with traction and its associated prolonged periods of immobility including pressure sores, infections and deep vein thromboses. It is these principles and findings that have shaped fracture fixation surgery over the last 30 years and seen a shift from non-operative management of these fractures to a greater propensity for surgical fixation (Broos & Sermon 2004). This has been promoted by a higher patient expectation and a desire for earlier return to activities of daily living, and facilitated by the design of better surgical devices for fracture fixation.

BONE HEALING

Depending on the biological and mechanical environment, potentially contributed to by the surgical fixation devices, bone can heal in two ways (Rahn 1987). The first is indirect bone healing, afforded by relative stability of the fixation device. This begins with haematoma and inflammation followed by callus formation that remodels into woven or lamellar bone. This is achieved by any device which holds the bone sufficiently to maintain length and prevent rotation and angular deformity, but still allowing a low level of displacement or micro-movement between fracture fragments thus providing a mechanical signal that stimulates the biological repair processes. Gross motion between fracture fragments leads to non-union and fibrocartilage tissue formation and should be avoided. Examples of fixation devices that provide relatively stable fixation include locked intra-medullary nails, plates used as bridging plates and external fixators as discussed below.

The second method is direct bone healing, and is facilitated in an environment of absolute stability provided by the fixation device. This results from internal remodelling that bypasses callus formation and allows contact healing between two vascular bone surfaces. This can be achieved by a device that prevents fracture surfaces displacing under physiological load. This requires anatomical reduction and inter-fragmentary compression. Inter-fragmentary compression is best achieved by a lag screw, or for large, dense bones, compression plate fixation as discussed below. The design and use of various surgical fixation devices relies on an understanding of bone healing and the loads and forces they are subjected to.

DIFFERENT IMPLANTS USED IN FRACTURE FIXATION SURGERY

Fractures vary in their pattern, and bones vary in their size, structure and strength. As a result, a wide variety of fixation devices has been developed and continues to be developed. More recent implants are made of biocompatible materials and have a low profile resulting in reduced rates of soft tissue irritation. They can also be contoured to suit individual anatomy. The successful application of these fixation devices lies in a thorough understanding of the individual fracture personality, its biology and the underpinning biomechanics of the fixation device.

In addition to the understanding of how the mechanical environment of fracture fixation shapes fracture healing, it is crucial to recognise how the type of implant affects the biology of the fracture healing. It is thought that adequate blood supply to bony fragments of the fracture through the soft tissues is of utmost importance for fracture healing to progress (Rüedi & Murphy 2000). Hence any fracture fixation surgery which further violates this blood supply in already tenuous devascularised bony fragments will adversely affect healing. This is one of the main reasons why external fixation is preferred where there is significant soft tissue damage, rather than internal fixation and its associated soft tissue dissection.

Any fixation device used in trauma surgery must be biologically inert, and not give rise to toxic reactions or local inflammatory changes (Gotman 1997). It is also important to avoid any electrolytic degradation and corrosion by avoiding implant of different materials at the same site. Metals currently used include stainless steel (316L), alloys of chromium, cobalt and molybdenum, and titanium (Ti-6Al-4V). Corrosion resistance of these materials relies on their passivation by a thin surface layer of oxide. Stainless steel is the least corrosion resistant and less inert, but easier to machine and cheaper. The cobalt chrome alloys are biologically very inert but are difficult to machine adding to their cost. Titanium has the favourable combination of high strength, light weight, high fatigue strength and low modulus of elasticity, and is biomechanically closer to bone than 316L stainless steel. This allows production of thinner plates and stronger intra-medullary nails.

More recently there has been interest in the use of biodegradable polymers e.g. polylactic acid (Hughes 2006). These have the advantage of being more flexible resulting in greater weight-bearing by the bone thus avoiding stress shielding, and they do not need to be removed. Their disadvantages include limited strength and risk of adverse biological response, and these have hindered the more widespread use of these materials.

Numerous devices are available for the fixation of fractures and these include wires, pins, screws, plates, intra-medullary nails and external fixators (Malik et al. 2009, Khan et al. 2010, Dheerendra et al. 2011, Haughton et al. 2012).

1. Pins

There is a variety of pins used in trauma surgery for the fixation of fractures (Kurup et al. 2008, Yosri et al. 2012). The pins may be smooth or threaded, and are available in a number of sizes. Threaded pins provide additional stability, as they minimise sliding of bone fragments, but are also more difficult to take out. Among the most commonly used are Kirschner wires, commonly called K-wires, and Steinman pins.

K-wires can be used to hold fragments of bone prior to rigid fixation, and for percutaneous pinning of small bone fractures. They are commonly used in hand and wrist fractures (Malik et al. 2009). At least two wires should be used and they should not be parallel (Figure 1).

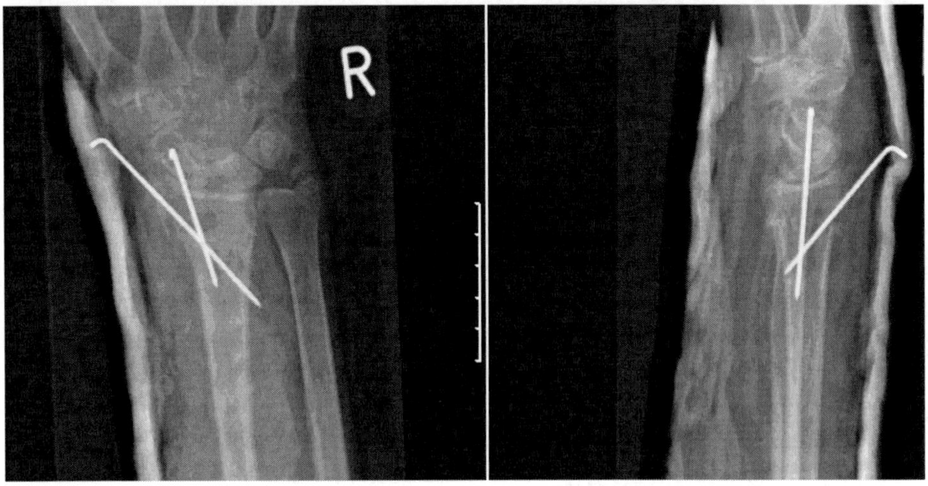

Figure 1. Antero-posterior and lateral radiograph of a distal radial fracture at the wrist stabilised with two Kirschner wires and a back-slab plaster.

They lack sufficient mechanical stability for use as the primary fixation device in long weight bearing bones. Steinman pins, are commonly used to apply skeletal traction, and are attached to traction devices.

2. Wires

In combination with pins or screws, wires can be used to create a tension band that converts distractive muscular forces to compressive forces at the fracture site. Wires are frequently used for the fixation of olecranon (Figure 2) and patella fractures. They are also used to reattach bone fragments e.g. greater trochanter or olecranon after elective osteotomies (Nork et al. 2001). The use of tension band wires requires tightening to achieve equal tension, and this can result in wire breakage or cut-through of bone. Many companies now manufacture wire tensioning and twisting instruments. The use of wires also relies on the making of holes for passing the wires that can be associated with complications. Wires in the form of cerclage wires, are also used to deal with periprosthetic fractures, for fixation of bone fragments and plate onto bone.

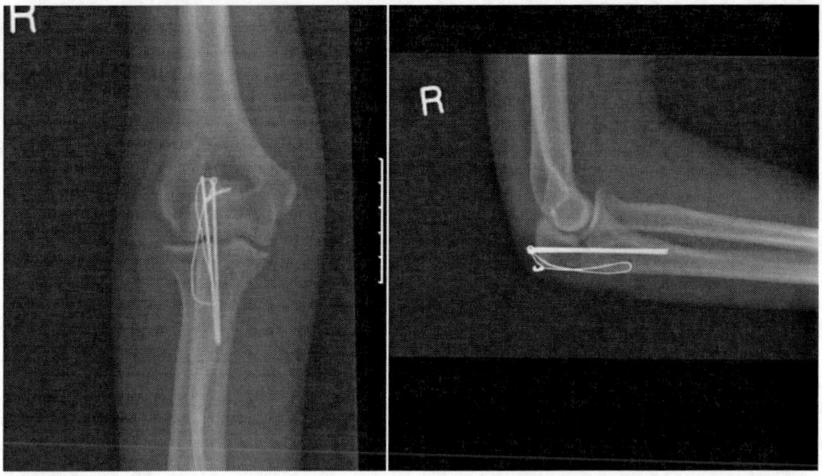

Figure 2. Antero-posterior and lateral radiograph of an olecranon fracture at the elbow fixed with tension band wiring.

3. Screws

A variety of screws are used in trauma surgery (Mudgal & Jupiter 2006). It is a device which converts rotational or torsional forces to compressive forces. Screws can be cancellous or cortical, self tapping or non-tapping, partial or fully threaded, locking or non-locking. They can be of different sizes from 1.5mm to 8.0 mm, based on the site of their application. The screw essentially consists of the screw head, the bulbous end and the part engaged by the screwdriver, and the shank or core, which can be of variable diameter and sizes. The distance between the threads is called the pitch. The factors that affect the holding power of the screw are its outer thread diameter, thread configuration and thread length. The choice of screw depends on the type of bone, fracture configuration, associated implant used and surgeon's preference.

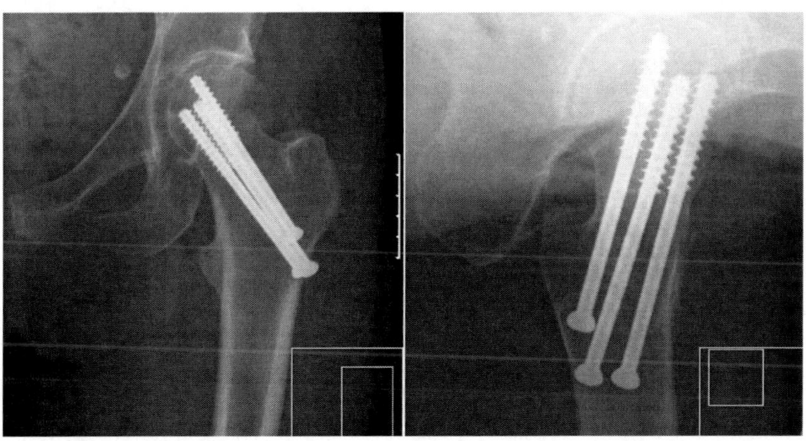

Figure 3. Antero-posterior and lateral radiograph of an intra-capsular fracture of the hip fixed with three cannulated screws.

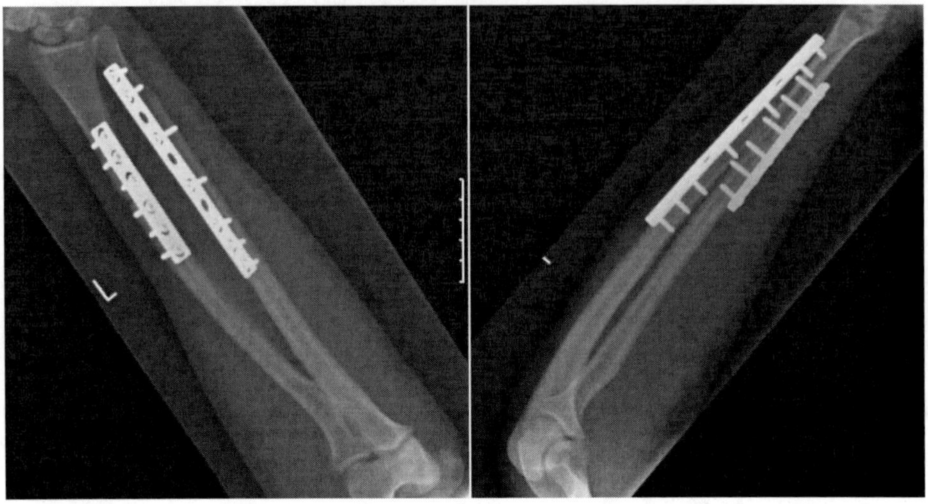

Figure 4. Antero-posterior and lateral radiograph of a radial and ulnar fracture of the forearm fixed with plates and screws.

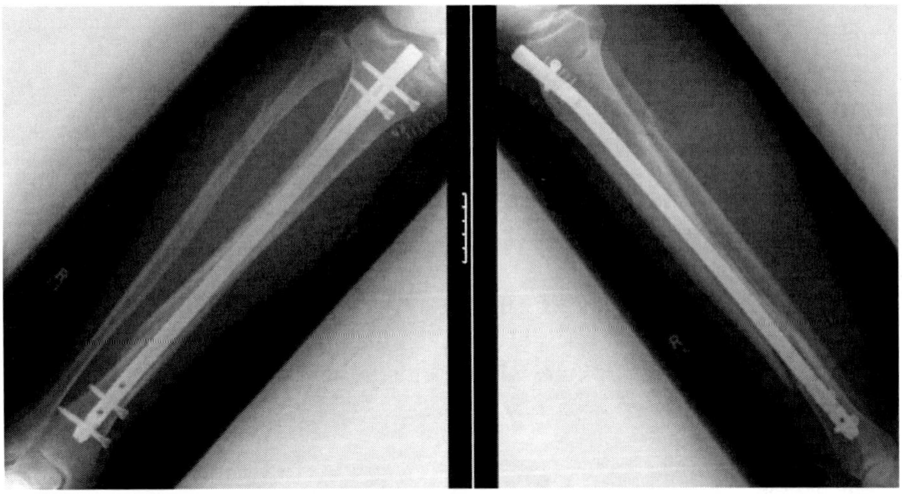

Figure 5. Antero-posterior and lateral radiograph of a tibial fracture of the lower leg fixed with an intra-medullary nail and locked with proximal and distal screws for rotary and axial stability.

They can be used in isolation to hold two fragments of bone together. If screws are used in isolation, an attempt should be made to insert them perpendicular to the fracture line to avoid shear forces (Figure 3). If the fixation relies on the lag principle, the hole in the proximal bone fragment is over-drilled to avoid engagement of the threads and this allows compression between the distal fragment engaging the screw threads and the screw head on the proximal fragment. Screws are commonly used in combination with plates (Figure 4) and nails or rods (Figure 5). Screw can be inserted using a torque screwdriver that allows a controlled and constant force to be applied.

4. Plates

Plates have screw holes that are counter-sunk to avoid prominence of the screw head. A variety of plates is available that can be used for fracture fixation to provide both relative stability and absolute stability (Egol et al. 2004). The way a plate is used determines its mechanical function. In the neutralisation mode, the plate functions to reduce the forces on an inter-fragmentary compression or lag screw. In the buttress mode, the plate acts to support the fracture fragment preventing displacement from forces. Plates can be used as bridging plates to span gaps where bone has been lost due to trauma or disease. In the compression mode, the screws are inserted offset from the centre and on tightening the bone fragments move closer together providing inter-fragmentary compression. Locking plates have threaded holes for the screw head to engage in and provide more durable fixation that is better for osteoporotic bone (Cornell et al. 2003). These locking plate systems avoid the need for bicortical fixation. The majority of these plates are made of stainless steel or titanium.

A plate is considered to provide relative stability if it allows appreciable inter-fragmentary movement under functional load. Fracture healing under conditions of relative stability takes place by callus formation. Bridging of the fracture with a stiff splint reduces mobility of the fracture fragments, which allows minimal displacement under functional load. A plate that provides rigid fixation, e.g. with inter-fragmentary compression, provides absolute stability of the fracture fragments diminishes the strain at the fracture site and allows direct healing without callus formation.

Rigid fracture fixation with plates and screws still has an important place and is desirable for fractures that involve an articular surface. Articular fractures require exact anatomic reduction and stable fixation to avoid development of abundant callus. This is important because incongruity of the joint surface and presence of callus formation at the articular surface lead to patient discomfort and often development of early and progressive osteoarthritis (Dirschl et al. 2004).

The use of plates does rely on a significant exposure that can compromise blood supply that is already disrupted from the fracture and possible associated soft tissue injury. If a plate is in total contact with a bone surface, it can act like a plug and stop radial perfusion, leading to necrosis of the bone. If the bone plate contact is reduced, as is increasingly the case with the newly developed plates, there will be less disruption to this radial perfusion of the bony fragment (Miclau & Martin 1997).

5. Intra-Medullary Nails

Intra-medullary devices act as an internal splint to stabilise long bone fractures (Hohaus et al. 2008) as shown in Figure 5. They neutralise varus and valgus forces, and allow axial compression. This can result in shortening in comminuted fracture if the nail is not locked. The locking option of a nail allows better rotational control. Nails can be solid or hollow, slotted or non-slotted. Solid nails are stiffer in bending, although these properties may be altered by changing the wall thickness. Reaming of bone allows better fixation of the nail and improves the transfer of load from the bone to the nail and stability (Pape & Giannoudis 2007). Slotted nails have less torsional stiffness than non-slotted ones.

Stiffness and strength are related to the diameter of the nail, and the strength of a nail determines its resistance to fatigue failure. The bending rigidity of the nail is proportional to the radius to the fourth power thus one large nail is stiffer than multiple smaller nails.

6. External Fixation

Another method of fracture stabilisation is with an external fixation (Ziran et al. 2008) as shown in Figure 6. This involves percutaneously placed transosseus pins and/or wires secured to external scaffolding in the form of bars and rings providing support and stabilising a fractured bone. There are a large number of variables that determine the stability provided by the external fixator construct and these include the number, location and diameter of the pins and connecting rods as well as the orientation of the construct.

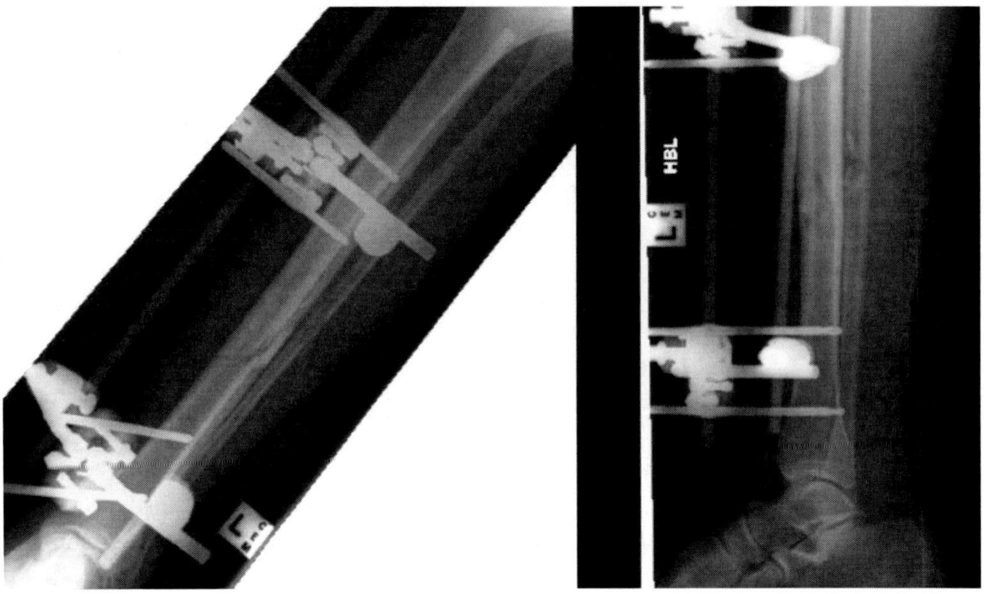

Figure 6. Antero-posterior and lateral radiograph of a tibial fracture of the lower leg fixed with an external-fixator.

External fixators cause less disruption to the soft tissues, and better preserve the blood supply to bone and periosteum (Claes et al. 1999). This makes fixators a useful tool in open fractures enabling satisfactory soft tissue management in the acute trauma setting with skin contusions and open wounds. They are also useful in peri-articular fractures as they allow restoration of the articular surface by ligamentotaxis and early mobilisation (Khan & Fahmy 2006, Bhamra et al. 2012). One major complication with the use external fixators is associated pin site infections. External fixators have a wide scope of use in trauma surgery as quick, life saving temporary fracture stabilisation devices in the multiple trauma patients.

CONCLUSION

Fractures are common injuries and there has been a greater trend over the last few years from non-operative management with traction to early surgical fixation. There are a number of fracture fixation devices available for the fixation of fractures and these devices could be used in a number of different ways depending on the nature of the fracture and associated injuries. Bone can heal in two ways; the first is indirect bone healing afforded by relative stability of locked intra-medullary nails, bridging plates and external fixators. The second method of bone healing is direct bone healing, and is facilitated in an environment of absolute stability provided by lag screws and compression plating.

REFERENCES

Al-Rashid M, Khan WS, Vermulapali K (2010). Principles of Fracture Fixation in Orthopaedic Trauma Surgery. *J. Perioper. Pract.* 20(3): 113-7.

Bhamra JS, Khan WS, Pastides P (2012). The use of the S-Quattro dynamic external fixator for the treatment of intra-articular phalangeal fractures: a review of the literature. *Open. Orthop. J.* 6(1): 54-59.

Broos PL, Sermon A 2004 From unstable internal fixation to biological osteosynthesis. A historical overview of operative fracture treatment. *Acta. Chirurgica Belgica* 104 396-400.

Claes L, Heitemeyer U, Krischak G, Braun H, Hierholzer G 1999 Fixation technique influences osteogenesis of comminuted fractures. *Clinical Orthopaedics & Related Research* 365 221-229.

Cornell CN, Lane JM, Poynton AR 2003 Orthopedic management of vertebral and long bone fractures in patients with osteoporosis. *Clinics in Geriatric Medicine* 19 433-455.

Dheerendra S, Khan WS, Barber J, Goddard N, Ahrens P (2011). Outcomes of locking plates in proximal humeral fractures: a systematic review. *Shoulder & Elbow*. 3: 74-84.

Dirschl DR, Marsh JL, Buckwalter JA et al. 2004 Articular fractures. *Journal of American Academy of Orthopaedic Surgeons* 12 416-423.

Donaldson LJ, Reckless IP, Scholes S, Mindell JS, Shelton NJ 2008 The epidemiology of fractures in England. *Journal of Epidemiology & Community Health* 62 174-180.

Egol KA, Kubiak EN, Fulkerson E, Kummer FJ, Koval KJ 2004 Biomechanics of locked plates and screws. *Journal of Orthopaedic Trauma* 18 488-493.

Gotman I 1997 Characteristics of metals used in implants. *Journal of Endourology* 11 383-389.

Haughton DN, Jordan D, Malahias M, Hindocha S, Khan WS (2012). Principles of hand fracture management. *Open Orthop*. J. 6(1): 43-53.

Hohaus T, Bula P, Bonnaire F 2008 Intramedullary osteosynthesis in the treatment of lower extremity fractures. *Acta Chirurgiae Orthopaedicae et Traumatologiae Cechoslovaca* 75 52-60.

Hughes TB 2006 Bioabsorbable implants in the treatment of hand fractures: an update. *Clinical Orthopaedics & Related Research* 445 169-174.

Khan WS, Fahmy NRM 2006 The S-Quattro in the management of intra-articular fractures of the fingers. *Journal of Hand Surgery* 31B 79-92.

Khan WS, Oragui E, Akagha E (2010). Common Fractures and Injuries of the Ankle and Foot: Functional Anatomy, Imaging, Classification and Management. *J. Perioper Pract.* 20(7): 249-58.

Kurup HV, Mandalia VM, Shaju KA, Singh B, Beaumont AR 2008 Late collapse of distal radius fractures after K-wire removal: is it significant? *Journal of Orthopaedic Traumatology* 9 69-72.

Malik AA, Yousaf N, Khan WS, Ihsan M, Ravenscroft M 2009 Common fractures of the wrist and hand, and their management. *Journal of Perioperative Practice* (in press).

Miclau T, Martin RE 1997 The evolution of modern plate osteosynthesis *Injury* 28 3-6.

Mudgal CS, Jupiter JB 2006 Plate and screw design in fractures of the hand and wrist *Clinical Orthopaedics & Related Research* 445 68-80.

Nork SE, Jones CB, Henley MB 2001 Surgical treatment of olecranon fractures *American Journal of Orthopaedics* 30 577-586.

Pape HC, Giannoudis P 2007 The biological and physiological effects of intramedullary reaming *Journal of Bone & Joint Surgery* 89B 1421-1426.

Rahn BA 1987 Direct and indirect bone healing after operative fracture treatment Otolaryngologic *Clinics of North America* 20 425-440.

Rüedi TP, Murphy WM 2000 AO principles of fracture management. Stuttgart, Germany: Thieme.

Tambe A, Rodriguez JC, Monk J, Chen C, Calthorpe D 2005 Orthopaedic trauma care: a two-tier system? *Injury* 36 771-774.

Yousri T, Tarassoli P, Whitehouse M, Khan WS, Monsell F (2012). Systematic Review of Randomized Controlled Trials Comparing Efficacy of Crossed Versus Lateral K-wire fixation in Extension type Gartland type III Supracondylar Fractures of the Humerus in Children. *Orthop. Trauma Rehab.* 14(5):397-405.

Ziran BH, Smith WR, Anglen JO, Tornetta III P 2008 External fixation: how to make it work. *Instructional Course Lectures* 57 37-49.

In: Perioperative Practice in Trauma and Orthopaedic Surgery ISBN: 978-1-63483-325-7
Editor: Wasim S. Khan

Chapter 16

COMMON FRACTURES OF THE WRIST AND HAND, AND THEIR MANAGEMENT

A. A. Malik, N. Yousaf, W. Khan*, M. Ihsan and M. Ravenscroft

Stockport NHS Foundation Trust, Stepping Hill Hospital, Stockport, UK

ABSTRACT

The wrist and hand are important in helping perform activities of daily living. Fractures of the wrist and hand are common injuries and, if inappropriately managed, can result in significant functional deficit. In this chapter some common fractures are discussed including Colles' fractures, Smith's fractures, Bennett's and Rolondo's fractures, scaphoid fractures, peri-lunate fracture dislocations, metacarpal fractures and phalangeal fractures.

Keywords: Fractures, wrist, hand, non-operative treatment, operative treatment

INTRODUCTION

In this chapter we discuss common fractures of the wrist and hand, and their management (Malik et al. 2010). The wrist and hand are important in helping perform activities of daily living (Khan et al. 2008). Fractures of the wrist and hand are common injuries and, if inappropriately managed, can result in significant functional deficit. These fractures can be treated non-operatively or operatively depending on the severity of the fracture.

* Corresponding Author: Mr W Khan, Clinical Lecturer, University College London Institute of Orthopaedics and Musculoskeletal Research, Royal National Orthopaedic Hospital, Stanmore, Middlesex, HA7 4LP, UK, Telephone number: +44 (0) 77791 025554, Fax number: +44 (0) 1707 655059, E-mail address: wasimkhan@doctors.org.uk.

Undisplaced fractures of the wrist and hand are generally managed non-operatively with immobilisation alone in a splint or plaster cast. There is a variety of splints and casts available depending on the nature of fracture. Initially only a partial plaster or backslab is usually applied that provides stability and also accommodates any associated soft tissue swelling following the injury; if there is no undue swelling, this is completed after a few days. Displaced fractures need to be realigned or manipulated before they are immobilised. This realignment or manipulation could be performed under local, regional or general anaesthesia. This may need to be supplemented with internal or external fixation, commonly Kirshner wires, if the fracture is unstable. All surgical procedures have the risk of associated complications such as infection, nerve or vascular injuries.

If no fixation is performed, the fracture requires close monitoring to ensure that the fracture position does not change. This often requires weekly fracture clinic appointments for check radiographs. Generally the splint or plaster is left in situ for three to six weeks. A fine balance however needs to be struck between leaving the splint or cast in situ for a sufficient period to allow the fracture to heal, and the risks of stiffness and decreased range of motion of the hand joints if the cast is not removed at the earliest opportunity.

A comprehensive review of all wrist and hand fractures is beyond the scope of this article. Below there is a section on the relevant bony anatomy of the wrist and hand, followed by a general overview of some common fractures.

Bony Anatomy

The forearm has two long bones, the radius and ulna. These articulate with each other at the proximal and distal radio-ulnar joints. Figure 1 shows an anteroposterior radiograph of the wrist and hand. The proximal wrist bones also articulate with distal radius.

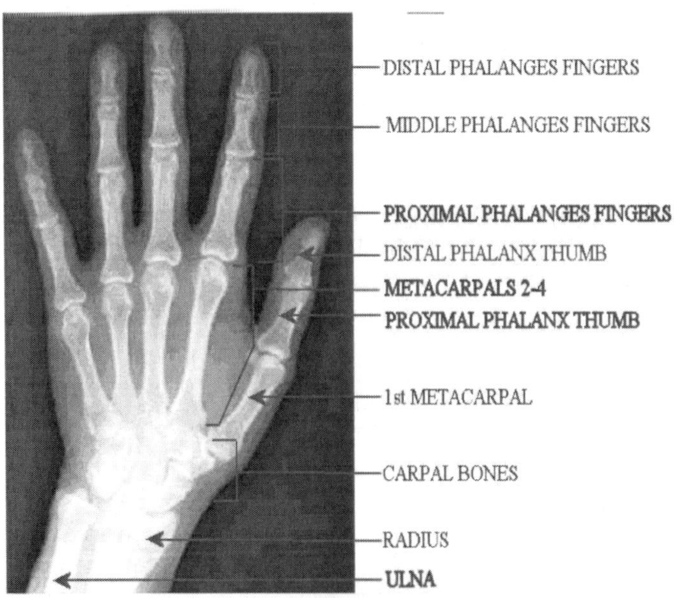

Figure 1. An anteroposterior radiograph showing the bones of the wrist and hand.

The wrist or carpus consists of eight small carpal bones in two rows. These are the scaphoid, lunate, triquetrum and pisiform in the proximal row, and trapezium, trapezoid, capitate and hamate in the distal row. These carpal bones in turn articulate with five metacarpals. Four of these five metacarpals form the support for the respective fingers with one supporting the thumb. The fingers in turn consist of three bones the proximal, middle and distal phalanges, and the thumb consists of two bones, the proximal and distal phalanges (Ellis 2006).

COLLES' FRACTURES

Colles' fractures were first described by Abraham Colles in 1814 before the advent of radiographs. Although originally described as an extra-articular distal radius fracture, the term Colles' fracture is now rather loosely used to describe any distal radius fracture with dorsal angulation. Typically it is a fracture of the distal 2.5cm of radius with dorsal angulation and displacement leading to a 'dinner-fork deformity' as shown in Figure 2. These fractures are more common with advancing age and even more so in osteoporotic women.

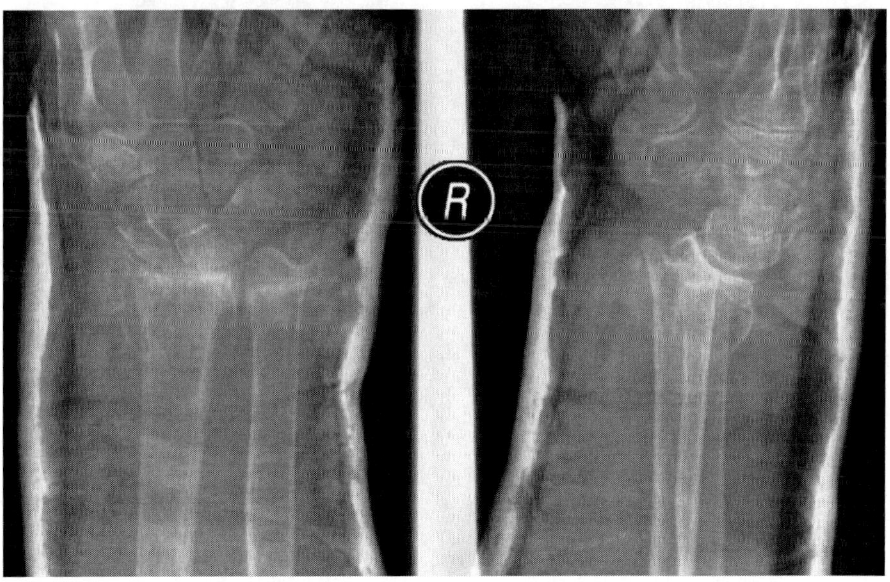

Figure 2. An anteroposterior and lateral radiograph of a Colles' fracture of the distal radius. An outline of the radiolucent white plaster can be seen around the forearm. The letter 'R' on the radiographs denotes that it is the right side being imaged.

The decision for operative management of these fractures needs careful patient assessment including age, hand dominance, level of activities, and fracture assessment including fracture pattern and any shortening and angulation (Fitz et al. 1999). Non-operative treatment is reserved for the undisplaced or minimally displaced fractures, and is generally in the form of a Colles' plaster cast. If the fracture is displaced it may warrant reduction before the plaster is applied. For fractures that are unstable, the reduction needs to be supplemented with some form of fixation. The principal methods of fixation are percutaneous pinning using

Kirshner wires as shown in Figure 3, external fixation and volar plate fixation. Unstable fractures with comminution need an aggressive approach and fixation may need to be supplemented with bone grafting (Young et al. 2003). The recent introduction of volar locking plates allows open reduction of the fracture fragments and internal fixation.

SMITH'S FRACTURES

This fracture is named after Robert Smith who first described the fracture in 1847. These fractures generally occur in younger patients and, unlike Colles' fractures that typically occur after falling on the extended wrist, these occur when landing on a flexed wrist. For this reasons it is often termed the 'reverse Colles' fracture.' It is also a distal radial extra-articular fracture but the angulation is volar. If there is an articular component to the fracture, the fracture is referred to as a Barton's fracture.

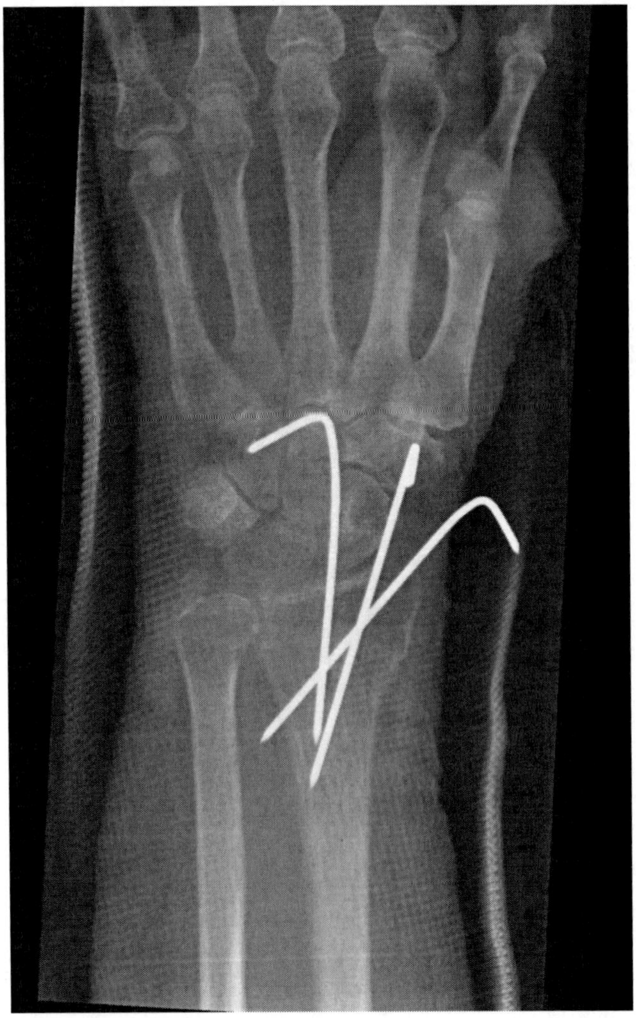

Figure 3. An anteroposterior radiograph of a Colles' fracture treated with a Kirshner wires.

Again careful evaluation is required to formulate either a non-operative or operative management plan. Non-operative treatment is reserved for the undisplaced or minimally displaced fractures, and is generally in the form of a plaster cast. If the fracture is displaced it may warrant reduction before the plaster is applied. The reduction is performed by manipulating the fracture in reverse to Colles' fracture manipulation (Bongers 1984). Fractures that are unstable necessitate open reduction and internal fixation, often with a volar plate as shown in Figure 4.

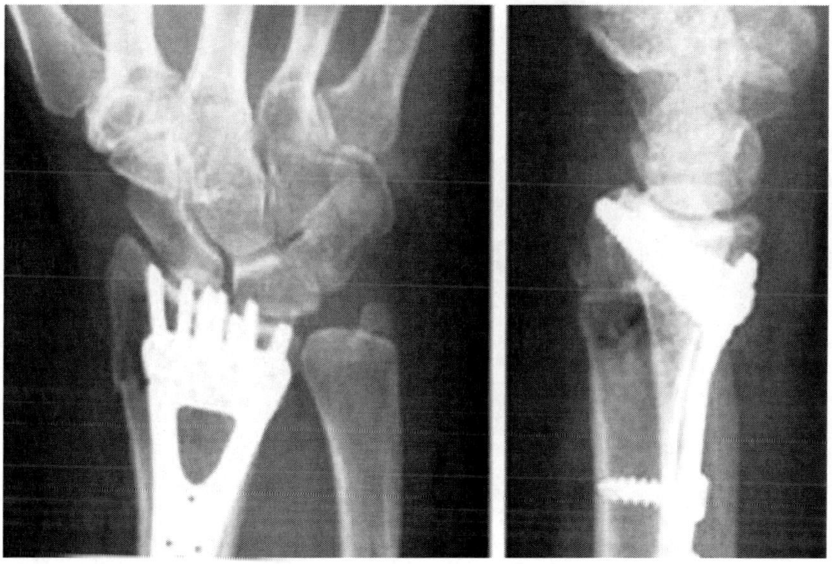

Figure 4. Anteroposterior and lateral radiographs of a Smith's fracture treated with a volar plate.

BENNETT'S AND ROLONDO'S FRACTURES

These are described as fracture dislocations of the base of first metacarpal i.e. at the base of the thumb (Siddiqui et al. 2012). Bennett's fracture was first described by Edward Bennett in 1882 and involves a partial articular fracture of the base of the metacarpal. If the fracture is a complete articular fracture, it is termed a Rolondo's fracture. Generally patients present with swelling and pain at the thumb base following injury. On examination, there is a reduced range of movement and carpo-metacarpal instability is frequently noted with gentle stress. Early treatment is essential given that thumb mobility is essential for hand function and if this joint develops arthritis, all movements will be severely affected.

Generally, patients with small avulsion fractures and minimal articular incongruity and instability can be managed with immobilization in a spica cast for at least five weeks with subsequent physiotherapy to help improve mobility. Evidence suggests that patients managed non-operatively retained good function following the injury (Milogević et al. 2005). These patients must however be carefully monitored with serial radiographs; the strong pull of the abductor pollicis longus frequently leads to displacement. If this happens, or if there is a large displaced unstable fragment to start with, open or closed reduction combined with internal fixation may be required. If more than 1 mm of articular displacement remains after closed reduction, it is also an indication for fixation. Studies have shown that patients treated with closed wire fixation, as shown in Figure 5, had significantly better results than patients treated with either plaster immobilisation or open wire fixation (Lemberger 1980). Good results have also been obtained with open reduction and lag screw fixation (Foster & Hastings 1987).

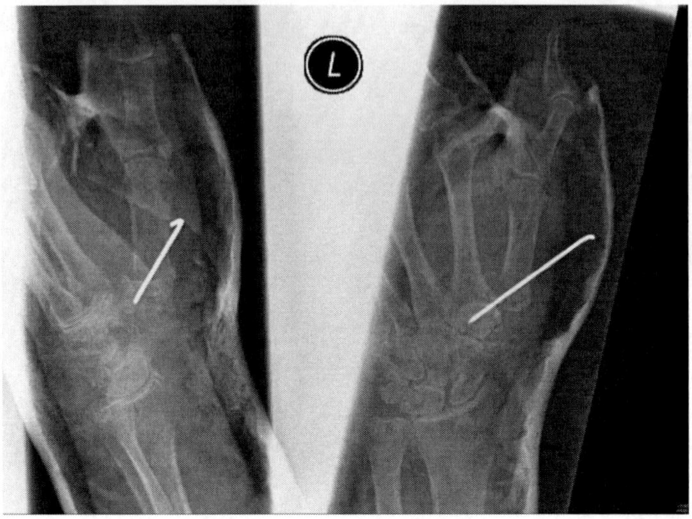

Figure 5. Pre-operative and post-operative radiographs of a Bennett's fracture treated with closed wiring.

SCAPHOID FRACTURES

The scaphoid accounts for about 70% of all carpal bone fractures (Leslie & Dickson 1981). Scaphoid fractures often occur in young and middle-aged adults following a fall on an outstretched hand.

Pain occurs primarily on the lateral side of the wrist, especially on dorsiflexion and abduction of the hand. On examination, there is tenderness in the anatomical snuff box and above the distal radius on the volar side.

Diagnosis is usually confirmed by obtaining specific scaphoid radiographs as shown in Figure 6, but the fracture may still be missed.

If clinical suspicion of fracture is high then a non-operative treatment plan should be initiated with the patient placed in a scaphoid splint or plaster, and the radiographs repeated in one to two weeks. An MRI scan has been shown to accurately diagnose scaphoid fractures (Gaebler et al. 1996).

There are various methods of treating scaphoid fractures. Undisplaced fractures are in the first instance generally managed non-operatively with fracture immobilisation in a scaphoid cast. The cast should include the proximal phalanx of thumb, and hold the wrist in 10 degrees flexion with slight radial deviation to provide compression at the fracture gap. Undisplaced fractures that fail to heal, and displaced fractures require open reduction and internal fixation as shown in Figure 7. This has gained popularity but remains technically demanding.

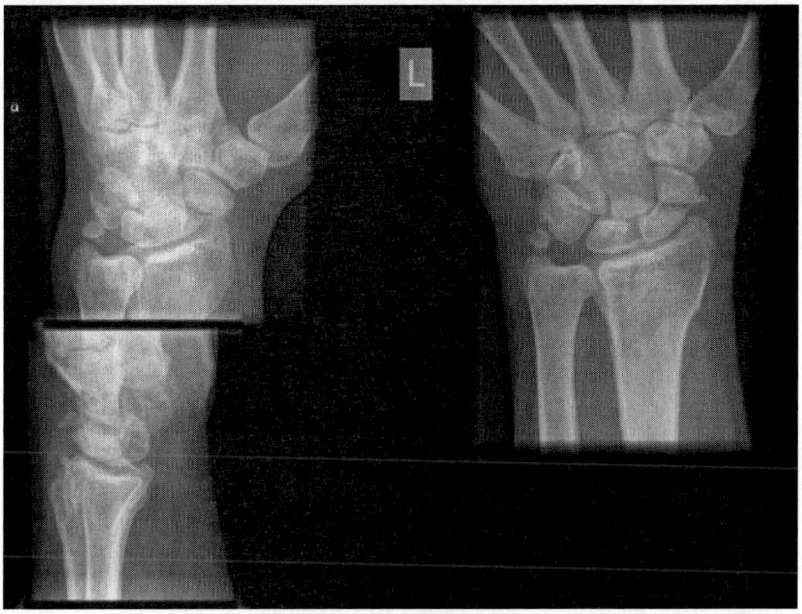

Figure 6. Pre-operative radiographs of a scaphoid fracture.

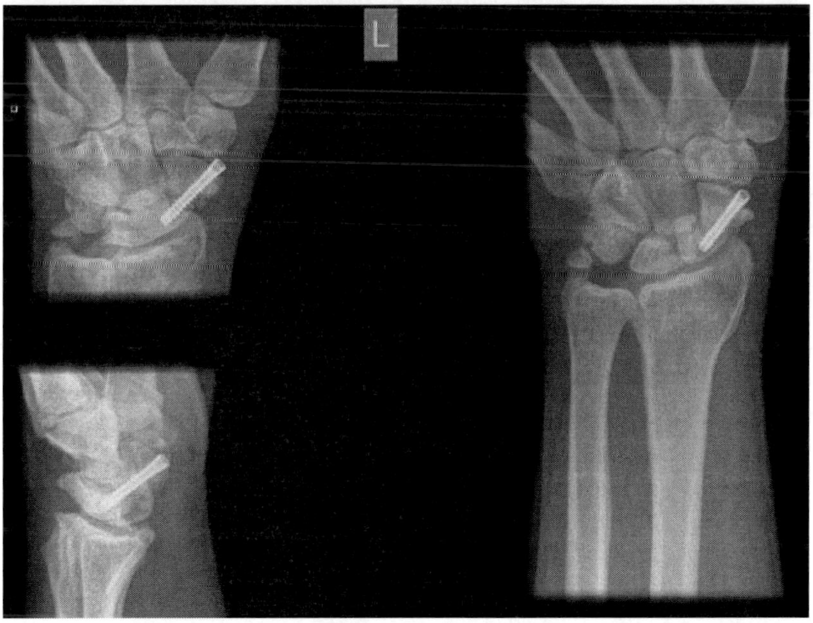

Figure 7. Post-operative radiographs of the scaphoid fracture treated with open reduction and internal fixation with a cannulated screw.

There are many approaches and fixation techniques described including the use of Herbert, AO cannulated or Acutrak screws (Meermans & Verstreken 2008). The scaphoid blood supply may be disrupted with the fracture predisposing the scaphoid to avascular necrosis. For this reason the role of bone grafting in treating the scaphoid fractures is gaining popularity (Ikeda et al. 2008). The fracture normally heals within eight to twelve weeks following fixation, and functional range of wrist movements and full grip strength can be achieved with physiotherapy. Studies have shown earlier healing and lower non-union rates with operatively treated fractures as compared to those treated non-operatively (McQueen et al. 2008).

Peri-lunate Fracture Dislocations

Peri-lunate fracture dislocations, as shown in Figure 8, are a common injury occurring mainly in the young male population following a fall on an outstretched hand or high-energy trauma. They can have devastating results if missed on initial presentation. They involve damage to the capsular ligamentous structures surrounding the lunate and, as a result, other carpal fractures and damage to the median nerve can occur.

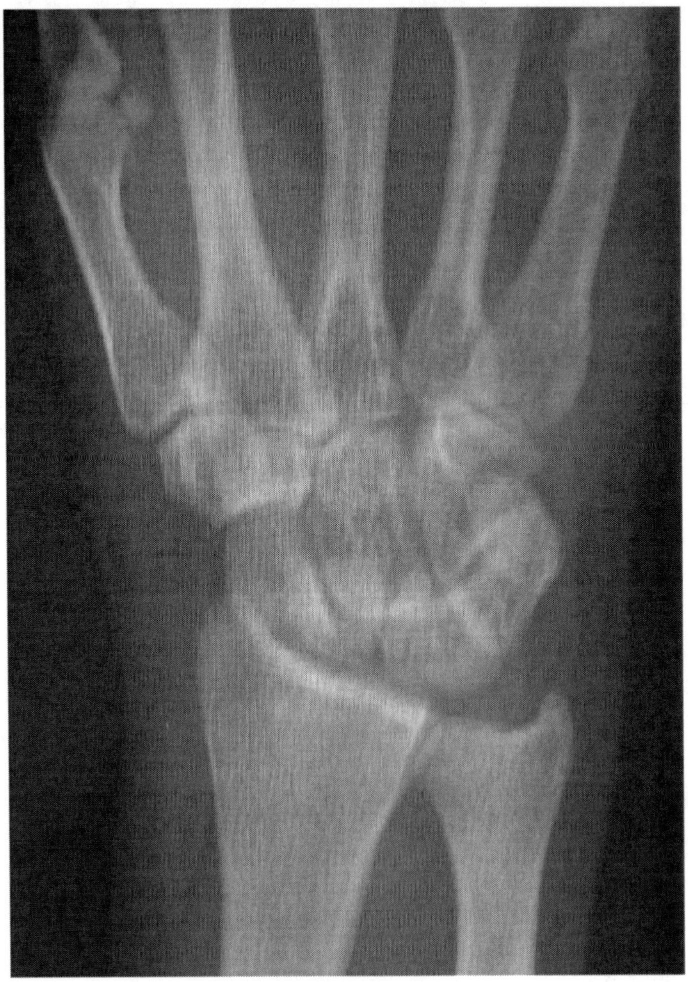

Figure 8. An anteroposterior radiograph of a peri-lunate fracture dislocation.

Peri-lunate fracture dislocation should be reduced as soon as possible. Following reduction, the patients can be placed a scaphoid cast with careful observation for further neurological symptoms or loss of reduction. If closed reduction is not possible, open reduction and internal fixation should be performed (Green & O'Brian 1978). Studies have shown that internal fixation decreases the risks of further dislocations, and allows a stable environment for ligament healing (Garcia-Elias 2004).

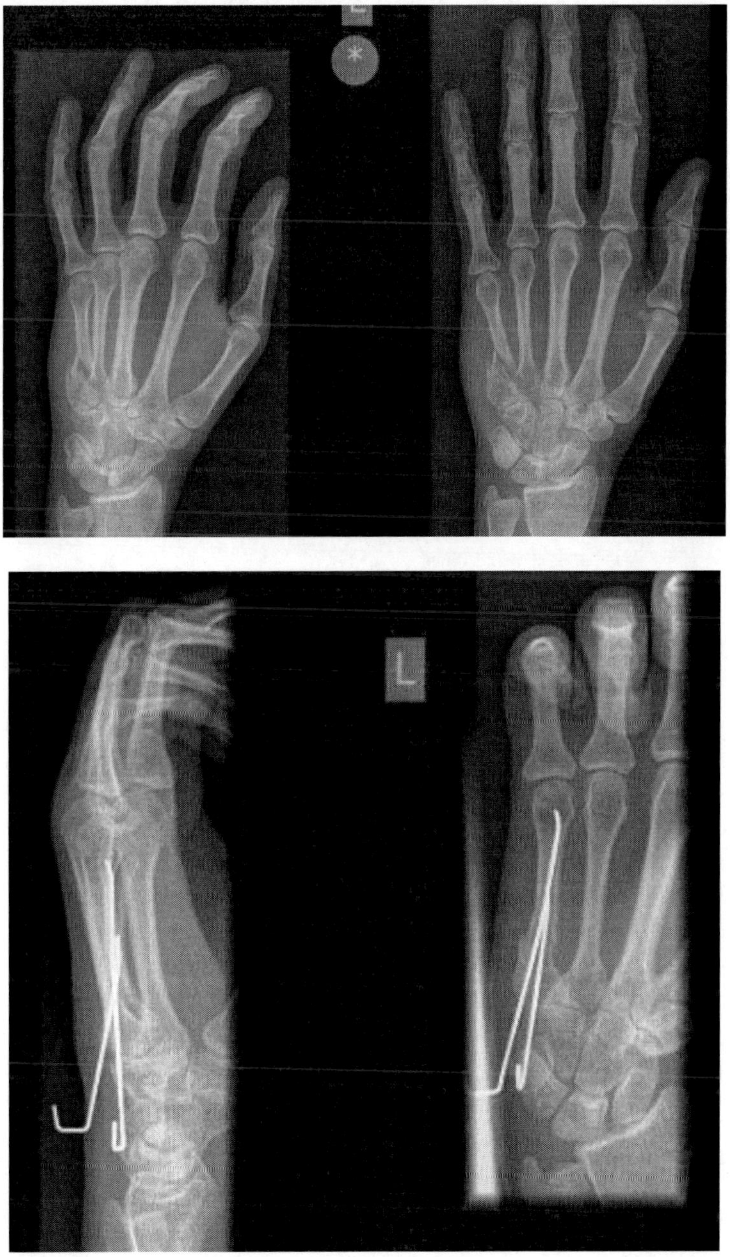

Figure 9. Pre-operative and post-operative anteroposterior and oblique radiographs of a fractured fifth metacarpal base treated with intramedullary Kirshner wires.

METACARPAL FRACTURES

Metacarpal fractures can be divided according to the location of the fracture line; this can be at the base, shaft, neck or head. Fracture pattern is an important consideration in the assessment of these fractures. Oblique or spiral fractures are more commonly associated with either shortening or rotation of the distal metacarpal fragment compared to transverse fractures. Rotation is difficult to assess radiologically and careful clinical assessment is crucial. Generally 10° of rotation is considered acceptable (Royle 1990). The goal in intra-articular metacarpal fractures is always to maintain the articular congruity.

The management of these fractures could be non-operative or operative (Haughton et al. 2012). If there is significant displacement or angulation, manipulation will be required to restore normal anatomy. Non-operative treatment may include manipulation followed by immobilisation in a plaster cast. The two types of casts are a short-arm volar cast and a short-arm cast extending to the proximal inter-phalangeal joints with a metacarpo-phalangeal extension. Patients should be reviewed with serial radiographs and evidence suggests that if good reduction is maintained, there is little stiffness and good hand movements return after removal of the plaster (Hofmeister et al. 2008). Operative methods include closed or open reduction followed by internal fixation (Omokawa et al. 2008). Fixation is usually achieved by Kirshner wire stabilisation with neighbouring metacarpals, intra-medullary Kirshner wire fixation as shown in Figure 9, or with screws with or without a plate as shown in Figure 10. Bone union is usually successfully achieved over a period of four to six weeks. Fifth metacarpal fractures are often treated surgically if angulation is more than 40 degrees (Sandner & Menke 2008).

PHALANGEAL FRACTURES

The phalanges can easily sustain injury, often as a result of sporting injuries, and need appropriate treatment to ensure that range of movement remains within functional levels (Khan & Fahmy 2006a, Khan et al., 2011, Bhamra et al. 2012). The digits consist of proximal, middle and distal phalanges, with the thumb consisting of only the proximal and distal phalanges. The phalange can be divided into the base, shaft, neck and head, with basal and head fractures usually consisting of an articular component. The flexor and extensor tendons create deforming forces on the fracture fragments resulting in displacement.

Undisplaced fractures tend to be stable and are generally treated with Zimmer splints, whereas displaced fractures tend to be unstable and require reduction (Maitra & Burdett-Smith 1992). If the fracture is unstable then either internal or external fixation is required (Khan & Fahmy 2006b). Methods used to fix fractures include Kirshner wires, screws with or without a plate as shown in Figure 11, and intraosseous wire fixation (Gorosh & Page 1989). For an extensive hand injury with open fractures and severe comminution, external fixation is favorable and has shown good results in terms of early healing (Windolf 2008).

Fractures of the distal phalanx often are associated with nail, nail bed and crush injuries and therefore this should formulate part of the initial assessment. If intra-articular fractures are due to avulsion of the extensor tendon, this is termed a Mallet finger. If the fracture is due to the avulsion of flexor digitorum profundus, it is called Jersey fracture. Mallet fingers can be treated in a mallet splint or, if there is a large avulsion fragment, surgical fixation (Tuttle et al. 2006).

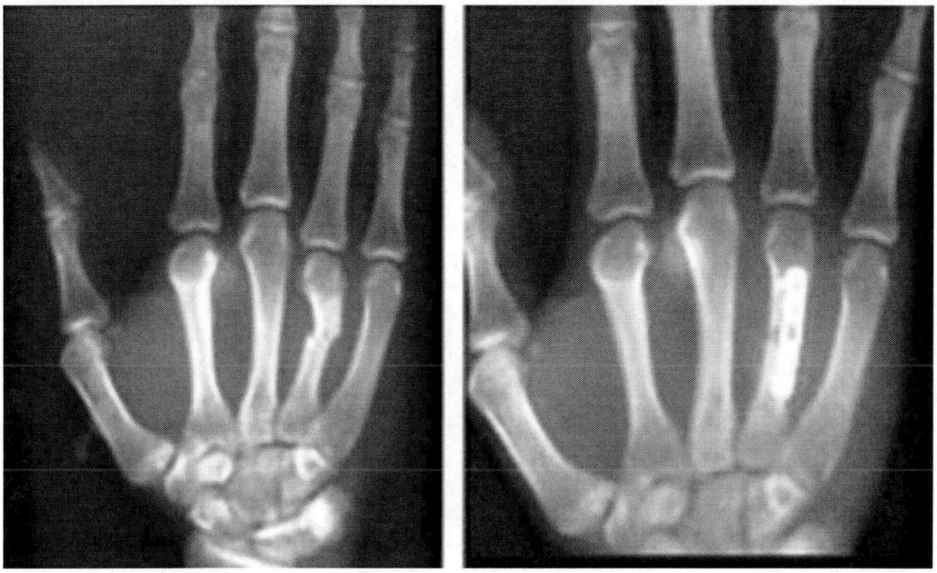

Figure 10. Pre-operative and post-operative anteroposterior radiographs of a fractured fourth metacarpal treated with a plate and screws.

In all fractures of the wrist and hand, it is important that an early decision is made regarding non-operative or operative treatment. It is also important to regularly review the patient, especially if the fracture is unstable or if it has not been fixed, so any displacements could be identified early before the fracture heals in an unsatisfactory position.

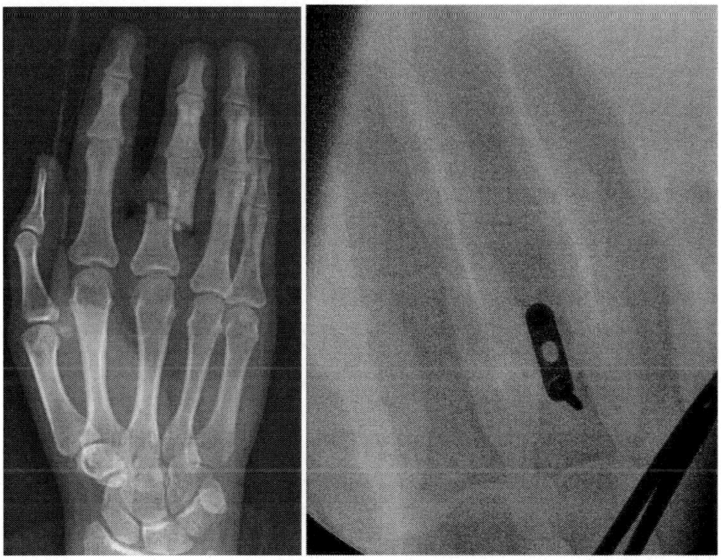

Figure 11. Pre-operative and post-operative anteroposterior radiographs showing a proximal phalangeal fracture treated with open reduction and internal fixation with a plate and screws.

Almost all fractures, whether operated or not, are managed in some form of immobilisation. A balance needs to be struck between prolong immobilisation to allow the fracture to heal, and early mobilisation that would allow the return of a good range of movement and strength. Further work is needed on identifying the optimum outcome measure to allow comparisons between different managements to be compared (Khan & Ravenscroft 2010, Khan et al., 2010, Mafi et al. 2012).

REFERENCES

Bhamra JS, Khan WS, Pastides P (2012). The use of the S-Quattro dynamic external fixator for the treatment of intra-articular phalangeal fractures: a review of the literature. *Open Orthop J.* 6(1): 54-59.

Bongers KJ 1984 Operative treatment of Smith's fracture *The Netherlands Journal of Surgery* 36 10-12.

Ellis H 2006 Clinical Anatomy: A Revision and Applied Anatomy for Clinical Students, 11th Ed, Blackwell publishing.

Foster RJ, Hastings II H 1987 Treatment of Bennett, Rolando, and vertical intraarticular trapezial fractures *Clinical Orthopaedics & Related Research* 214 121-129.

Fritz T, Wersching D, Klavora R, Krieglstein C, Friedl W 1999 Combined Kirshner wire fixation in the treatment of Colles fracture. A prospective, controlled trial *Archives of Orthopaedics & Trauma Surgery* 119 171-178.

Gaebler C, Kukla C, Breitenseher M et al., 1996 Magnetic resonance imaging of occult scaphoid fractures *Journal of Trauma* 41 73-76.

Garcia-Elias M 2004 *Perilunate injuries including fracture dislocations*. In: Berger RA, Weiss APC, Hand Surgery, Philadelphia, Lippincott Williams & Wilkins.

Gorosh J, Page BJ 1989 Treatment of phalangeal fractures of the hand with intraosseous wire fixation *Orthopaedic Reviews* 18 800-806.

Green DP, O'Brian ET 1978 Open reduction of carpal dislocations: indications and operative techniques *Journal of Hand Surgery* 3A 250-265.

Haughton DN, Jordan D, Malahias M, Hindocha S, Khan WS (2012). Principles of hand fracture management. Open Orthop J. 6(1): 43-53.

Hofmeister EP, Kim J, Shin AY 2008 Comparison of 2 Methods of Immobilization of Fifth Metacarpal Neck Fractures: A Prospective Randomized Study *Journal of Hand Surgery* 33A 1362-1368.

Ikeda K, Osamura N, Tomita K 2008 Percutaneous screw fixation without bone graft for cystic-type scaphoid fractures *Journal of Trauma* 65 1453-1458.

Khan W, Fahmy N 2006a The S-Quattro in the management of sports injuries of the fingers *Injury* 37 860-868.

Khan W, Fahmy N 2006b The S-Quattro in the management of acute intraarticular phalangeal fractures of the hand *Journal of Hand Surgery* 31 79-92.

Khan WS, Jain R, Dillon B et al., 2008 The 'M2 DASH'-Manchester-modified Disabilities of Arm Shoulder and Hand score *Hand* 3 240-244.

Khan WS, Ravenscroft MA (2010). Patient Evaluation Measure and Michigan Hand Outcome Measure- Statistical Analyses and Practical Feasibility. International Journal of Medical and Biological Frontiers; 17(1-2): 80-94.

Khan WS, Dheerendra S, Ravenscroft MA (2010). The Disabilities of the Arm, Shoulder and Hand Questionnaire and its Manchester-Modified version. International Journal of Medical and Biological Frontiers; 17(1-2): 69-79.

Khan WS, Smitham P, Fahmy NRM (2011). A modified technique of using the S-Quattro external finger fixation system- A case study. Ortop Traumatol Rehabil. 13(4): 399-402.

Lemberger U 1980 Long-term results of treatment of Bennett fractures *Handchirurgie* 12 245-246.

Leslie IJ, Dickson RA 1981 The fractured carpal scaphoid. Natural history and factors influencing outcome *Journal of Bone & Joint Surgery* 63B 225-230.

Mafi P, Mafi R, Hindocha S, Griffin M, Khan WS (2012). A systematic review of dynamometry and its role in hand trauma assessment. Open Orthop J. 6(1): 95-102.

Maitra A, Burdett-Smith P 1992 The conservative management of proximal phalangeal fractures of the hand in an accident and emergency department *Journal of Hand Surgery* 17B 332-336.

Malik AA, Yousaf N, Khan WS, Ihsan M, Ravenscroft M (2010). Fractures of the Wrist and Hand. J Perioper Pract. 20(2): 48-54.

McQueen MM, Gelbke MK, Wakefield A, Will EM, Gaebler C 2008 Percutaneous screw fixation versus conservative treatment for fractures of the waist of the scaphoid: a prospective randomized study *Journal of Bone & Joint Surgery* 90B 66-71.

Meermans G,Verstreken F 2008 Percutaneous transtrapezial fixation of acute scaphoid fractures *Journal of Hand Surgery* 33B 791-796.

Milogević I, Sudjić V, Bumbasirević V et al., 2005 Nonoperative treatment of fractures of the base of the first metacarpal bone- Bennett fracture *Acta chirurgica Iugoslavica* 52 67-71.

Omokawa S, Fujitani R, Dohi Y, Okawa T, Yajima H 2008 Prospective Outcomes of Comminuted Periarticular Metacarpal and Phalangeal Fractures Treated Using a Titanium Plate System *Journal of Hand Surgery* 33A 857-863.

Royle SG 1990 Rotational deformity following metacarpal fracture *Journal of Hand Surgery* 15B 124-125.

Sandner A.M, Menke H 2008 Results of antegrade intramedullar Kirschner-wire pinning of subcapital fracture of the fifth metacarpal bone using Foucher's technique *Handchirurgie Mikrochirurgie Plastische Chirurgie* 40 336-341.

Siddiqui NA, Ahmad ZM, Khan WS (2012). A Review of Current Management of Metacarpal Base Fractures. Orthop Traumatol Rehabil. 14(4): 305-14.

Tuttle HG, Olvey SP, Stern PJ 2006 Tendon avulsion injuries of the distal phalanx *Clinical Orthopaedics & Related Research* 445 157-168.

Windolf J, Siebert H, Werber KD, Schädel-Höpfner M 2008 Treatment of phalangeal fractures: recommendations of the Hand Surgery Group of the German Trauma Society *Der Unfallchirurg* 111 331-338.

Young CF, Manu AM, Checketts RG 2003 Seven-year outcome following Colles' type distal radial fracture. A comparison of two treatment methods *Journal of Hand Surgery* 28B 422-426.

In: Perioperative Practice in Trauma and Orthopaedic Surgery ISBN: 978-1-63483-325-7
Editor: Wasim S. Khan

Chaper 17

COMMON FRACTURES AND INJURIES OF THE ANKLE AND FOOT

Wasim S. Khan**, Emeka Oragui and Edwin Akagha
University College London Institute of Orthopaedics
and Musculoskeletal Science,
Royal National Orthopaedic Hospital,
Stanmore, Middlesex, London, UK

ABSTRACT

The ankle and foot are functionally important and complex joints. Bony fractures and ligamentous injuries are common. In this chapter we will discuss the functional anatomy, imaging, classification and the management of common ankle and foot injuries including ankle fractures, achilles tendon ruptures, Lisfranc joint injuries, calcaneo fractures and fractures of the metatarsals and phalanges.

Keywords: Fracture, ankle, foot, Lisfranc, calcaneum, metatarsal

INTRODUCTION

In this chapter, we will review the classification, diagnosis and management of common ankle and foot fractures and injuries (Khan et al. 2010). Fractures and injuries of the wrist and hand, and ankle and foot make up over 50% of trauma and orthopaedic workload (van Staa et al. 2001). We have covered common wrist and hand fractures and injuries in another chapter, and this chapter deals with common ankle and foot fractures. This includes ankle fractures,

* Corresponding Author: Mr Wasim S Khan, Clinical Lectrurer, University College London Institute of Orthopaedics and Musculoskeletal Science, Royal National Orthopaedic Hospital, Stanmore, Middlesex, London, HA7 4LP, UK, Telephone number: +44 (0) 7971 190720, Fax number: +44 (0) 20 8570 3864, E-mail address: wasimkhan@doctors.org.uk.

achilles tendon ruptures, Lisfranc joint injuries, calcaneo fractures and fractures of the metatarsals and phalanges.

Ankle Fractures

The ankle joint can be viewed functionally as the mortise and tenon joint found in woodwork with the tibia and fibula forming a mortise-like cavity that receives the tenon like talus (Figure 1) (Nannaparaju et al. 2014). Stability of the joint is due to the congruity of the osseous structures and associated ligaments. The tibial plafond articulates with the talus and forms the roof of the mortise. The medial malleolus articulates with the medial talus and the lateral malleolus binds the lateral aspect of the joint. The medial malleolus is supported by the strong deltoid ligament that consists of a superficial and deep portion. The lateral aspect of the joint is reinforced by the lateral complex which consists of lateral collateral ligaments and a syndesmosis. The ankle syndesmosis consists of an anterior and posterior tibio-fibular ligament at the level of the plafond and an interosseous ligament located 1cm above the tibial plafond and is a condensation of the interosseous membrane (Lundberg et al. 1989).

Pain, bruising, swelling and an inability to weight bear suggest a fracture or ligamentous injury. Lateral and mortise view radiographs should be performed.

Classification Systems of Ankle Injuries

Different classification methods have been devised to characterise ankle injuries; the two most common being the Lauge-Hansen (Lauge-Hansen 1950) and Danis-Weber (Weber 1972) systems.

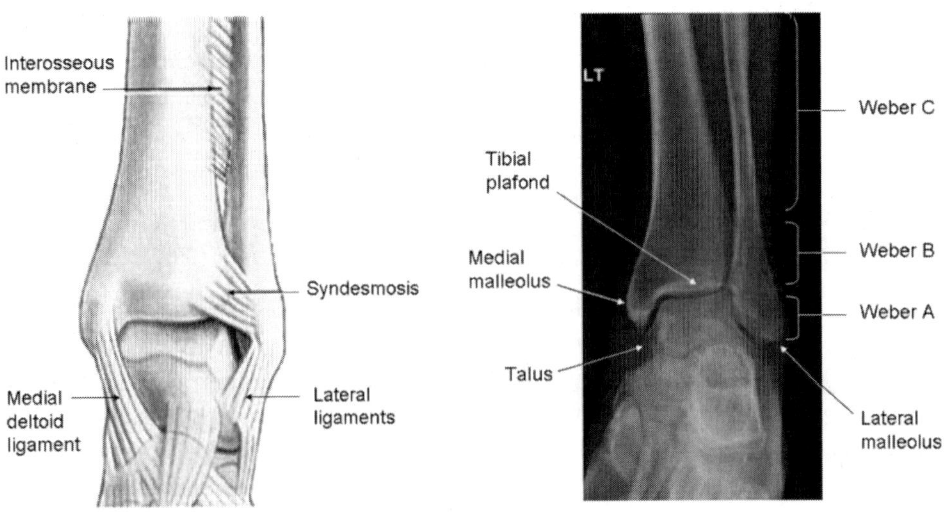

Figure 1. Antero-posterior images of the left ankle showing the ligamentous structures (line drawing) and bony structures (radiograph) that form the joint, and the location of the syndesmosis with associated Weber B fractures.

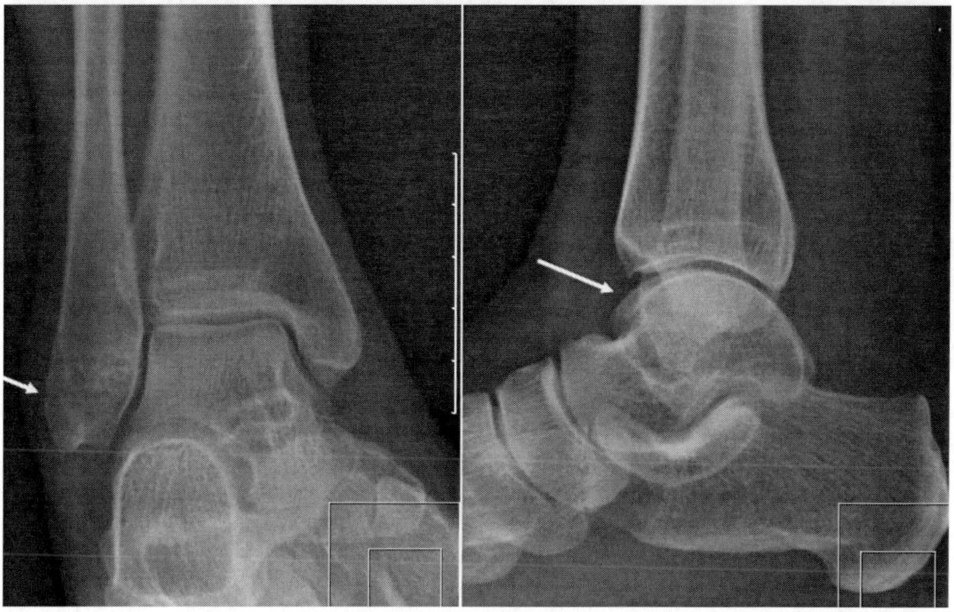

Figure 2. An antero-posterior and lateral radiograph of the right ankle showing a Weber A fracture (arrows).

The Lauge-Hansen classification resulted from work on cadavers in which forces were applied to a rigid foot and the resultant pattern of injuries observed. Failure is either a bony fracture or ligamentous disruption.

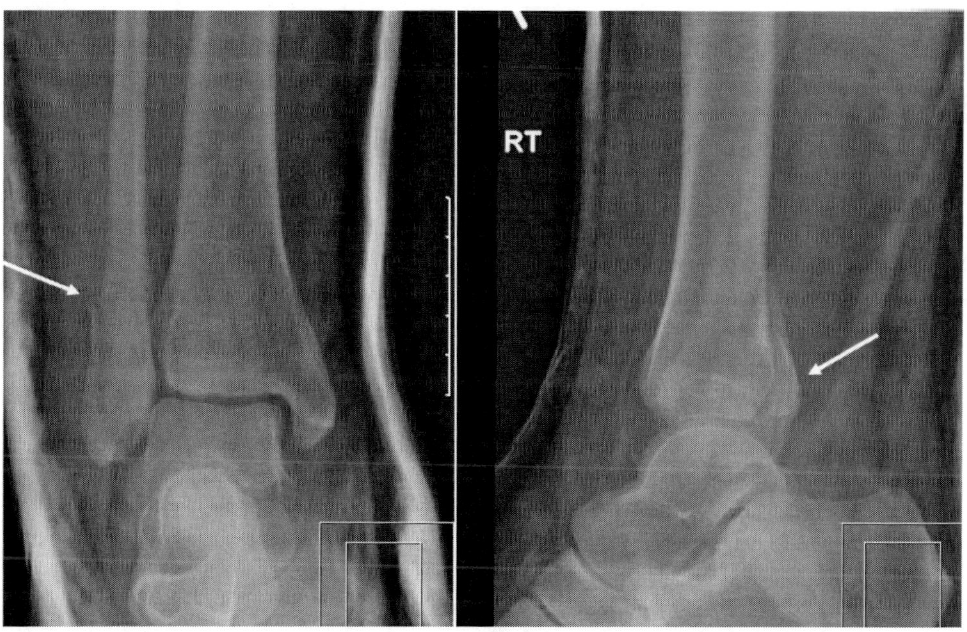

Figure 3. An antero-posterior and lateral radiograph of the right ankle showing a Weber B fracture. The first arrow is pointing at the Weber B fracture of the lateral malleolus and the second arrow is pointing at a fracture of the posterior malleolus that involves less than 25% of the articular surface.

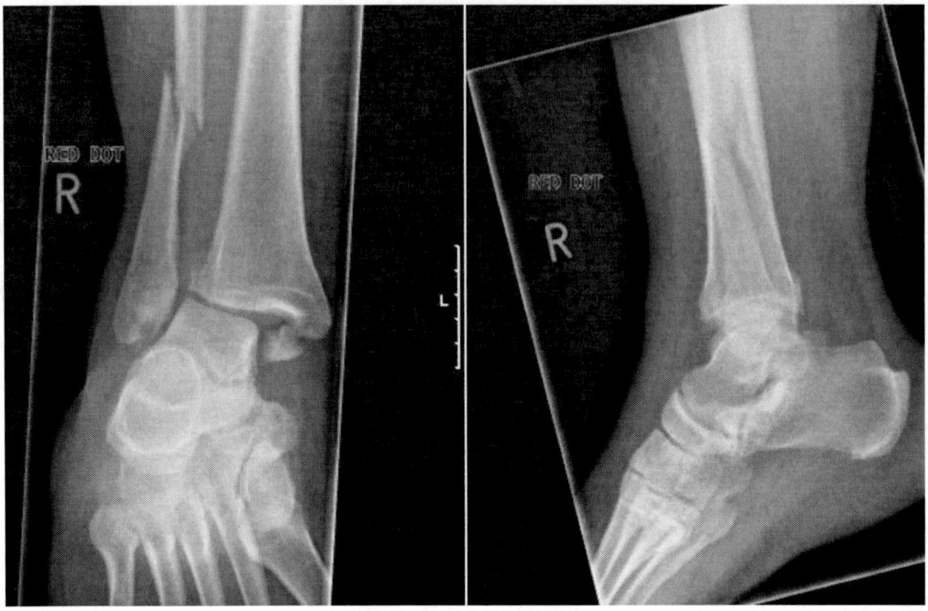

Figure 4. An antero-posterior and lateral radiograph of the right ankle showing a Weber C fracture and an associated fracture of the medial malleolus. There is also subluxation of the ankle joint.

Lauge-Hansen uses a two-word nomenclature where the first word describes the position of the foot at the time of injury and the second word describes the direction of the deforming force. There are five types of Lauge-Hansen fracture each with progressive stages of injury, supination adduction, supination external rotation, pronation external rotation, pronation abduction and pronation dorsiflexion. This classification was initially proposed to guide the closed reduction of ankle fractures by reversing the injury mechanism. It is useful in describing the pathomechanics of ankle injuries and inferring their stability (Michelson et al. 2007). The Weber classification system is based on the belief that the lateral structures are the main stabilising structures of the ankle joint and the degree of the disruption of these structures determines the need for and degree of operative correction (Michelson et al. 1996). In Weber type A injuries the level of lateral malleolar injury is distal to tibial plafond (Figure 2). The injury is at level of tibial plafond in type B injuries (Figure 3), and proximal to tibial plafond in type C injuries (Figure 4).

MANAGEMENT OF ANKLE FRACTURES

Stability of the fractured ankle is the main determinant of prognosis and management. Stable fractures can be managed non-operatively and unstable fractures fare better with operative stabilisation (Micheslon 1995). Stable fractures are immobilised with a below-knee back slab and elevated. The plaster is completed once the swelling has subsided and is left for approximately six weeks with the patient non-weight bearing. The patient is followed up in clinic with repeat radiographs to ensure satisfactory healing.

Displaced bimalleoler or trimalleolar fractures, talar shift and syndesmotic widening are indications for operative fixation (See Case study 1). The various operative treatment modalities are discussed by the authors in a previous review paper (Al-Rashid et al. 2010). Lateral malleolar fractures are managed with an inter-fragmentary lag screw and a third tubular plate used as a neutralisation plate as shown in Figure 5 and Figure 6. A bridging plate with locking screws may be used in severely comminuted fractures (Micheslon 1995). Proximal fibular fractures without shortening can be managed with a syndesmosis screw alone, where the screw holds the tibiofibular joint stable while the sysndesmosis heals. Medial malleolar fractures are usually fixed with one or two 3.5mm partially threaded cancellous screws (Baird & Jackson 1987) as shown in Figure 6. Medial deltoid ligament injuries are usually only repaired if they prevent reduction of the joint, although this is rare.

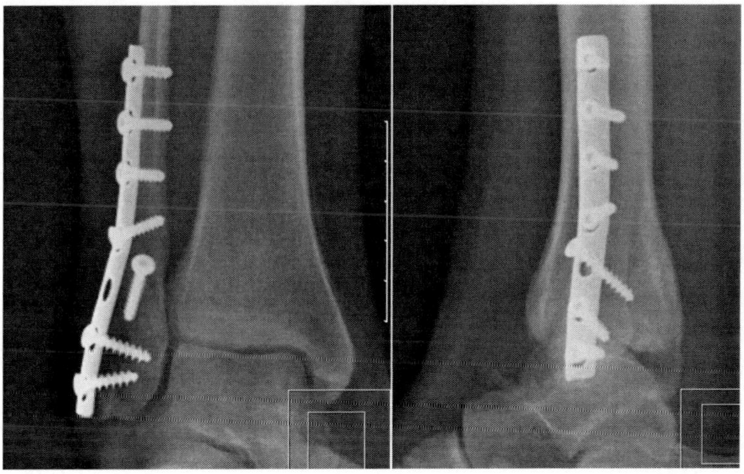

Figure 5. An antero-posterior and lateral radiograph of the right ankle showing fixation of the Weber B fracture shown in Figure 3. The fracture has been fixed with a lag screw and a plate with six additional screws. The fracture of the posterior malleolus has been left.

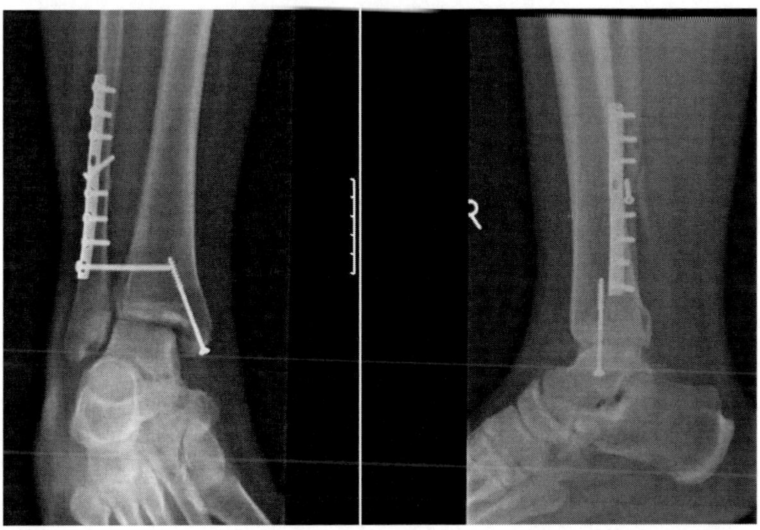

Figure 6. An antero-posterior and lateral radiograph of the right ankle showing fixation of the Weber C fracture shown in Figure 4. The lateral and medial malleoli have both been fixed. There is also a syndesmosis screw stabilising the tibiofibular syndesmosis.

Posterior malleolar fractures that involve less than 25% of the joint surface, as shown in Figure 2, can be left alone (van den Bekerom et al. 2009). Those involving greater than 25%, should be reduced and fixed with lag screws through a posterolateral or anterior approach.

Where there is a suspicion of a syndesmotic injury, the proximal fibula fracture should be fixed and the stability of the mortise tested. Any instability requires insertion of a 4.5mm syndesmotic screw from lateral to medial and should purchase three or four cortices (Micheslon 1995) as shown in Figure 6.

Following surgery, patients are immobilised in a below knee back-slab which is converted to a full cast once the swelling subsides. The patient is non-weight bearing for approximately six weeks, or longer if there are concerns about bone quality or fracture fixation. Removal of metalwork is not routinely performed unless indicated by infection or pain from prominent metalwork. Removal of syndesmosis screws is controversial with some surgeons removing them before weight bearing and others leaving them unless they cause symptoms.

Delayed surgery for an old fracture dislocation is a difficult undertaking due to soft-tissue contractures and malunited fractures. Previous studies have shown that if anatomic reduction is achieved, results with delayed surgery can be as good as those obtained with immediate surgery (Khan et al. 2007).

Achilles Tendon Ruptures

The Achilles tendon has evolved to become a structure prone to injury (Malvankar & Khan 2011). The achilles tendon attaches the gastrocnemius and soleus muscles to the calcaneum. Injury to the tendon may result in a partial or complete tear usually occurring two inches above the calcaneum. The mechanism of injury usually involves eccentric loading on a dorsiflexed ankle with the knee extended, such as when jumping or running.

Complete tears usually occurs in middle-aged patients often during the performance of sport or activity they are unaccustomed to, whereas partial tears are much less common and typically occur in the younger competitive athlete. Systemic conditions such as gout and the use of medications such as steroids and certain antibiotics are risk factors. Diagnosis is made by history and examination findings which may include the presence of a defect over the area and a positive Simmond's test where squeezing of the calf does not result in plantar flexion of the foot. An ultrasound or magnetic resonance scan may help in cases of ambiguity.

Management of Achilles Tendon Injuries

Bhandari et al., (2002) performed a systematic review and meta-analysis of literature and found that operative fixation is associated with a lower re-rupture rate of 4% compared with 13% for non-operative management. Operative repair of the tendon is generally performed in active patients with a complete rupture. Although operative fixation is also associated with an earlier return to sport and activity, the incidence of complications including wound infection and breakdown because of the tenuous blood supply is significant at 26% for open procedures and 8% for minimally invasive procedures (Bhandari et al. 2002). Minimally invasive surgical repair techniques are associated with reduced perioperative morbidity, faster recovery times, shorter hospital stays and improve functional outcomes when compared with open procedures (Maffuli et al. 2009).

Conservative management may be indicated in all other cases of complete rupture and for partial ruptures (see Case study 2). An equinus cast is applied with the foot in extreme plantar-flexed position, and is changed serially over six to eight weeks with the foot gradually brought out of equinus. Weight bearing is usually commenced at six weeks. Gradual strengthening by physiotherapy is recommended for optimal results. The rehabilitation protocol is determined by a number of factors including the injury, the quality of the repair, the patient's age, medical and social history, and sporting endeavours (Strom & Casillas 2009).

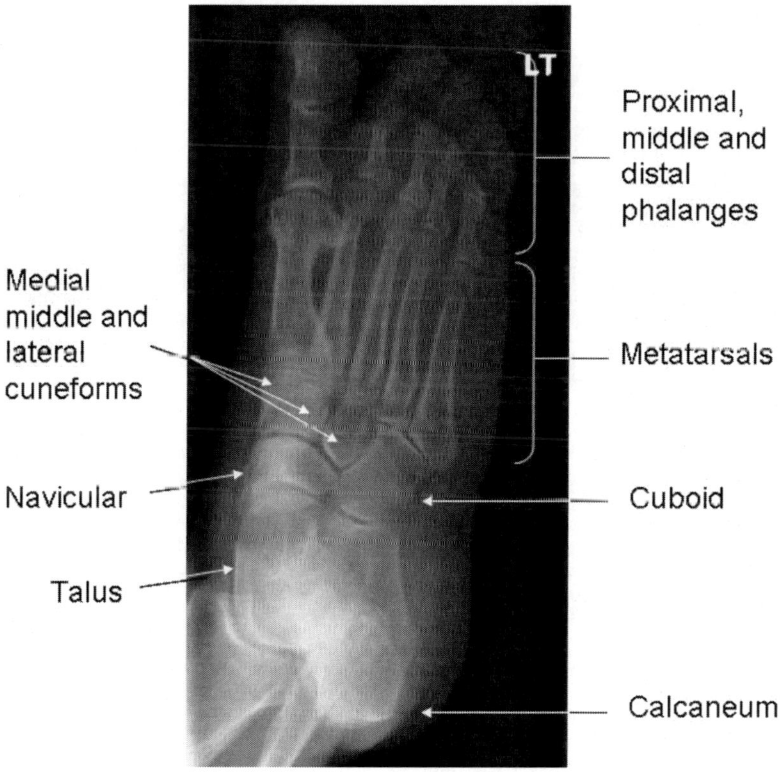

Figure 7. An oblique radiograph of the left foot showing the bony structures.

LISFRANC JOINT INJURIES

Jacques Lisfranc de St Martin (1790-1847) was a French Surgeon in the Napoleonic army who developed a method of quick amputation through the taros-metatarsal joint that did not involve any osteotomy. The eponymous name Lisfranc injury was later given to describe any injury that occurred at this joint. The Lisfranc ligament is a thick ligament arising from the medial aspect of the first cuneiform and attaching to the base of the second metatarsal (Figure 7 and Figure 8). The Lisfranc ligament is the only significant attachment between the first and second ray at the mid-tarsal level, therefore dysfunction leads to an unstable joint with severe pain and instability.

The mechanism of injury is usually a direct blow or axial loading of the metatarsal with rotation in a hyper-flexed foot. Low energy injuries occur in athletes and higher energy injuries occur in road traffic and industrial accidents (Vuori & Aro 1993).

A relevant mechanism of injury, and findings of swelling and erythema over the medial aspect of the mid-foot aide diagnosis. Instability on abduction and pronation stress testing of the forefoot may be evident.

IMAGING OF THE LISFRANC JOINT

Greater than 2mm spacing between the second metatarsal and medial cuneiform or the second and first metatarsal on antero-posterior radiographs suggests instability (Figure 8). A positive 'Fleck sign', avulsion of the lateral aspect of the medial cuneiform or medial aspect of the base of the second metatarsal suggests a Lisfranc injury.

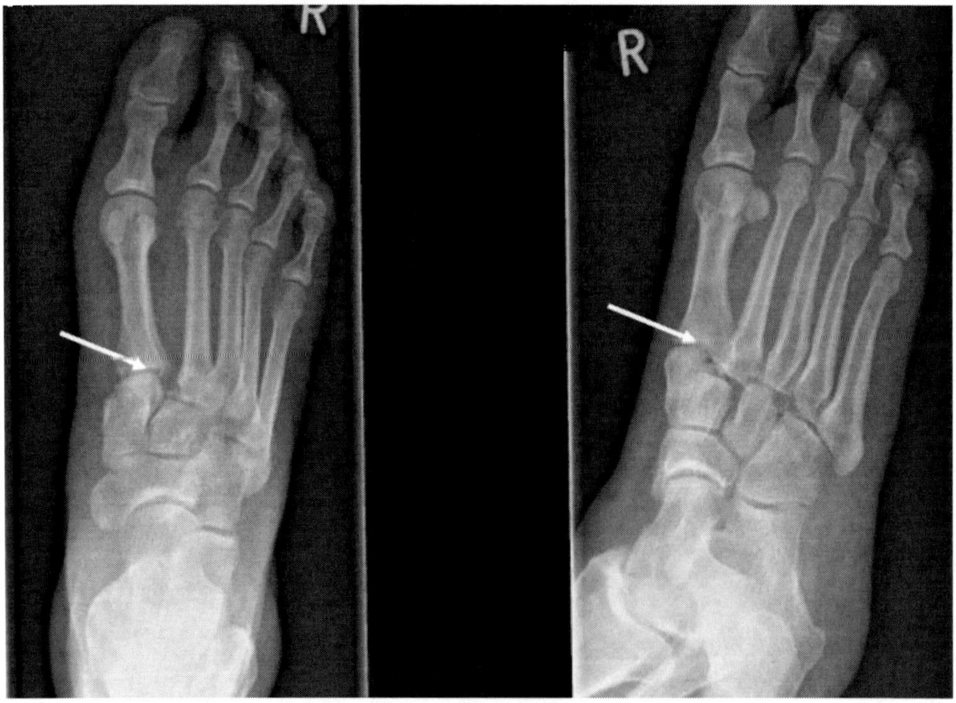

Figure 8. An antero-posterior and oblique radiograph of the right foot showing a Lis-franc injury with widening of the gap between the fractured second metatarsal base and medial cuneiform (arrows).

Any dorsal displacement of the taros-metatarsal joints or plantar displacement of greater than 1mm on lateral radiographs suggests an unstable Lisfranc injury (Hatem 2008). If the diagnosis is uncertain abduction stress testing under fluoroscopic control (Coss et al. 1998) or a CT of the foot will clinch the diagnosis.

MANAGEMENT OF LISFRANC JOINT INJURIES

Injuries with no radiographic evidence of instability can be treated conservatively with closed reduction. Operative stabilisation is indicated if there is evidence of instability, neurovascular compromise, open fracture or compartment syndrome. Closed reduction and percutaneous pinning is suitable for injuries with greater than 2mm of displacement but less than 15 degrees of talo-metatarsal angulation. Open reduction is required for displacement of greater than 2mm and 15 degrees of talo-metatarsal angulation (Kuo et al. 2000). It may also be indicated in the young competitive athlete with lesser degrees of displacement.

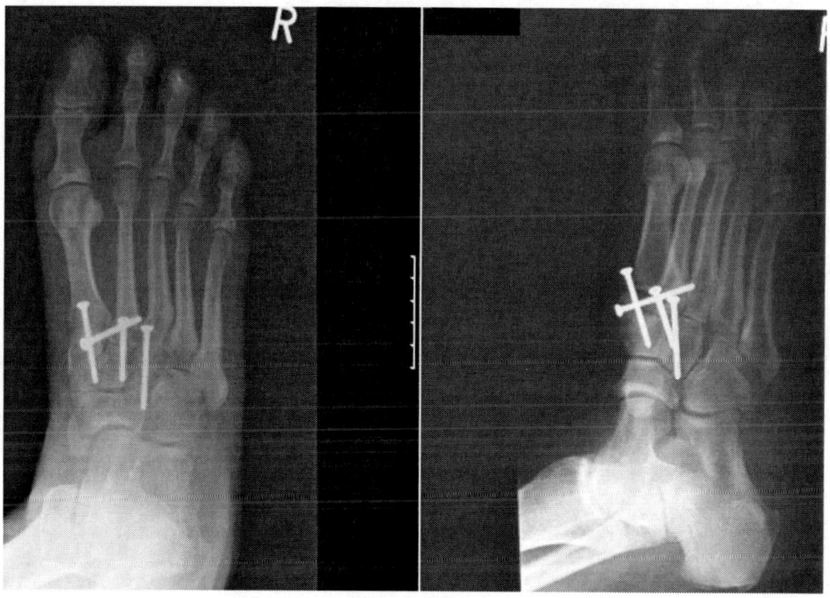

Figure 9. An antero-posterior and oblique radiograph of the right foot showing the Lis-franc injury from Figure 8 reduced and fixed with screws.

The principles of treatment involve stabilising or debriding osteochondral defects, reducing medial joints and stabilising the rays from a medial to a lateral direction. Stabilisation involves any combination of screws, plates and K-wires (Figure 9). Open fractures are usually treated with external fixation. Post-operative rehabilitation of all Lisfranc injuries involves non-weight bearing in a cast for six weeks followed by weight bearing in a cast for a further six weeks. Delayed presentation of unstable injuries manifests as severe pain, instability or early onset arthritis. Treatment is symptomatic but may require a taros-metatarsal joint fusion.

CALCANEO FRACTURES

These infrequent injuries create a major socioeconomic burden. In 1945, Bankart noted that 'the results of crush fractures of the os calcis are rotten' and the results have not improved significantly since then (Gougoulias et al. 2009).

The calcaneum is important in maintaining vertical posture and normal walking. Its tough outer cortical bone is surrounded by softer cancellous bone, allowing it to resist bending, tensile and compressive forces. The superior surface articulates with the talus via a posterior, middle and anterior facet, whereas its anterior surface articulates with the cuboid bone. The achilles tendon inserts into the posterior tuberosity. Below the middle talar facet is the sustentaculum tali which serves as attachment of several other ligaments and laterally the peroneus longus tendon attaches to a tubercle called the peroneal trochlea. Intra-articular fractures are usually the result of axial loading of the calcaneum following a fall from a height or a motor vehicle accident. Extra-articular fractures usually result from twisting injuries or may be the result of a direct blow. There is a relevant history and the patient complains of a painful and swollen ankle and inability to weight bear.

Imaging of Calcaneo Fractures

Radiographs form the principle diagnostic tool. Antero-posterior images may show a lateral wall bulge of the calcaneus. On the lateral view a reduction in Bohler's angle (Bohler 1931) or an increase in Gissane's angle (Gissane 1945) is highly suggestive of an intra-articular fracture with displacement. Bohler's angle subtends two lines drawn from the superior margin of the posterior facet to the superior margin of the anterior process, and the superior margin on the posterior facet to the superior margin of the tuberosity. A reduction from the normal angle of 20-40 degrees suggests an intra-articular fracture. The crucial angle of Gissane subtends a line drawn along the border of the posterior facet and a line drawn along the anterior process. It is normally 100-130 degrees and an increase in the angle suggests depression of the posterior facet.

Classification of Calcaneo Fractures

A number of classification systems based on the radiographic appearance have been devised. The Essex-Lopresti classification (Essex-Lopresti 1993) distinguishes extra-articular fractures from intra-articular ones. For intra-articular fractures the calcaneum impacts the ground and a primary fracture line develops and runs from plantar-medial to dorso-lateral. This results in an antero-medial sustentacular fragment and a postero-lateral tuberosity fragment. A secondary fracture line may then develop. If this extends posterior a large 'tongue-type' postero-lateral fragment results, whereas if it begins at the crucial angle of Gissane and extends postero-dorsally, a depressed fragment containing the majority of the posterior facet results (Figure 10). The Sanders classification is a prognostic classification system based on CT appearances of the posterior facet (Sanders 1993)· The coronal CT image that shows the posterior facet in widest profile is chosen and the posterior facet is divided into three equal portions by two vertical lines. A third line marks the border of the sustentaculum. The lines are labelled A to C from lateral to medial. Fractures in the more medial zones are more difficult to visualize and subsequently more difficult to repair. Type I fractures are non-displaced and Type II are two-part fractures. Type III are three-part or split depression fractures and Type 4 are comminuted fractures.

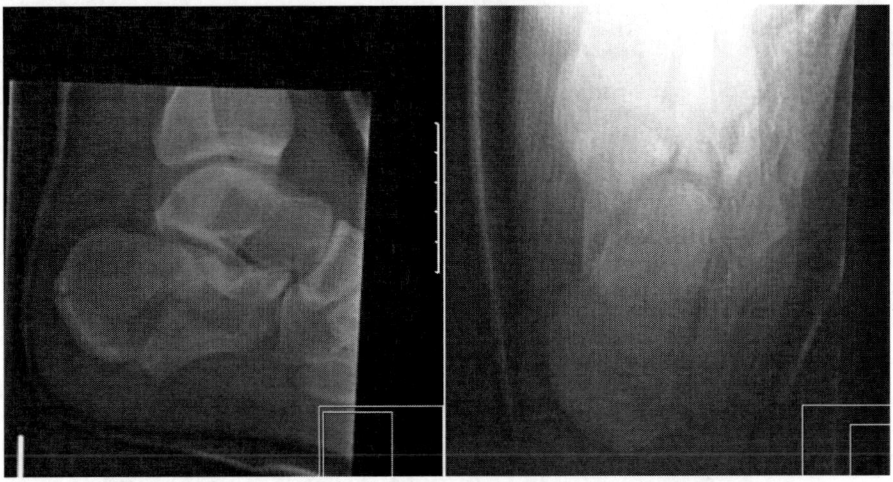

Figure 10. A lateral and axial radiograph of the calcaneum showing a calcaneal fracture.

MANAGEMENT OF CALCANEO FRACTURES

In a recent systematic review of randomised trials, the results of operative and non-operative treatment showed no difference in residual pain, but favoured surgical management on ability to return to the same work and to wear the same shoes as before the fracture. Surgery reduced the need for subsequent subtalar fusion, but it is unclear whether general health outcome measures, injury specific scores and radiographic parameters improved after operative treatment, and whether the benefits of surgery outweigh the risks that include deep infection and subtalar arthritis (Gougoulias et al. 2009).

Undisplaced extra-articular fractures make up a third of these fractures and can generally be treated non-operatively with elevation, cast immobilisation and early range of movement exercises (Schepers et al. 2008). Sanders type I fractures do well with non-operative management. Displaced fragments may be amenable to closed or semi-open reduction with Steinman pins. Surgery can be performed within the first 24 hours if swelling has been controlled or after a week or so once the swelling subsides. Exceptions include large displace fragments and those that involve the achilles tendon which should be treated by open reduction and internal fixation.

Displaced intra-articular fractures are generally treated by operative stabilisation (Potter & Nunley 2009). A lateral, medial or combined approach can be used. Sanders type II and III fractures should be treated with open reduction and internal fixation. The principles are to achieve congruency of the posterior facet, restore the normal height and width of the calcanuem, free any enclosed peroneal tendon, reduce the calcaneo-cuboid joint and neutralise any varus deformity. Outcomes of Sanders type IV injuries are poor and some clinicians manage them conservatively whilst others opt for primary fusion of all or some of the calcaneal joints (Sanders et al. 1993). Surgery should be avoided in diabetic patients, smokers who refuse to stop immediately, those with limited ambulation and repeat 'jumpers' such as those with psychiatric issues

METATARSAL AND PHALANGEAL FRACTURES

Fractures to the metatarsal bones and phalanges of the foot are common injuries and are due to direct trauma, excessive rotational forces or repetitive stress. They are usually minimally displaced and respond well to conservative treatment either by splint age or a walker boot with early mobilisation (Schenck & Heckman 1995). If displaced or unstable they are stabilised with K-wires (Figure 11 and Figure 12) as seen in Case study 3.

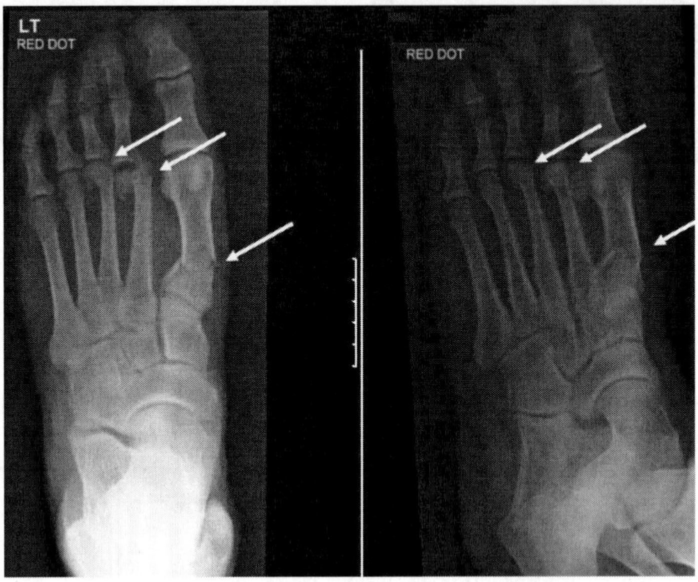

Figure 11. An antero-posterior and oblique radiograph of the right foot showing fractures of the first, second and third metatarsals (arrows)

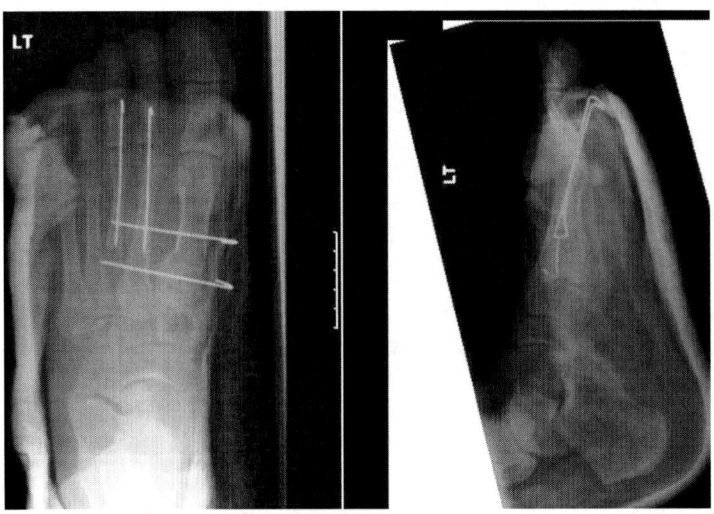

Figure 12. An antero-posterior and oblique radiograph of the right foot shown in Figure 11 after fixation of the fractures of the first, second and third metatarsals with three K-wires.

Fractures of the fifth metatarsal are common injuries worthy of special mention. It is important that a distinction is made between the more benign proximal tuberosity fractures (Figure 13) and Jones' fractures that occur at the metaphyseal-diaphyseal junction (Figure 14). The lateral cord of the plantar fascia and the peroneus brevis tendon attach to the plantar and lateral aspect of the tuberosity respectively.

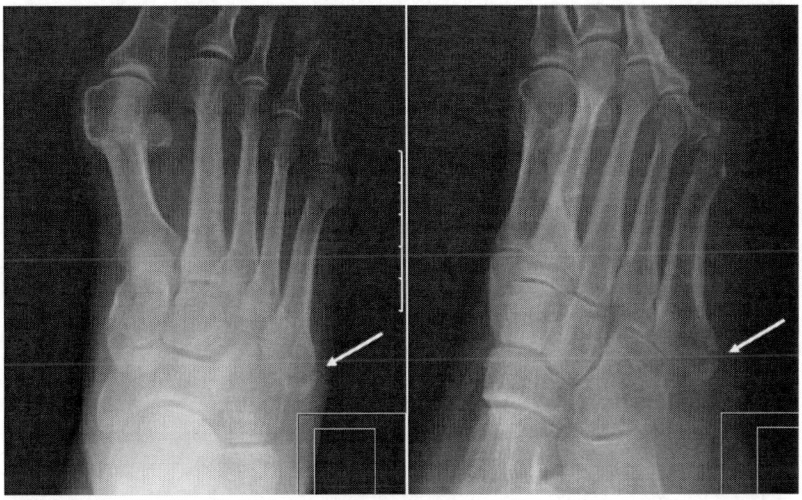

Figure 13. An antero-posterior and oblique radiograph of the right foot showing a tuberosity fracture at the base of the fifth metatarsal (arrows).

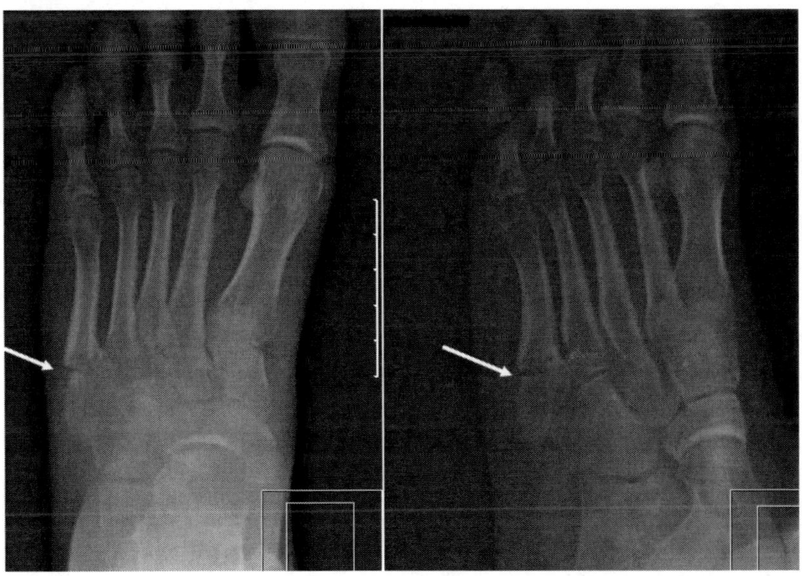

Figure 14. An antero-posterior and oblique radiograph of the left foot showing a Jones' fracture at the metaphyseal-diaphyseal junction at the base of the fifth metatarsal (arrows).

Avulsion fractures of the tuberosity are due to the pull of the lateral cord and peroneus brevis tendon following a twisting injury. The tuberosity receives blood from multiple metaphyseal vessels and branches of the nutrient artery and healing occurs easily with conservative management. In a large series of 288 tuberosity fractures, we have previously shown that these fractures heal well if managed symptomatically and none of them required surgery (Khan et al. 2006).

Jones' fractures were first described by Sir Robert Jones (1857-1933), an Orthopaedic Surgeon from London who himself sustained this injury dancing and these fractures have taken the eponymous name (Jones 1902). These fractures at the metaphyseal-diaphyseal junction occur within 1.5 cm of the tuberosity and can be acute fractures or stress fractures. A review of Jones' original case examples shows that the some radiographs meet the criteria of stress fractures. These fractures require prolong immobilisation and have a high propensity for delayed union and non-union. The treatment of choice for acute fractures is immobilisation of the limb in a below knee non-weight bearing plaster for six to eight weeks. Fractures with delayed union may eventually heal if treated non-operatively, although this may take up to 20 weeks. An active athlete will benefit from early surgery. Fractures with symptomatic non-union require surgery. Surgical procedures fall into two categories, medullary curettage and inlay grafting, and axial closed intra-medullary screw fixation (Khan et al. 2005).

Conclusion

The ankle and foot are functionally important and complex joints. The spectrum of injuries seen vary from stable injuries that can be managed non-operatively to unstable injuries that require surgical fixation. It is important to appreciate the functional anatomy and have an understanding of the imaging and classification systems used to decide on the appropriate management.

References

Al-Rashid M, Khan WS, Vermulapali K 2010 Principles of fracture fixation in orthopaedic trauma surgery *Journal of Perioperative Practice* 20 113-117.

Baird RA, Jackson ST 1987 Fractures of the distal part of the fibula with associated disruption of the deltoid ligament. Treatment without repair of the deltoid ligament *Journal of Bone and Joint Surgery* 69 1346-1352.

Bankart ASB 1942 Fractures of the os calcis *Lancet* 2 175.

Bhandari M, Guyatt GH, Siddiqui F et al., 2002 Treatment of acute Achilles tendon ruptures: a systematic overview and metaanalysis *Clinical Orthopaedics & Related Research* 400 190-200.

Bohler L 1931 Diagnosis, pathology, and treatment of fractures of the calcaneus *Journal of Bone and Joint Surgery* 13 75-89.

Coss HS, Manos RE, Buoncristiani A, Mills WJ 1998 Abduction stress and AP weightbearing radiography of purely ligamentous injury in the taros-metatarsal joint *Foot and Ankle International* 19 537-41.

Essex-Lopresti P 1993 The mechanism, reduction technique, and results in fractures of the os calcis *Clinical Orthopaedics* 290 3-16.

Gissane W 1947 Discussion on "Fractures of the os calcis." In Proceedings of the British Orthopaedic *Association Journal of Bone and Joint Surgery* 829 254-255.

Gougoulias N, Khanna A, McBride DJ, Maffulli N 2009 Management of calcaneal fractures: systematic review of randomized trials *British Medical Bulletin* 92 153-167.

Hatem SF 2008 Imaging of lisfranc injury and midfoot sprain *Radiology Clinics of North America* 46 1045-1060.

Jones R 1902 Fracture of the base of the fifth metatarsal bone by indirect violence *Annal of Surgery* 35 697-700.

Khan WS, Agarwal M, Warren-Smith C 2005 Management of fractures of the base of the fifth metatarsals distal to the tuberosity *The Foot Journal* 15 141-145.

Khan WS, Jain R, Agarwal M, Warren-Smith C 2006 Fractures of the base of the fifth metatarsal- a review of 322 patients *The Surgery Journal* 1 65-68.

Khan WS, Malik AA, Agarwal M, Dalal R 2007 Delayed open reduction and internal fixation of a neglected ankle fracture dislocation *International Journal of Clinical Practice* 61 594-595.

Kuo RS, Tejwani NC, Digiovanni CW et al., 2000 Outcome after open reduction and internal fixation of Lisfranc joint injuries *Journal of Bone and Joint Surgery* 82A 1609-1618.

Lauge-Hansen N 1950 Fractures of the ankle. II. Combined experimental-surgical and experimental-roentgenologic investigations *Archives of Surgery* 60 957-985.

Lundberg A, Goldie I, Kalin B et al., 1989 Kinematics of the ankle/foot complex: plantarflexion and dorsiflexion *Foot and Ankle* 9 194 200.

Maffulli N, Longo UG, Oliva F et al., 2009 Minimally invasive surgery of the achilles tendon Orthopaedic *Clinics of North America* 40 491-498.

Malik AA, Yousaf N, Khan W, Ihsan M, Ravenscroft M 2010 Fractures of the wrist and hand *Journal of Perioperative Practice* 20 48-54.

Malvankar S, Khan WS (2011). Evolution of the Achilles tendon: the athlete's Achilles heel? *Foot* (Edinb). 21(4): 193-7.

Micheslon JD 1995 Current Concepts Review; Fractures about the ankle *Journal of Bone and Joint Surgery* 77A 142-152.

Michelson JD, Ahn UM, Helgemo SL 1996 Ankle motion following simulated supination-external rotation fracture *Journal of Bone and Joint Surgery* 78A 1024-1031.

Michelson JD, Magid D, McHale K 2007 Clinical utility of a stability-based ankle fracture classification system *Journal of Orthopaedic Trauma* 21 307-315.

Miller SD 2000 Controversies in ankle fracture treatment. Indications for fixation of stable Weber type B fractures and indications for syndesmosis stabilization *Foot and Ankle Clinics* 5 841-851.

Nannaparaju MR, Khan WS, Vemulapall K. The Biomechanics of the Ankle Joint, pp 111-8, In Advances in Medicine and Biology, Volume 77, Editor Berhardt LV, 2014, Nova Science Publishers, New York.

Potter MQ, Nunley JA 2009 Long-Term Functional Outcomes After Operative Treatment for Intra-Articular *Fractures of the Calcaneus Journal of Bone and Joint Surgery* 91A 1854-1860.

Sanders R, Fortin P, DiPasquale T, Walling A 1993 Operative treatment in 120 displaced intraarticular calcaneal fractures *Clinical Orthopaedics* 290 87-95.

Schenck RC Jr, Heckman JD 1995 Fractures and Dislocations of the Forefoot: *Operative and Nonoperative Treatment Journal of the American Academy of Orthopaedic Surgeons* 3 70-78.

Schepers T, Ginai AZ, Van Lieshout EM, Patka P 2008 Demographics of extra-articular calcaneal fractures: including a review of the literature on treatment and outcome *Archives of Orthopaedics and Trauma Surgery* 128 1099-1106.

Strom AC, Casillas MM 2009 Achilles tendon rehabilitation *Foot and Ankle Clinics* 14 773-782.

van den Bekerom MP, Haverkamp D, Kloen P 2009 Biomechanical and clinical evaluation of posterior malleolar fractures. A systematic review of the literature *Journal of Trauma* 66 279-284.

van Staa TP, Dennison EM, Leufkens HG, Cooper C 2001 Epidemiology of fractures in England and Wales Bone 29 517-522.

Vuori JP, Aro HT 1993 Lisfranc joint injuries: trauma mechanisms and associated injuries Journal of Trauma 35 40-45.

Weber B G 1972 *Die Verletzungen des Oberen sprunggelenkes, 2nd Ed,* Verlag Hans Huber, Bern, Stuttgart, Wien.

CASE STUDIES

Case study 1

Mr DT, a 57 year old painter decorator fell off his ladder at work and was brought to A&E by ambulance with a closed fracture subluxation of his right ankle. He had not sustained any other injuries and had a past medical history of ischemic heart disease and chronic obstructive airways disease. On examination he had no distal neurovascular compromise. He had radiographs of his ankle performed to determine the exact nature of his injury and showing a Weber C fracture subluxation (Figure 4). In view of the unstable nature of the ankle injury a decision was made to treat the injury operatively following informed consent. The patient was operated on later that day under general anaesthetic, six hours after he had last eaten and drank. He had open reduction and internal fixation of his ankle (Figure 6) under tourniquet control at 300 mmHg and using an image intensifier. The patient was placed supine on the operating table with a sandbag under the ipsilateral buttock.

A lateral incision was made and the fibula fracture was identified. The fracture was held reduced with a lag screw applied across the fracture site. An eight-hole dynamic compression plate was applied across the fracture site acting as a neutralisation plate with three proximal and three distal bicortical screws. A medial incision was then made and the medial malleolus fracture was reduced. In view of the small size of the fragment, it was stabilised with one partially threaded cancellous screw. As the ankle remained unstable on stressing the syndesmosis, a syndesmosis screw was inserted from the fibula engaging the tibia. The wounds were then washed and closed. The skin was closed with non-absorbable sutures and a plaster backslab applied.

Postoperatively the patient was advised to continue with elevation to help reduce the swelling and allowed to partially weight bear. At one week follow-up, the plaster backslab was completed as the swelling had subsided and a check x-ray performed. At two weeks follow-up, the sutures were removed, the plaster reapplied and a further check x-ray performed. At six weeks follow-up, the patient had the syndesmosis screw removed under local anaesthetic and was allowed to commence full weight bearing mobilisation. In view of the restricted range of movement in his ankle he was referred for physiotherapy. At final follow-up six months following surgery, the patient had resumed a full range of movement in his ankle and had resumed his occupation. His metalwork was not causing him any problems and there are no plans to remove it.

Case study 2

Mrs GT, a 37 year old retail manager experienced sudden pain in the back of her right ankle when playing badminton and fell to the ground. She attended A&E and was diagnosed with a right sided achilles tendon rupture; she had a palpable gap in her achilles tendon and a positive Simmond's sign. She was otherwise fit and well and not on any medication. A radiograph of the ankle showed no fractures. Following a detailed discussion regarding the pros and cons of operative and nonoperative management, the patient opted for nonoperative management of her injury. This was because the patient was not a keen sportsperson and had only just started playing badminton. Her decision was also determined by the fact that she would have to stay in a plaster for the same length of time whether she was operated on or not.

The patient was placed in an equinus cast that was changed every two weeks. After eight weeks the plaster was removed and the patient allowed to commence mobilisation unaided. She was referred for physiotherapy and was doing well at six months follow-up. She had not resumed any sporting activities due to a change in her employment and social circumstances.

Case study 3

Mr AK, a 22 year old student sustained a crush injury to his left foot when a car wheel drove over it at slow speed. He presented to A&E with a painful swollen foot. He had not sustained any other injuries and had no significant past medical history. On examination he had a swollen foot with no wounds and no distal neurovascular compromise. Radiographs of his foot showed fractures of the first, second and third metatarsals (Figure 11). In view of the unstable nature of the foot injury a descision was made to manage the fractures with manipulation under anaesthetic and K-wire fixation (Figure 12) following informed consent. As the foot was swollen, he was admitted for elevation, analgesia and observation. The swelling subsided five days following admission and he was operated on under general anaesthetic, using a tourniquet at 300 mmHg and an image intensifier. The patient was placed supine on the operating table.

Fractures of the first second and third metatarsals were manipulated to a satisfactory position. Stab incisions were made at the medial aspect of the foot proximal and distal to the first metatarsal fracture, and at the plantar aspect of the foot at the site of the second and third metatarsal heads. Blunt dissection was performed to bone to avoid injury to neurovascular structures. Two K-wires of 1.8mm diameter were used to stabilise the first metatarsal fracture by engaging into the second and third metatarsals. Two further retrograde K-wires were then used to stabilise the second and third metatarsal fractures. The K-wires were then cut, dressings applied and the patient placed in a plaster backslab.

Postoperatively the patient was advised to continue with elevation to help reduce the swelling and advised to non-weight bear. At one week follow-up, the plaster backslab was completed as the swelling had subsided and a check x-ray performed. At six weeks follow-up, the patient had the plaster and K-wires removed in the fracture clinic and was allowed to commence full weight bearing mobilisation. He was referred for physiotherapy. At final follow-up six months following surgery, the patient was not limited in his activities of daily living and had made a complete recovery.

In: Perioperative Practice in Trauma and Orthopaedic Surgery ISBN: 978-1-63483-325-7
Editor: Wasim S. Khan

Chapter 18

ACUTE COMPARTMENT SYNDROME

W. S. Khan**, A. A. Malik, A. Chaudhry,
M. Ihsan and N. P. Cullen
Royal National Orthopaedic Hospital, Stanmore, Middlesex, UK

ABSTRACT

Acute compartment syndrome is a life and limb threatening condition.

Clinical assessment is the diagnostic cornerstone of compartment syndrome but pressure monitoring also has a role in equivocal cases, in unconscious or uncooperative patients, and patients with nerve blocks and other forms of regional and epidural anaesthesia. A high degree of suspicion and early decompression of all compartments at risk are important for a satisfactory outcome.

Keywords: Acute compartment syndrome, patient positioning, pressure monitoring

INTRODUCTION

This chapter outlines the pathophysiology, diagnosis and management of acute compartment syndrome (Malik et al. 2009, Mabvuure et al. 2012, Donaldson et al. 2014). Compartment syndrome has been defined as ‘a condition where the circulation and function of tissues within a closed space are compromised by an increase of pressure within that space’ (Matsen 1975). The closed space could be an osteo-fascial compartment of a limb that contains muscles and neurovascular structures and are lined with tough fibrous tissue called fascia, or it could be the abdominal cavity.

Richard von Volkmann first described compartment syndrome in 1881 leading to the eponymous naming of the forearm contracture. In 1926, Jepson described the management of

---

* Corresponding Author: Mr WS Khan, Clinical Lecturer, University College London Institute of Orthopaedics and Musculoskeletal Research, Royal National Orthopaedic Hospital, Stanmore, Middlesex, HA7 4LP, UK, Telephone number: +44 (0) 77791 025554, Fax number: +44 (0) 1707 655059, E-mail address: wasimkhan@doctors.org.uk.

the syndrome through fascial decompression. Further work was done by Bywaters et al., in 1941 on patients having suffered crush injuries during the London Blitz.

Compartment syndrome is seen most commonly after trauma, but is not necessarily only associated with fractures or indeed closed fractures (McQueen et al. 2000). The fractures most commonly associated with compartment syndrome are tibial fractures and forearm fractures (Newton & Love 2007). It is also seen following burns due to constriction of the skin and soft tissue swelling (Namias 2007), and following intra-operative patient malpositioning (Wilde 2004). Acute compartment syndrome is a surgical emergency that requires urgent recognition and treatment to avoid ischaemic contractures, amputation, multi-organ failure or death. The potential to produce long-term disability in a patient also has important medicolegal implications, particularly as the complications are avoidable.

PATHOPHYSIOLOGY

A rising compartment pressure leads to increased interstitial tissue pressure, collapse of thin-walled veins and decreased capillary blood flow. If not addressed, this increase in pressure subsequently leads to ischaemia, and ischaemia leads to further cellular injury and inflammation further increasing the compartment pressure. Eventually the metabolic demands of the tissue are no longer met and necrosis sets in. Cellular hypoxia results in anaerobic respiration and rhabdomyolysis. Left untreated, this can lead to renal failure, multi-organ failure and death. In patients with early compartment syndrome, hyperbaric oxygen therapy may reduce the number of cells at risk from ischemia. Animal experiments and preliminary human studies have suggested benefits of such therapy but more data is needed before this could be used in routine clinical practice (Greensmith 2004).

Research has shown that compartment syndrome lasting for longer than 12 hours can produce chronic functional deficits, contractures, muscle weakness and sensory changes, but if decompression is performed in less than 6 hours a full recovery is likely (Matsen 1975, McQueen et al. 1996, Mullet et al. 2001). It is difficult however to clinically determine the time of onset of compartment syndrome.

AETIOLOGY

An application of external pressure or an increase in internal volume within the compartment can result in a progressive increase in the pressure within the compartment and subsequent impairment in tissue perfusion (Khan et al. 2007). Application of external pressure could be from tight dressings, casts and tourniquets, or from pressure on malpositioned limbs intra-operatively. Increase in internal volume within the compartment could be from bleeding due to injury or coagulopathy, swelling, venous obstruction or incorrect administration of intravenous fluids (Roberge & McLane 1999). Compartment syndrome may also be seen in patients with eclampsia and nephrotic syndrome.

Lower leg compartment syndrome can occur due to external pressure during the lithotomy position. Compartment syndrome has been described in gynaecological, urological or abdominal operations performed in the Lloyd-Davis position. Pressure in the anterior compartments of the lower legs reaches 30mmHg when the legs are placed in the lithotomy position for over four hours. The pressure is further increased with Trendelenburg positioning (Chase et al. 2000). Obesity and long operation times have also been associated with gluteal compartment syndrome (Bostanjian et al. 2003).

More research is needed to determine clear guidelines on patient positioning during surgery (Beraldo & Dodds 2006). Nevertheless, a heightened awareness of positioning the patient on the operating table, attention to intra-operative padding and limiting the duration of the operation are all important factors that can lead to prevention of this intra-operative complication. Removing the limbs from the stirrups and placing them in the supine position allows the pressure in the compartments to return to normal and should be considered in all surgical procedures lasting more than four hours (Chase et al. 2000). There is still debate on the intra-operative use of pulse oximetry to detect hypoperfusion in the limb and the appropriate use of sequential compression devices and anti-thromboembolic stockings.

Clinical Diagnosis

Evaluation of a patient with suspected compartment syndrome is of utmost importance given the potential for limb and life threatening damage (Köstler et al. 2004). The diagnosis relies on a careful history and examination, and requires a high index of suspicion. Particular attention should be paid to the mechanism of injury, the energy involved, the presence of fractures, crush injuries, vascular insults and coagulopathies. The classical signs used to aid the diagnosis of compartment syndrome are pain, pallor, paraesthesia, paralysis, pulselessness, pressure and poikilothermia. This should however only be used as a guide rather than an absolute as the presence or absence of one or more of these is not conclusive. Patients typically exhibit pain out of proportion to the clinical situation, pain on passive stretching of the muscle compartment, altered sensation, muscle weakness, and tense and tender compartments (Olson & Glasgow 2005).

It must be stressed that the diagnosis of compartment syndrome in most cases should be solely made on clinical grounds and delay to obtain further information through other investigations should not delay treatment. Although simple blood biochemistry may be useful e.g. creative kinase levels to assess muscle breakdown and clotting studies to assess coagulopathy, there are few imaging studies of value in the diagnosis of compartment syndrome. The symptoms may be confused with deep vein thrombosis and a Doppler ultrasound scan may be useful.

Compartment Pressure Measurement

In 1976, Mubarak et al., described compartment pressure monitoring to aid the diagnosis of compartment syndrome. Certain patient groups cannot be adequately assessed clinically and require compartment pressure measurements. These include unconscious or uncooperative patients, patients with distracting injuries, young children where history may be difficult to obtain. Patients who have undergone certain anesthetic techniques, such as nerve blocks and other forms of regional and epidural anesthesia, that have been reported to contribute to a delay in diagnosis, also benefit from pressure measurements (Olsen & Glasgow 2005). There are various techniques available for the measurements and monitoring of compartment pressures. These include the Whitesides method that uses a needle, plastic tubes and a mercury manometer (Whitesides et al. 1975). The solid state transducer has a multiperforated tip that prevents blocking and improves reliability, and a pressure transducer that allows continuous monitoring (McDermott et al. 1984). Moed & Thorderson in 1993 compared various methods of measuring compartment pressure and found good results with a side ported needle and slit catheters compared with straight needles. Predictably various devices make use of such a needle including the Stryker portable intra-compartmental pressure monitor. In the absence of such equipment transducer tip catheters, infusion techniques or central venous pressure monitors may be used (Boody & Wongworawat 2005). Possible future developments include noninvasive compartment measurement devices including near-infrared spectroscopy and laser Doppler flowmetry (Singh et al. 2004). Another important consideration in measuring compartment pressures is accurate tip placement. The lower leg is one of the commonest sites for compartment syndrome following tibial fractures and contains four compartments. The anterior compartment is most susceptible to compartment syndrome followed by the deep posterior compartment (McQueen et al. 1996). The perfusion of the compartment depends on the difference between the diastolic blood pressure and the compartment pressure. Normal interstitial tissue pressure is 0-10mmHg but this can rise significantly in compartment syndrome. The difference between diastolic blood pressure and compartment pressure is called the delta pressure. Studies have suggested that a delta pressure of less than 30mmHg is an indication for an urgent decompression of the fascial compartment (Matsen & Clawson 1975, McQueen & Court-Brown 1996).

MANAGEMENT

Immediate management involves identification of external compressive forces, and circumferential or constricting casts and dressings should be released entirely to alleviate pressure on the compartment.

The limb should be placed at heart level. If the limb is elevated above this, blood flow to the limb may be reduced increasing ischaemia (Matsen et al. 1980). Early assessment of hypovolaemia, metabolic acidosis and myoglobinaemia is also necessary to prevent impending renal failure.

This may be done by administration of intravenous fluids and supplemental oxygen, regular blood biochemistry and urinalysis. It is important to maintain normotension as hypotension reduces perfusion pressure and leads to tissue injury. However these measures should not delay definitive treatment of compartment syndrome and rather should be performed adjunctively. If the clinical symptoms do not improve, definitive treatment involves fasciotomy, with orthopaedic and vascular management of other injuries e.g. fracture fixation, to relieve the pressure within the compartment. Adequate decompression should not be compromised by cosmesis.

Upper Limb

The commonest presentation of compartment syndrome in the upper limb is in the forearm following a supracondylar humeral fracture (Seiler et al. 2000). It was following such a fracture that a patient developed a contracture that was initially described by Volkmann in 1881. There are four compartments in the forearm: the deep and superficial volar compartments, the dorsal extensor compartment and the mobile wad compartment. The volar compartments are more often affected. In addition there are six dorsal extensor compartments at the wrist with the carpal tunnel and compartments containing flexor carpi ulnaris, flexor carpi radialis and palmaris longus tendons passing on the volar aspect of the wrist. In the forearm, fasciotomy of all compartments can be performed using two incisions, volar and dorsal. The volar incision follows the volar surgical approach to the radius, and the dorsal incision begins 2cm distal to the lateral epicondyle and is carried to the wrist. If necessary these can be extended proximally and distally to involve the upper arm and hand. The hand contains ten separate compartments (Boles et al. 2000) that may be released with a carpal tunnel release and two dorsal incisions. Further individual digital incisions may also be necessary.

Lower Limb

Thigh compartment syndrome is uncommon due to the large potential for accommodating fluid volumes and the possibility for extravasation of blood outside the compartment given that the fascia bounding the compartment blends with the muscles around the hip joint.

Tibial fractures are commonly encountered fractures and a frequent cause of compartment syndrome in the lower leg (DeLee & Stiehl 1981). The compartments in the lower leg consist of the anterior, lateral, superficial posterior and deep posterior compartments. Compartment syndrome of the deep posterior compartment also has associations with compartment syndrome of the foot. In the lower leg, all four compartments can be reached by the use of two incisions, medial and lateral and at least 15cm. The lateral incision is made midway between the anterior tibia and fibula and allows release of the anterior and medial compartments. The medial incision is based 2cm behind the posterolateral border of the tibia and fasciotomy here allows release of the deep and superficial posterior compartments (Singh et al. 2004).

The existence of nine foot compartments and the frequent presence of associated foot fractures and other complicating injuries producing pain, swelling and paraesthesia necessitate multiple compartment pressure measurements. The approaches for compartment decompression generally include two dorsal incisions for decompression of the forefoot compartments, one medial incision for decompression of the calcaneal, medial and superficial compartment and a lateral incision for decompression of the lateral compartments (Fulkerson et al. 2003).

Post-operatively, the limb needs to be elevated and regular inspections are necessary for the open wounds. Primary closure of wounds is uncommon and generally secondary closure is carried out (Wiger et al. 1998), but this may be difficult due to skin retraction and swelling.

Split skin grafts may also be used if wound edges cannot be approximated, and this has been shown to have fewer complication rates when compared to primary or secondary would closure (Johnson et al. 1992).

ABDOMEN

Abdominal compartment syndrome is defined as an intra-abdominal pressure of greater than 20mmHg with evidence of organ dysfunction (Malbrain et al. 2007). Abdominal compartment syndrome may be due to a primary abdominal cause e.g. gross intra-abdominal or retroperitoneal haemorrhage, severe gut oedema and intestinal obstruction, or a secondary cause e.g. pathology outside the abdomen. A massive fluid resuscitation, as often seen following trauma, has been associated with secondary abdominal compartment syndrome (Balogh et al. 2007). The presentation is usually of abdominal pain and distension. Increased intra-abdominal pressure causes venous stasis and reduced arterial perfusion of all intra- and extra-abdominal organs resulting in ischemia, hypoxia and necrosis (Lerner 2008). Respiratory, cardiovascular, renal, intestinal and cerebral decompensation can also occur, and multiorgan failure has a mortality rate of 60-70%. The diagnosis can be confirmed by the measurement of intra-abdominal pressure, either by a Foley catheter into the bladder or a naso-gastric tube in the stomach. It occurs most commonly following major trauma and complex surgical procedures, but can also occur in their absence (Harrisson et al. 2008).

An early multidisciplinary approach is essential in the management of this complex condition to ensure a good outcome. Definitive treatment is decompression at laparotomy.

Sudden release of the abdominal compartment syndrome may lead to an ischaemic reperfusion injury causing acidosis, cardiac dysfunction and cardiac arrest.

Primary closure of the abdominal wall is generally not possible due to tissue loss and retraction of the abdominal wall. Reconstruction is generally delayed until infection and swelling have resolved. Recent developments in negative suction wound dressings, bioprosthetics and new surgical techniques like component separation result in less donor site morbidity. There is however still a place for local and distant flaps (Libberecht et al. 2007).

Prevention and recognition of abdominal compartment syndrome are crucial to avoid additional morbidity and mortality. Abdominal compartment syndrome complicates current resuscitation methods and new strategies for resuscitating critically ill patients need to be explored in addition to more accurate monitoring of intra-abdominal pressure (Cheatham 2008).

COMPLICATIONS

Patients need to be carefully observed and monitored for complications of compartment syndrome. Complications can be divided into systemic and local. Systemic complications include metabolic acidosis, reperfusion injury, acute renal failure, systemic inflammatory response syndrome, acute respiratory distress syndrome, multi-organ failure and death. Local complications include infection, contracture, neurological deficit and amputation (Matsen et al. 1980, Olson & Glasgow 2005).

CONCLUSION

Acute compartment syndrome is a life and limb threatening condition that could result from external pressure e.g. on a malpositioned anaesthetised patient, or from intra-compartmental rises in pressure e.g. from bleeding or swelling associated with fractures. Clinical assessment is the diagnostic cornerstone of compartment syndrome. Compartment pressure monitoring can confirm the diagnosis in suspected patients and may have a role in the diagnosis in unconscious or uncooperative patients, and patients with nerve blocks and other forms of regional and epidural anesthesia. Research suggests that a delta pressure of 30mmHg or less is an accepted level to perform a fasciotomy. A high degree of suspicion and early decompression of all compartments at risk are important for a satisfactory outcome.

REFERENCES

Balogh Z, Moore FA, Moore EE, Biffl WL 2007 Secondary abdominal compartment syndrome: a potential threat for all trauma clinicians. *Injury* 38 272-279.

Beraldo S, Dodds SR 2006 Lower limb acute compartment syndrome after colorectal surgery in prolonged lithotomy position. *Diseases of the Colon & Rectum* 49 1772-1780.

Boody AR, Wongworawat MD 2005 Accuracy in the measurement of compartment pressures: a comparison of three commonly used devices. *Journal of Bone and Joint Surgery* 87 2415-2422.

Boles CA, Kannam S, Cardwell AB 2000 The forearm anatomy of muscle compartments and nerves. *American Journal of Roentgenology* 174 151-159.

Bostanjian D, Anthone GJ, Hamoui N, Crookes PF 2003 Rhabdomyolysis of gluteal muscles leading to renal failure: a potentially fatal complication of surgery in the morbidly obese. *Obesity Surgery* 13 302-305.

Bywaters EG, Delory GE, Rimington C, Smiles J 1941 Myohaemoglobin in the urine of air raid casualties with crushing injury. *Biochemistry Journal* 35 1164-1168.

Chase J, Harford F, Pinzur MS, Zussman M 2000 Intraoperative lower extremity compartment pressures in lithotomy-positioned patients. *Diseases of the Colon & Rectum* 43 678-680.

Cheatham ML 2008 Intraabdominal pressure monitoring during fluid resuscitation. *Current Opinion in Critical Care* 14 327-333.

DeLee JC, Stiehl JB 1981 Open tibia fracture with compartment syndrome. *Clinical Orthopaedics & Related Research* 160 175-184.

Donaldson J, Haddad B, Khan WS (2014). The Pathophysiology, Diagnosis and Current Management of Acute Compartment Syndrome. The Open Orthop J. 8: 185-93.

Fulkerson E, Razi A, Tejwani N 2003 Review: acute compartment syndrome of the foot. *Foot & Ankle International* 24 180-187.

Greensmith JE 2004 Hyperbaric oxygen therapy in extremity trauma *Journal of the American Academy of Orthopaedic Surgeons* 12 376-384.

Harrisson SE, Smith JE, Lambert AW, Midwinter MJ 2008 Abdominal compartment syndrome: an emergency department perspective. *Emergency Medical Journal* 25 128-132.

Jepson PN 1926 Ischaemic contracture: experimental study. *Annals of Surgery* 84 785-795.

Johnson SB, Weaver FA, Yellin AE, Kelly R, Bauer M 1992 Clinical results of decompressive dermotomy-fasciotomy. *American Journal of Surgery* 164 286-290.

Sobajo C, Khan WS, Sochart DH 2007 A diagnostic dilemma: a patient presenting with a painful swollen leg. *The Cardiolgy Journal* 3 24-26.

Köstler W, Strohm PC, Südkamp NP 2004 Acute compartment syndrome of the limb. *Injury* 35 1221-1227.

Lerner SM 2008 Review article: the abdominal compartment syndrome. *Alimentary Pharmacology &Therapeutics* 28 377-384.

Libberecht K, Colpaert SD, Van Hee R et al., 2007 New developments in abdominal wall reconstruction after abdominal compartment syndrome decompression. *Acta Clinica Belgica Supplements* 1 220-224.

Mabvuure NT, Malahias M, Hindocha S, Khan WS, Juma A (2012). Acute Compartment Syndrome of the Limbs: Current Concepts and Management. *Open Orthop J.* 6: 535-43. PMID: 23248724.

Malbrain ML, De laet I, Cheatham M 2007 Consensus conference definitions and recommendations on intra-abdominal hypertension (IAH) and the abdominal compartment syndrome (ACS)- the long road to the final publications, how did we get there? *Acta Clinica Belgica Supplements* 1 44-59.

Malik AA, Khan WS, Chaudhry A, Ihsan M, Cullen NP (2009). Acute Compartment Syndrome- A Life and Limb Threatening Surgical Emergency. *J Perioper Pract.* 19(5): 137-42.

Matsen FA 3rd 1975 Compartmental syndrome. An unified concept. *Clinical Orthopaedics & Related Research* 113 8-14.

Matsen FA 3rd, Clawson DK 1975 The deep posterior compartmental syndrome of the leg. *Journal of Bone & Joint Surgery* 57A 34-39.

Matsen FA 3rd, Winquist RA, Krugmire RB Jr 1980 Diagnosis and management of compartmental syndromes. *Journal of Bone & Joint Surgery* 62A 286-291.

McDermott AGP, Marble AE, Yabsley RH 1984 Monitoring acute compartment pressures with the STIC catheter. *Clinical Orthopaedics* 190 192-198.

McQueen MM, Christie J, Court-Brown CM 1996 Acute compartment syndrome in tibial diaphyseal fractures. *Journal of Bone & Joint Surgery* 78B 95-98.

McQueen MM, Court-Brown CM 1996 Compartment monitoring in tibial fractures: the pressure threshold for decompression. *Journal of Bone & Joint Surgery* 78B 99-104.

McQueen MM, Gaston P, Court-Brown CM 2000 Acute compartment syndrome: who is at risk? *Journal of Bone & Joint Surgery* 82B 200-203.

Mubarak SJ, Hargens AR, Owen CA, Garetto LP, Akeson WH 1976 The wick catheter technique for measurement of intramuscular pressure. *Journal of Bone & Joint Surgery* 58A 1016-1020.

Moed BR, Thorderson PK 1993 Measurement of intracompartmental pressure: a comparison of the slit catheter, side-ported needle, and simple needle. *Journal of Bone & Joint Surgery* 75A 231-235.

Mullet H, Al-Abed K, Prasad CVR, O'Sullivan M 2001 Outcome of compartment syndrome following intramedullary nailing of tibial diaphyseal fractures *Injury* 32 411-413.

Namias N 2007 Advances in burn care. *Current Opinions in Critical Care* 13 405-410.

Newton EJ, Love J 2007 Acute complications of extremity trauma. *Emergency Medicine Clinics of North America* 25 751-761.

Olson SA, Glasgow RR 2005 Acute compartment syndrome in lower extremity musculoskeletal trauma. *Journal of the American Academy of Orthopaedic Surgeons* 13 436-444.

Roberge RJ, McLane M 1999 Compartment syndrome after simple venupuncture in an anticoagulated patient. *Journal of Emergency Medicine* 17 647-649.

Seiler JG 3rd, Casey PJ, Binford SH 2000 Compartment syndromes of the upper extremity. *Journal of the Southern Orthopaedic Association* 9 233-247.

Singh S, Trikha SP, Lewis J 2004 Acute compartment syndrome. *Current Orthopaedics* 18 468-476.

Volkmann R 1881 Die ischaemischem muskellamungen und kontrakturen. *Zentralblatt für Chirurgie* 8 801.

Whitesides TE, Haney TC, Morimoto K, Harada H 1975 Tissue pressure measurements as a determinant for the need of fasciotomy. *Clinical Orthopaedics* 113 43-51.

Wiger P, Tkaczuk P, Styf JJ 1998 Secondary wound closure following fasciotomy for acute compartment syndrome increases intramuscular pressure. *Orthopaedic Trauma* 12 117-121.

Wilde S 2004 Compartment syndrome: the silent danger related to patient positioning and surgery. *British Journal of Perioperative Nursing* 14 546-550.

In: Perioperative Practice in Trauma and Orthopaedic Surgery ISBN: 978-1-63483-325-7
Editor: Wasim S. Khan

Chapter 19

SURGICAL MANAGEMENT OF FRACTURED NECK OF FEMUR

Atif A. Malik, Peter Kell, Wasim S. Khan* and Paul Dunkow

Blackpool Victoria Hospital, Whinney Heys Road, Blackpool, UK

ABSTRACT

Fractured necks of femur are becoming increasingly common with an ageing population. These fractures could be divided into intra-capsular and extra-capsular fractures. The management of these fractures varies significantly depending on the patient and fracture configuration including location and displacement. In this chapter we discuss the surgical management of these fractures.

Keywords: Surgery, fracture, neck of femur, intra-capsular, extra-capsular

INTRODUCTION

In this chapter we discuss the surgical management of fractured neck of femur (Malik et al. 2009). The fractured neck of femur is the classically described fracture in osteoporotic elderly patients. Further, the fracture has a strong predominance in post-menopausal women and although relatively uncommon in both children and young adults, where present in this age group it is usually the result of significant trauma. In elderly patients, with an already weakened bone, even minimal trauma may be sufficient to cause fracture and as such a fractured neck of femur is often referred to as a fragility fracture.

---

* Corresponding Author: Mr Wasim S Khan, Clinical Lecturer, University College London Institute of Orthopaedics and Musculoskeletal Science, Royal National Orthopaedic Hospital, Stanmore, Middlesex, London, HA7 4LP, UK, Telephone number: +44 (0) 7791 025554, Fax number +44 (0) 20 8570 3864, E-mail address: wasimkhan@doctors.org.uk.

The femur is the largest and strongest bone in the body. Proximally it forms the hip joint by articulating with the acetabulum of the pelvis whereas distally it articulates with the tibia, fibula and patella at the knee joint. The proximal third of the femur can be divided into specific regions and the key to understanding the management of the fractured neck of femur lies in understanding the anatomy of these specific regions.

The head of femur is a hemi-spherical structure, extending upwards and medially from the neck. The surface is smooth and covered with articular cartilage to articulate with the cup shaped acetabulum. The neck of femur however is a flattened pyramid of bone connecting the head to the body of the femur. It is widest at the base and runs at an angle of about 125° from the shaft to the head (Rockwood et al. 2001). The joint capsule inserts onto the neck near the base. The greater and lesser trochanters are prominent processes and it is here that muscles involved in movement of the hip joint attach. The area between the two trochanters is termed the inter-trochanteric region.

Distally the shaft of femur is an almost cylindrical region of the bone, curved slightly to be convex anteriorly and concave, and slightly flattened, posteriorly.

The blood supply to the head of the femur arises from the Profunda Femoris Artery (a branch of the Femoral Artery) and can be divided into three routes of supply (Snell 2003): Firstly and most importantly, vessels running in the retinaculum of the joint capsule that enter the femur at the base of the neck. The place of entry of these blood vessels into the femur is particularly important when considering fractures as any fracture above the level where these vessels enter the femur may lead to vascular insufficiency of the proximal head. Secondly, the intramedullary vessels that run within the bone. And finally the artery of the ligamentum teres femoris, a small nutrient artery which runs in the ligament which connects the head of the femur to the acetabulum. This only minimally contributes to the blood supply in elderly patients and in fact may be absent.

There are two main mechanisms of injury leading fractures in this region, either a rotational injury at the hip joint which tends to give rise to intra-capsular fractures or direct impact injury to the lateral aspect of the hip, leading to extra-capsular fractures (Rockwood et al. 2001, Felciano 2004). Intra-capsular fractures may result in disruption in the blood supply from vessels derived from both the capsule and the intramedullary vessels, leaving only the minimal supply of the ligamentum teres (Snell 2003). Intra-capsular fractures are additionally complicated by the nature of the bone within the capsule as intra-articular bone has only thin periosteum and no soft tissue contact hindering callus formation (Feliciano 2004). Further bleeding from the fracture site into the capsule results in a haemarthrosis, increasing intra-capsular pressure and further hindering healing. These factors lead to a high risk of avascular necrosis (AVN).

Intra-capsular fractures are further sub-classified into sub-capital (at the level between the head and the neck of the femur), transcervical (through the neck of the femur) and baso-cervical (at the level between the neck and the body of the femur). Baso-cervical fractures are technically extra-capsular, but as they often extend into the transcervical region and the associated soft tissue damage can involve disruption of the capsule. This means that they are often treated as intra-capsular fractures. A method of classifying intra-capsular fractures is with Garden's classification giving four groups (Garden 1964) as shown in Figure 1.

In practice, the real question to be answered affecting the subsequent management of the patient is to whether the fracture is undisplaced or displaced. The answer effectively groups Garden's 1 and 2 fractures separately from the displaced Garden's 3 and 4 fractures.

However with extra-capsular fractures, due to the site of the break, the blood supply from the capsule remains intact (Snell 2003). This gives a much more reliable blood supply to the head to allow for healing and avoiding the other complications mentioned of an intra-capsular fracture. Once an accurate assessment of both the patient and the type of fracture is made, a surgical management plan can be initiated. Intra-capsular fractures are generally (though obviously not solely) treated in one of five ways namely non-operatively, hemi-arthroplasty, a dynamic compression hip screw (DHS), cannulated hip screws or a intra-medullary hip screw (Haidukewych 2004, Leighton 2007, Lee 2008). In extremely fit and active elderly patients who enjoy a reasonable quality of life, there is also a case for primary total hip replacement (Gebhard 1992). Given the severe compromise in the blood supply to the femoral head femoral neck fractures, and the potential for restoration of blood flow following reduction, it is generally advised to proceed with reduction and fixation of femoral neck fractures as soon as possible (Arnoldi 1972, Arnoldi 1977, Strömqvist 1984).

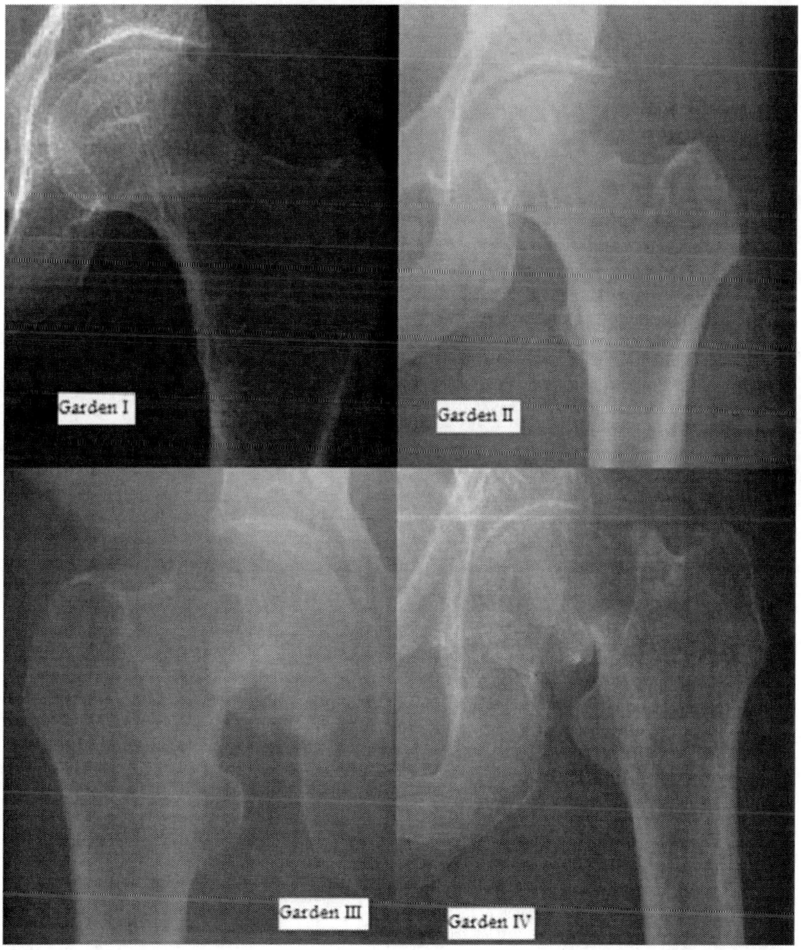

Figure 1. Garden classification with Grade I: Incomplete fracture with minimal displacement, Grade II: Complete, but undisplaced, Grade III: Complete and partially displaced, and Grade IV: Complete and displaced.

Undisplaced intra-capsular fractures generally require cannulated hip screws or a 2 hole DHS. There is a however an ever present risk of AVN which approaches 20% and therefore there is a reasonable chance that this group of patients may require further intervention at some time in the future (Linde 1986, Nikolopoulos 2003). In patients who perhaps may be non-compliant to medical advice or who have significant other health problems and where a further procedure would be medically unsafe, hemi-arthroplasty may be more prudent as a primary definitive procedure rather than cannulated screw/ DHS.

Where cannulated hip screws are used, the fracture is fixed by passing several (usually three) cannulated screws across the fracture site, creating a compression force holding the head onto the neck. This technique can be performed either percutaneously or through a minimal incision. This requires that the fracture be anatomically reduced prior to the commencement of surgery, on a fracture table where the fracture can be manipulated into the correct position under x-ray guidance.

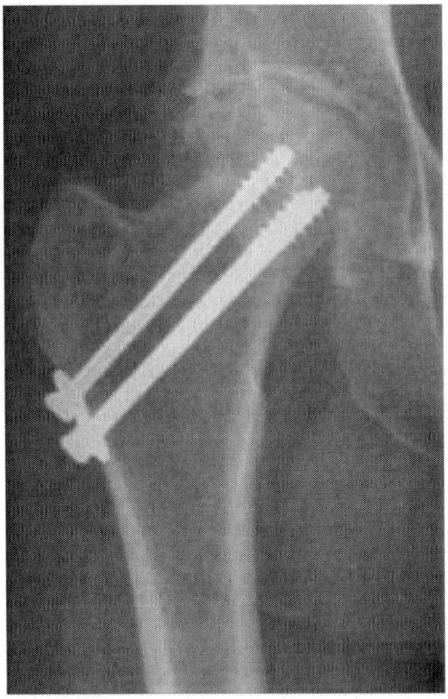

Figure 2. Avascular necrosis following cannulated screw fixation.

Displaced intra-capsular fractures almost always require a hemi-arthroplasty due to the high risk of AVN (Frihagen 2007) (Figure 2). The hemi-arthroplasty is used to replace the femoral head with a prosthesis. The exception to this is in the younger patient where it is preferable to attempt a cannulated screw fixation in order to preserve the patients natural hip. With the high risk of AVN (up to 40%) in this group, this needs to be carried out quickly in order to minimise the disruption of the blood supply to the femoral head (Nikolopoulos 2003). Although the risk of failure may seem high, in the younger patient, this percentage is deemed acceptable given that the alternative is to take out a young patients natural hip joint and replace it with a prosthesis with its own set of problems.

Generally the prosthesis used in the majority of hip hemi-arthroplasty is the cemented Thompsons prosthesis. However other fixation techniques have been employed namely a stable "press fit" between the femoral canal/ implant and also stimulating bone to grow on or into the prosthesis e.g., the Austin- Moore (Figure 3).

The use of cement offers definite advantages in the treatment of hip fracture patients. Cementing the prosthesis in place offers immediate interface stability between implant and bone. This is generally associated with reduced pain compared to a un-cemented prostheses, and there is no need to restrict weight bearing post-op, allowing faster rehabilitation. The decreased bone density and expanded canal of older, osteoporotic patients may prevent achievement of the mechanical stability that is required for a fixation dependent on in-growth of bone or a press-fit fixation.

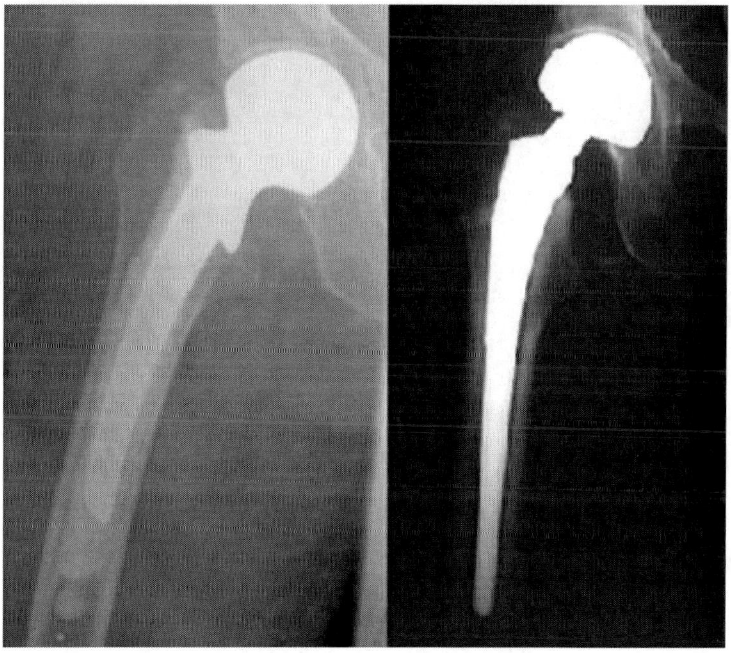

Figure 3. Cemented Unipolar Hemiarthroplasty and Uncemented Bipolar Hemiarthroplasty

Uncemented prostheses are usually used in relatively ill patients who already have poor mobility (i.e., bed to chair). The uncemented technique is a much faster operation minimising the risks of anaesthetic, and also eliminating the cardiovascular risk of cement, and the already poor mobility of the patient reduces the impact of a period of non-weight bearing on the rehabilitation of the patient.

The other distinction to comprehend when working with hemi-arthroplasty implants is the difference between uni-polar and bipolar implants. The majority of hemi-arthroplasty implants are of a uni-polar nature i.e. the stem and head of the prosthesis are one complete unit. There have, however, been reports of problems with acetabular wear, particularly in younger patients with longer lifespans and greater activity levels than the typically described older, osteoporotic fractured neck of femur patient. Gilberty & Bateman first reported the use of a bipolar prosthesis. In a bipolar prosthesis the head is separate from the stem and also consists of a large metallic acetabular cup containing a polyethylene component with an articular cavity into which the metallic femoral head is locked into place. This allows for two articular sites giving a greater range of movement and reducing wear on the acetabulum (Nottage 1990, LaBelle 1990). The other advantage of this design is that, should the patient require a total hip replacement in the future, the head of the bipolar hemi-arthroplasty can be removed and, providing the stem remains stably fixed in the femoral canal, the stem can be re-used for the total hip replacement, greatly simplifying what would be a difficult revision procedure.

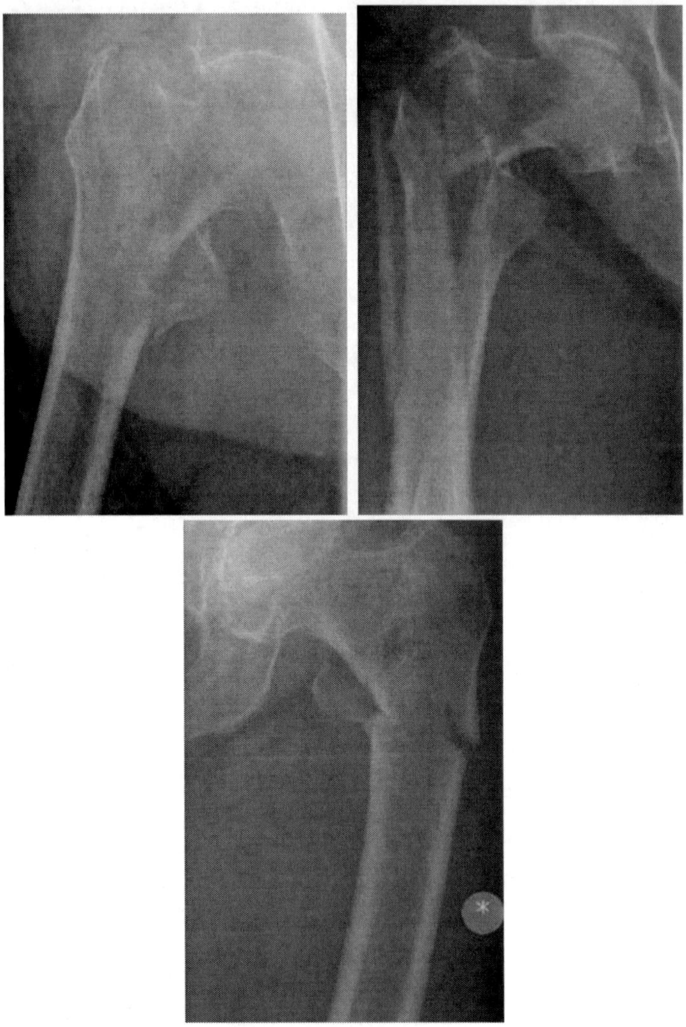

Figure 4. Extra-capsular fractures can be inter-trochanteric, inter-trochanteric with sub- trochanteric extension or sub-trochanteric.

The surgical approaches most commonly used for hemi-arthroplasty are either the antero-lateral approach or the posterior approach. In both of these the patient is positioned on their side on the operating table, with the injured side up. Both approaches have their exponents, however the evidence is divided as to whether or not there is any benefit of one over the other, and so it usually comes down to surgical preference (Juttmann 1991, Keene 1993, Lu-Yao 1994).

Extra-capsular fractures (Figure 4) may be either inter-trochanteric or sub-trochanteric. Inter-trochanteric fractures are usually treated with a dynamic hip screw (DHS). Sub-trochanteric fractures may be thought of as fractures of the shaft of the femur, rather than true neck of femur fractures and are classified as either transverse or spiral/oblique. Spiral fractures are usually treated with a long plate DHS, and transverse fractures with an intra-medullary nail (Kraemer 1996).

Dynamic hip screws are used for fixation of fractures of the inter-trochanteric region, and may also be used in both base of cervical fractures and occasionally in Garden 1 or 2 fractures. Occasionally this device is used with the addition of a derotation pin or screw (Lee 2008, Abalo 2008, Chen 2008). The screw is a large cancellous lag screw that glides freely in a metal sleeve. The sleeve is continuous with a side plate that is fixed to the lateral cortex of the femoral shaft with screws. Weight bearing causes the femoral head to become impacted onto the femoral neck producing dynamic compression of the fracture. The shaft of the lag screw slides down the sleeve maintaining reduction of the fracture as compression occurs.

Dynamising the fracture site stimulates bone healing, and the impaction produces a stable fixation, often allowing immediate weight-bearing, simplifying the rehabilitation procedure (Koval 1996). The lag screw has little resistance to torsion, therefore the torque required to insert it can spin the femoral head, causing vascular damage. In those cases where there is a risk of rotation of the head the use of a derotation wire or screw is recommended (Figure 5).

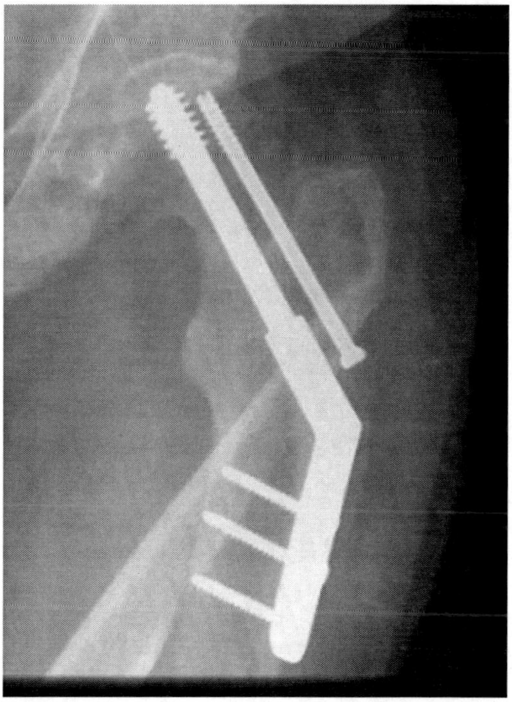

Figure 5. Dynamic hip screw fixation with de-rotation screw.

In those inter-trochanteric fractures in which there is sub-trochanteric extension, or in spiral sub-trochanteric fractures a long plate DHS may be used (Trafton 1987, Mullaji 1993). In this prosthesis the plate is lengthened to extend well past the fracture site in order to provide a stable fixation. The application of a DHS requires that the fracture be anatomically reduced prior to the commencement of surgery (Figure 6). This is best achieved on a fracture table where the fracture can be manipulated into the correct position under x-ray guidance.

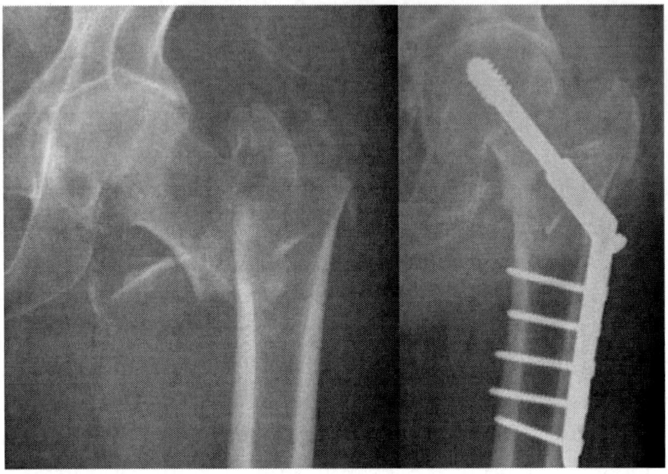

Figure 6. Long plate dynamic hip screw for subtrochanteric fracture.

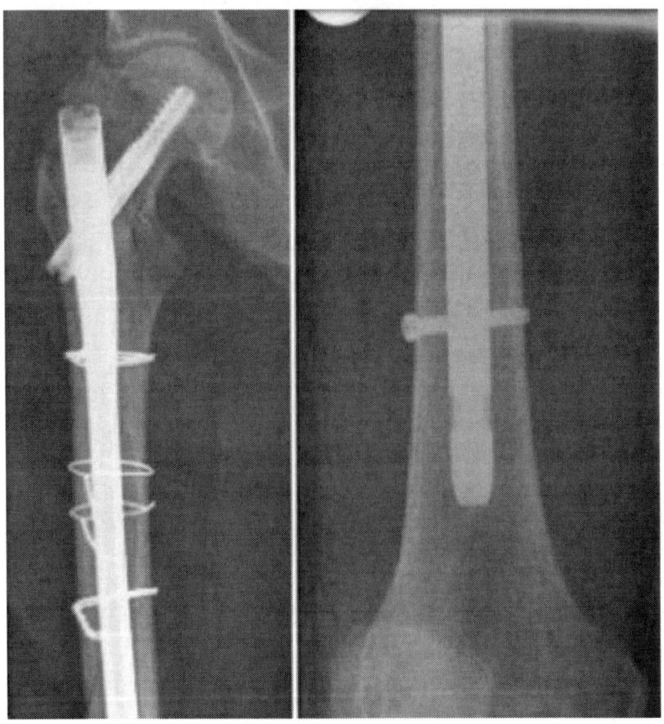

Figure 7. Gamma nail fixation.

Where there is any extension of the fracture into the sub-trochanteric region or in those fractures with severe comminution of the medial cortex, a long intra-medullary device such as a Gamma nail can be used (French 1998) as shown in Figure 7. Here the patient is positioned supine on the operating table and the nail is inserted into the femur in an ante-grade fashion. The point of entry is either through the greater trochanter, or through the piriformis fossa. The nail is passed down the shaft of the femur and a lag screw is passed through the nail into the head, along the neck of the femur. Proximal and distal lag screws are then inserted percutaneously under x-ray guidance. This gives a stable fixation to a fracture by holding it both proximally and distally in what is otherwise a unstable fracture (having lost its medial buttress) and therefore difficult to fix.

With this technique it is important to have an intact inter-trochanteric region as there is a risk of shattering the proximal fragment during the insertion of the nail and in these cases it is often more appropriate to use a long plate DHS.

Conclusion

This is a by no means a definitive guide to the fractured neck of femur, a topic which covers thousands of pages in hundreds of textbooks, and many more journal articles. It is intended simply as a quick overview of the current thinking in managing, what is a very common condition. Of course each fracture pattern is different and treatment should be initiated by assessing the patient as a whole and the optimum method of fixing each individual fracture.

References

Abalo A, Dossim A, Ouro Bangna AF, Tomta K, Assiobo A, Walla A. 2008. Dynamic hip screw and compression plate fixation of ipsilateral femoral neck and shaft fractures. *J. Orthop. Surg* (Hong Kong). Apr; 16(1):35-8.

Arnoldi CC, Lemperg RK. 1977. Fracture of the femoral neck. II. Relative importance of primary vascular damage and surgical procedure for the development of necrosis of the femoral head. *Clin. Orthop.*;129:217–222.

Arnoldi CC, Linderholm H. Fracture of the femoral neck. I. 1972. Vascular disturbances in different types of fractures, assessed by measurements of intraosseous pressures. *Clin. Orthop.*;84:116–127.

Chen CY, Chiu FY, Chen CM, Huang CK, Chen WM, Chen TH. 2008. Surgical treatment of basicervical fractures of femur-a prospective evaluation of 269 patients. *J. Trauma.* Feb;64(2):427-9.

Feliciano D, Mattox K, Moore E. 2004. *Trauma 5th Ed.* McGraw Hill Professional.

French BG, Tornetta P. 1998. Use of an interlocked cephalomedullary nail for subtrochanteric fracture stabilization. *Clin. Orthop.*; 348:95–10.

Frihagen F, Nordsletten L, Madsen JE. 2007. Hemiarthroplasty or internal fixation for intracapsular displaced femoral neck fractures: randomised controlled trial. *BMJ.* Dec 15; 335(7632):1251-4.

Garden RS. Stability and union in subcapital fractures of the femur. 1964. *J. Bone Joint Surg. Br.*; 46:630-47.

Gebhard-J-S. Amstutz-H-C. Zinar-D-M. Dorey-F-J. A comparison of total hip arthroplasty and hemiarthroplasty for treatment of acute fracture of the femoral neck. 1992. *Clin.-Orthop*. Sep (282):123-31.

Haidukewych GJ, Rothwell WS, Jacofsky DJ, Torchia ME, Berry DJ. 2004. Operative treatment of femoral neck fractures in patients between the ages of fifteen and fifty years. *J. Bone Joint Surg. Am.* Aug; 86-A(8):1711-6.

Juttmann JW, Quist J, Kroesen JH. 1991. Which approach for femoral head replacement? *Neth. J. Surg*; 43:258–260.

Keene GS, Parker MJ. 1993. Hemiarthroplasty of the hip—the anterior or posterior approach? A comparison of surgical approaches. *Injury*;24:611–613.

Koval KJ, Friend K, Aharonoff GB, Zukerman JD. 1996. Weightbearing after hip fracture: a prospective series of 596 geriatric hip fracture patients. *J. Orthop. Trauma*;10(8):526–530.

Kraemer WJ, Hearn TC, Powell JN, Mahomed N. 1996. Fixation of segmental subtrochanteric fractures: a biomechanical study. *Clin. Orthop.*; 332:71–7.

LaBelle LW, Colwill JC. 1990. Swanson AB. Bateman bipolar hip arthroplasty for femoral neck fractures. A five- to ten-year follow-up study. *Clin. Orthop.*; 251:20–25.

Lee YS, Chen SH, Tsuang YH, Huang HL, Lo TY, Huang CR. 2008. Internal fixation of undisplaced femoral neck fractures in the elderly: a retrospective comparison of fixation methods. *J. Trauma.*; 64(1):155-62.

Lee YS, Chen SH, Tsuang YH, Huang HL, Lo TY, Huang CR. 2008. Internal fixation of undisplaced femoral neck fractures in the elderly: a retrospective comparison of fixation methods. *J. Trauma.* Jan; 64(1):155-62.

Leighton RK, Schmidt AH, Collier P, Trask K. 2007. Advances in the treatment of intracapsular hip fractures in the elderly. *Injury*. Sep;38 Suppl 3:S24-34.

Linde F. Andersen E. Hvass I. Madsen F. Pallesen R. 1986. Avascular femoral head necrosis following fracture fixation. *Injury*. May; 17(3):159-63.

Lu-Yao GL, Keller RB, Littenberg B, Wennberg JE.1994. Outcomes after displaced fractures of the femoral neck. A meta-analysis of one hundred and six published reports. *J. Bone Joint Surg.*; 76A:15–25.

Malik AA, Kell P, Khan WS, Ihsan KM, Dunkow P (2009). A Review of the Surgical Management of Neck of Femur Fracture. *J. Perioper. Pract*. 19(3): 100-4.

Mullaji AB, Thomas TL. 1993. Low-energy subtrochanteric fractures in elderly patients: results of fixation with the sliding screw plate. *J. Trauma*; 34:56–61.

Nikolopoulos KE, Papadakis SA, Kateros KT, Themistocleous GS, Vlamis JA, Papagelopoulos PJ, Nikiforidis PA. 2003. Long-term outcome of patients with avascular necrosis, after internal fixation of femoral neck fractures. *Injury*. Jul;34(7):525-8.

Nottage-WM. 1990. Comparison of bipolar implants with fixed-neck prostheses in femoral-neck fractures; *Clin.-Orthop*. Feb (251): 38-43.

Rockwood C, Bucholz R, Heckman J, Green D. 2001. *Rockwood & Green's Fractures in Adults 5th Ed.* Lippincott, Wilkins & Williams.

Snell RS. 2003. *Clinical Anatomy by Regions 8th Ed*. Lippincott, Wilkins & Williams.

Strömqvist B, Hansson LI, Ljung P, et al.. 1984. Pre-operative and postoperative scintimetry after femoral neck fracture. *J. Bone Joint Surg.*; 66B:49–54.

Trafton PG. 1987. Subtrochanteric-intertrochanteric femoral fractures. *Orthop. Clin. North Am.*; 18:59–71.

In: Perioperative Practice in Trauma and Orthopaedic Surgery ISBN: 978-1-63483-325-7
Editor: Wasim S. Khan

Chapter 20

SURGERY IN ELDERLY PATIENTS WITH HIP FRACTURES

J. White, P. Smitham and W. S. Khan*
University College London Institute of Orthopaedic and Musculoskeletal Sciences,
Royal National Orthopaedic Hospital, Stanmore, Middlesex, UK

ABSTRACT

Hip fracture is a major cause of morbidity, mortality and loss of independence for the elderly. Surgical fixation of the fractured hip remains the standard of care to allow for early mobilisation and a return to independence. Operative management in this population carries its own set of problems. The altered physiological state of the older person, often coupled with significant co-morbidity, can present challenges for the anaesthetist, the surgeon and the rest of the perioperative team. This chapter provides an evidence-based review of these important perioperative factors associated with hip fractures in the older person and their management.

Keywords: Hip fractures, elderly, co-morbidity, pain, venous thromboemboli

INTRODUCTION

This chapter discusses the evidence for managing hip fractures in elderly patients (White et al. 2011). Hip fractures are frequent injuries amongst older patients with osteoporosis and account for about 76,000 cases in the UK per year according to the National Hip Fracture Database (NHFD 2010). A review that examined the extensive hip fracture literature published in the English language between 1980 and 2009 concerning hip fracture prevalence trends suggested that hip fractures will remain a serious global health issue (Marks 2010). Hip fractures are a major cause of morbidity, mortality and loss of independence in the elderly.

* Corresponding Author: Mr WS Khan, Clinical Lecturer, University College London Institute of Orthopaedics and Musculoskeletal Science, Royal National Orthopaedic Hospital, Stanmore, Middlesex, London, HA7 4LP, UK, Telephone number: +44 (0) 7791 025554, E-mail address: wasimkhan@doctors.org.uk.

These fractures pose a major public healthcare burden and continue to consume large portions of healthcare resources.

Surgical fixation of fractured hips remains the standard of care to allow early mobilisation and a return to independence. Timely surgery limits the period of recumbence and helps to prevent pressure sores, urinary tract infections, deep vein thrombosis and pulmonary complications including atelectases, pneumonia and pulmonary emboli. Surgical intervention is considered superior in medically-fit elderly patients (Parker et al. 2000, Beaupre et al. 2005), and ideally this should be completed within 48 hours for the majority of patients with hip fracture (Egol & Strauss 2009). Even in the absence of co-morbidity, the altered physiological state of the older person can present challenges for the anaesthetist and the rest of the perioperative team. Operative management in this population carries its own set of problems and implications, and these are discussed below.

Fractures of the neck of femur could be divided into extracapsular and intracpsular fractures. Extracapsular fractures are generally treated with fixation using a dynamic hip screw or intramedullary nailing. Although undisplaced intracapsular fractures are also generally treated with fixation using cannulated screws, there is controversy regarding the optimal management of displaced intraarticular fractures. Although most elderly patients with displaced intraarticular fractures are managed with a hemiarthroplasty and do well, there is increasing evidence to suggest that a total hip replacement improves patient functional outcomes for healthy, independent, elderly patients compared with hemiarthroplasty and should be considered as the treatment of choice for these patients as it is more predictable, durable and cost-effective in the longer-term (Schmidt et al. 2005, Malik et al. 2009, Dheerendra et al. 2010, Lowe et al. 2010). A detailed discussion on the surgical management of these fractures is beyond the scope of this chapter.

PREOPERATIVE MEDICAL CONSIDERATIONS

The key difference between elderly patients and their younger contemporaries is a loss of functional reserve and a general decline in organ function (Muravchick 2000). Although age is not an independent risk factor for post-operative complications, the perioperative period is filled with increased risk secondary to the higher incidence of co-existing disease in the elderly. Older patients may present with an array of co-morbidities involving any organ system and these must be evaluated and optimised prior to surgery to improve the post-operative outcome. This highlights the crucial roles played by both anaesthetists and geriatricians in the perioperative management of this challenging patient population.

The risk of postoperative complications in the elderly hip fracture patient is proportional to the number of co-morbidities present. Roche et al. (2005), in a prospective cohort study of 2,448 geriatric patients with hip fracture, evaluated the relationship between preoperative co-morbidity and the risk of postoperative complications and mortality. The authors found that the presence of three or more preoperative co-morbidities is the strongest predictor of increased mortality at 30 days postoperatively, followed by respiratory disease and malignancy. The most common postoperative complications were chest infection (9%) and cardiac failure (5%). These findings underline the importance of effective medical assessment and optimisation in the perioperative period.

A number of studies have sought to identify specific co-morbidities predictive of increased postoperative mortality. Mortality data at 30 days (Nettleman et al. 1996), six months (de Luise et al. 2008) and one year post-injury (Penrod et al. 2008) have identified a history of congestive cardiac failure (CCF), chronic obstructive pulmonary disease (COPD) and and/or malignancy as strong positive predictors. Nettleman et al. (1996), in a retrospective analysis of 390 elderly patients with hip fracture, found that 63% of inpatient mortalities were cardiovascular in nature.

The American Association of Anaesthetists Grading

The American Society of Anaesthetists (ASA) developed a grading system (I to V) to classify patients according to their physical status, thus serving as an indicator of anaesthetic and surgical risk. A normal, healthy individual with minimal risk is deemed ASA class I, whereas a moribund patient who is not expected to survive 24 hours regardless of surgery is designated ASA class V. The majority of elderly patients will be ASA class II or greater (AAGBI 2001).

The ASA score is a useful predictor of long term mortality after hip fracture (Michel et al. 2002, Richmond et al. 2003, Bjorgul et al. 2010). In a prospective study of 1,635 patients with hip fracture, Bjorgul et al. (2010) demonstrated that survival rates vary significantly between ASA classes. Over a five to ten year period postoperatively, survival for ASA I was 8.5 years versus only 1.6 years for ASA IV. Use of the ASA classification to predict postoperative mortality risk can be further enhanced by complementing it with the Short Potable Mental Status Questionnaire (SPMSQ) for assessing cognitive function. Soderqvist et al. (2009), in a prospective cohort study of 1,944 patients aged 66 or older, revealed that the combination of ASA score and SPMSQ provides greater information about survival times compared with the ASA score alone.

In addition to mortality the risk of medical complications can be predicted using the ASA class. In a retrospective analysis of 197 elderly patients with hip fracture, Donegan et al. (2010) reported that medical complications were more common in those with ASA classes III and IV compared with ASA class II. Furthermore, patients classed as ASA IV were over seven times more likely to have medical complications compared with those in class II. These complications are numerous, and in a retrospective study of 8,930 patients aged 60 or over with hip fracture, Lawrence et al. (2002) listed cardiac and pulmonary complications as most frequent (8% and 4% respectively). Other complications included gastrointestinal bleeding (2%), venous thromboembolism (1%), and transient ischaemic attack or stroke (1%). In another series of 1,010 patients evaluated by Ranhoff et al. (2010), the most common complications were anaemia requiring transfusion, delirium and urinary tract infections.

Surgical Complications

Surgical complications include superficial wound infections, deep joint infections, hip dislocations, periprosthetic fractures, failure of fracture fixation, neurovascular injuries and leg length discrepancies (Hall et al. 2009). Most of these complications will need further surgical interventions. Although no study has determined a link between age and complications, the number of co-morbidities is proportional to the risk of postoperative complications (Roche et al. 2005) and elderly hip fracture patients are more likely to have co-morbidities. The reduced functional reserve and general decline in organ function seen in the elderly patients (Muravchick 2000) makes it more difficult for them to cope with the increased physiological demands of the complication and the possible surgical intervention that it may require.

Postoperative Pain Control

The provision of adequate analgesia for hip fracture patients is essential, not only to allow for effective ambulation postoperatively, but also to help prevent complications. The pain induced by trauma and surgery leads to decreased mobility, and this in turn leads to reduced respiratory effort causing atelectasis and pneumonia. Decreased mobility also predisposes to urinary tract infections, deep vein thromboses and pulmonary emboli. Poor postoperative pain control can lead to a vicious cycle in which the pain itself is compounded by the patient's own anxieties, thus limiting progress even further.

Although some evidence exists regarding the most appropriate analgesia for patients with hip fracture, better analgesic control for the elderly need to be discovered (Beaupre et al. 2005). Poorly controlled pain however, increases the length of hospital stay, delays mobilisation, and reduces long-term functional ability (Morrison et al. 2003). It is likely that complications arise secondary to impaired cognition, medical co-morbidities, and altered drug metabolism and pharmacokinetics. These factors make effective pain control in the older population far more complex than their younger counterparts.

Acutely, postoperative pain management with intravenous morphine can be safely achieved using the same protocol as for younger patients. There appears to be no difference in the incidence of morphine-related complications or sedation (Aubrun et al. 2002). Several days postoperatively however, opioid requirements amongst elderly patients drop in comparison (Gagliese et al. 2000). It is important that regular pain assessments are made to allow for adequate dosing adjustments, in addition to a baseline assessment upon arrival to hospital. Furthermore, special consideration must be given to cognitively-impaired patients, whose pain control is often suboptimal due to self-reporting of less pain. Behavioural pain indicators do not however differ between congnitively-impaired and cognitively-intact patients, supporting the use of behavioural assessments in the cognitively-impaired (Horgas et al. 2009). Another strategy to ameliorate this may be the adoption a standardised protocol for pain management (Adunsky et al. 2002).

Regional analgesia via the epidural route may provide a novel technique for managing acute postoperative pain in elderly hip fracture patients, although more research is needed. Foss et al. (2005) examined the effect of four days postoperative epidural infusion of bupivacaine and morphine versus placebo in 60 elderly hip fracture patients. Epidural analgesia was found to be significantly superior in managing postoperative pain during all basic physical functions compared with controls. Despite the improved pain relief, there was no significant difference in scores for recovery of physical independence. These findings demonstrate that epidural analgesia provides enhanced pain control over standard regimens, but further studies are needed to elicit whether this improvement translates into enhanced recovery.

PRESSURE ULCER PREVENTION

The development of pressure sores after hip surgery is a common occurrence, with a reported incidence ranging from 9% to 55% (Gunningsberg et al. 2000, Baumgarten et al. 2003). It carries a great burden of morbidity as patients that develop pressure ulcers are at increased risk of developing nosocomial infections and other hospital complications, as well as enduring a significantly longer hospital stay (Allman et al. 1999). The assessment and management of a pressure ulcer requires a systematic, comprehensive and multidisciplinary approach. Assessment of an elderly hip fracture patient includes the patient's comorbidities, functional state, nutritional status, and degree of social and emotional support (Jaul 2010). Vigilant nursing care can reduce this risk, through visual inspection, frequent turning, and the application of topical preparations. Furthermore, the implementation of heel protection and pressure-relieving mattresses can provide additional benefit. In a prospective randomised controlled trial assessing the benefits of an interface pressure-decreasing mattress, Hofman et al. (1994) found that the incidence and severity of pressure ulcers were significantly reduced compared with a standard hospital mattress (24% versus 68%).

Currently there is no research evidence that high-tech pressure-relieving mattresses are more effective than low-tech foam mattresses for the prevention of pressure ulcers. There is also a lack of evidence regarding the benefit of heel protection devices. Professional consensus recommends their use, but further research is needed.

VENOUS THROMBOEMBOLISM PREVENTION

Hip fracture is a major risk factor for venous thromboembolism (VTE) throughout the perioperative period. Other significant risk factors include malignancy, coagulopathy, immobility, previous VTE, obesity, stroke, atherosclerosis, and ASA grade ≥ 3 (Beksac et al. 2006). Advanced age is weakly associated with the development of VTE (Abad Rico et al. 2010). Incidence rates for deep vein thromboses range from 36% to 60% (Ennis 2003), whilst those of pulmonary embolism range from 4% to 24% (Egol and Strauss 2009). Fatal pulmonary emboli occur in 1% to 13% of cases (Ennis 2003).

Despite extensive research on an optimal thromboprophylaxis strategy, there remains no agreement on a standard protocol (Chahal et al. 2013). The Pulmonary Embolism Prevention (PEP) trial (2000) assessed the effect of aspirin versus placebo for VTE prophylaxis in 13,365 patients with hip fracture. Treatment with aspirin reduced the risk of both symptomatic deep vein thromboses and pulmonary emboli when compared with placebo (29% and 43% respectively). There was an increased transfusion requirement in patients assigned aspirin, however mortalities due to bleeding were comparable between study groups. Based on the findings, the authors concluded that treatment with aspirin decreases the incidence of deep vein thromboses and pulmonary emboli by a third perioperatively and should be used routinely in patients with hip fracture.

A retrospective study by Ennis (2003) of 1,000 consecutive hip fractures compared the use of aspirin with the low-molecular-weight heparin (LMWH), enoxaparin. Although there was no significant difference in deep vein thrombosis rates between the treatment groups, there was one case of fatal pulmonary embolism in those treated with aspirin and no pulmonary emboli recorded with enoxaparin. Considering its short half-life, predictability and favourable safety profile, the author concluded that enoxaparin, and thus LMWH, was an ideal form of thromboprophylaxis.

A total of 32 trials covering 3,614 adult hip fracture cases have shown that unfractionated heparin and LMWH protect against VTE (Handoll et al. 2002, Eriksson & Lassen 2003). In a Cochrane review by Handoll et al. (2002) however, there was insufficient data to confirm a protective effect against pulmonary emboli. No significant differences were established between unfractionated heparin and LMWH. Eriksson & Lassen (2003) found that fondaparinux (factor Xa inhibitor) conferred a relative reduction in the risk of VTE (including pulmonary emboli) of 96% when compared with placebo. The incidence of symptomatic VTE was also found to be significantly lower in patients treated with fondaparinux and there was no increase in the incidence of clinically significant bleeding.

Turpie et al. (2002) reported a meta-analysis of four randomised, double-blind trials comparing the prophylactic effects of fondaparinux and enoxaparin in 7,344 cases of hip fracture. Fondaparinux was shown to confer a significantly greater protective effect against VTE than enoxaparin, with an odds reduction of 55%. It was also shown to significantly reduce the incidence of proximal deep vein thromboses with a reduction of 57%. The risk of clinically relevant bleeding was low and did not differ significantly between the treatment groups. In a retrospective study by Shorr et al. (2007) of 144,806 patients who had undergone major orthopaedic surgery, including that for hip fracture, the benefits of fondaparinux were further clarified. Patients receiving fondaparinux experienced fewer VTE events (1.5%) compared to enoxaparin (2.1%), dalteparin (2.1%) and unfractionated heparin (4.2%).

Post-discharge, there remains a risk of delayed thromboembolic events, thus justifying the need for extended thromboprophylaxis (Anand & Buch 2007). Prolonged treatment with fondaparinux over a 4-week period can reduce the risk of DVT by 96% and the risk of symptomatic VTE by 89% compared with perioperative (1-week) treatment (Kwong 2004). The American College of Chest Physicians recommends the routine use of fondaparinux, LMWH, or unfractionated heparin for patients undergoing hip fracture surgery. Their guidelines also recommend against the use of aspirin alone for thromboprophylaxis and encourage the use of physical methods of anticoagulation for patients with a high bleeding risk or as an adjunct to chemoprophylaxis (Geerts et al. 2008).

Postoperative Confusion/Delirium

Postoperative delirium is characterised by a disturbance of consciousness and temporary abnormalities in cognition and perception. It is a common problem in the elderly hip fracture patient with a postoperative incidence ranging from 5% to 61% (Edelstein et al. 2004, Gustafson et al. 1988). Risk factors for delirium include advanced age, pre-fracture cognitive and functional impairment, pre-existing cerebrovascular and other brain diseases, indoor injury, communication difficulties and social isolation (Duppils & Wikblad 2001, Juliebo et al. 2009). Precipitating factors for delirium comprise perioperative falls in blood pressure, postoperative infections and malnutrition (Edlund et al. 2001). Perioperative risk factors associated with postoperative delirium include intraoperative blood loss, electrolyte abnormalities and a postoperative haematocrit <30% (Mercantonio et al. 1998). Neither intraoperative haemodynamic instability nor route of anaesthesia is associated with increased postoperative delirium (Mercantonio et al. 1998). A randomised controlled trial by Sieber (2009) did demonstrate however that the depth of sedation achieved with propofol during spinal anaesthesia does influence the subsequent development of delirium. In the trial, 114 individuals were randomised and the results showed that there were far fewer cases of delirium in the light sedation group versus the deep group (19% versus 40% respectively). The authors concluded that limiting the depth of sedation during spinal anaesthesia is a safe, effective and economical and should be widely instituted.

Unfortunately, postoperative delirium has received little attention in the perioperative literature, despite its considerable morbidity and mortality. Over two decades ago, it had shown to significantly increase the length of hospital stay and postoperative complications such as urinary incontinence, feeding difficulties and pressure sores (Gustafson et al. 1988). Patients experience reduced ambulation and rehabilitation, with a decline in their activities of daily living, prefracture walking level and ultimately their independence. Finally, patients suffer an increased rate of mortality or are placed into a nursing home (Gustafson et al. 1988, Mercantonio et al. 2001, Edelstein et al. 2004).

Management strategies towards postoperative delirium are therefore necessary to prevent and/or lessen the impact on patient outcomes. Careful and frequent assessment of a patient's mental status and cognitive function are important as is addressing any risk factors present. Precipitating factors need to be avoided and if delirium does present itself, treatment needs to focus on supportive care and identifying the underlying causes. Specific measures include adequate postoperative analgesia, careful drug selection and management within a multidisciplinary framework. Mercantonio et al. (2001) conducted a randomised controlled trial assessing the effects of regular geriatrics input on postoperative delirium in 126 elderly hip fracture patients. Geriatrics consultation was shown to significantly decrease the incidence of postoperative delirium by a third, with a relative risk of 0.64. There was an even greater reduction in cases of severe delirium, although length of stay did not vary significantly between intervention groups. In a similar study by Lundstrom et al. (2007), postoperative care on either an orthopaedic ward or geriatric ward was compared in 199 patients. Less patients treated on the geriatric ward developed delirium, and if so, their delirium lasted for a shorter period of time. Furthermore, intervention patients developed fewer complications such as pressure ulcers, nutritional deficits, urinary tract infections, sleeping problems and falls.

CONCLUSION

Based on the literature we have reviewed, hip fractures are common injuries and are a major cause of morbidity, mortality and loss of independence for the elderly._Although surgical fixation of the fractured hips remains the standard of care, operative management carries its own set of problems. The altered physiological state of the older person, often coupled with significant co-morbidity, can present challenges for the anaesthetist and the rest of the perioperative team. It is important that an evidence-based approach is utilised to help ensure the patient, who has been optimised perioperatively, has appropriate management of pain, pressure ulcers, venous thromboemboli, delirium and confusion. The appropriate assessment and evidence-based management of these patients should lead to an improved outcome.

References

Abad Rico JI, Llau Pitarch JV, Rocha E 2010. *Overview of Venous Thromboembolism Drugs* 2010 70 (S2) 3-10.

Allman RM, Goode PS, Burst N, Bartolucci AA, Thomas DR 1999 Pressure ulcers, hospital complications, disease severity: impact on hospital costs and length of stay Advances in Wound Care: *The Journal for Prevention and Healing* 12 (1) 22-30.

Anaesthesia and Perioperative care of the Elderly 2001 [online] Available from: http://www.aagbi.org/publications/guidelines/docs/careelderly01.pdf [Accessed Sept. 2010]

Anand S, Buch K 2007 Post-discharge symptomatic thromboembolic events in hip fracture patients. *Annals of the Royal College of Surgeons of England* 89 (5) 517-520.

Baumgarten M, Margolis D, Berlin JA, Strom BL, Garino J, Kagan SH, Kavesh SH, Carson JL 2003 Risk factors for pressure ulcer among elderly hip fracture patients. *Wound Repair and Regeneration* 11 (2) 96-103.

Beaupre LA, Jones CA, Saunders LD, Johnston DW, Buckingham J, Majumdar SR 2005 Best practices for elderly hip fracture patients. A systematic overview of the evidence. *Journal of General Internal Medicine* 20 (11) 1019-1025.

Beksac B, Gonzalez Della Valle A, Salvati EA 2006 Thromboembolic disease after total hip arthroplasty: who is at risk? *Clinical Orthopaedics and Related Research* 453 211-224.

Bjorgul K, Novicoff WM, Saleh KJ 2010 American Society of Anaesthesiologist Physical Status score may be used as a comorbidity index in hip fracture surgery. *Journal of Arthroplasty* 25 (6 Suppl) 134-137.

Chahal GS, Saithna A, Brewster M, Gilbody J, Lever S, Khan WS, Foguet P (2013). A Comparison of Complications Requiring Return to Theatre in Hip and Knee Arthroplasty Patients Taking Enoxaparin versus Rivaroxaban for Thromboprophylaxis. *Orthop. Trauma Rehab.* 15(2): 125-9.

de Luise C, Brimacombe M, Pedersen L, Sorensen HT 2008 Comorbidity and mortality following hip fracture: a population-based cohort study. *Aging Clinical and Experimental Research* 20 (5) 412-418.

Dheerendra S, Khan WS, Saeed MZ, Goddard NJ (2010). Recent Developments in Total Hip Replacements: Cementation, Articulation, Minimal-Invasion and Navigation. *J. Perioper Pract.* 20(4): 133-8.

Donegan DJ, Gay AN, Baldwin K, Morales EE, Esterhai JL Jr, Mehta S 2010 Use of medical comorbidities to predict complications after hip fracture surgery in the elderly. *Journal of Bone and Joint Surgery* (American Volume) 92 (4) 807-813.

Duppils GS, Wikblad K 2000 Acute confusional states in patients undergoing hip surgery: a prospective observational study *Gerontology* 46 (1) 36-43.

Edelstein DM, Aharonoff GB, Karp A, Capla EL, Zuckerman JD, Koval KJ 2004 Effect of postoperative delirium on outcome after hip fracture *Clinical Orthopaedics and Related Research* (422) 195-200.

Edlund A, Lundstrom M, Brannstrom B, Bucht G, Gustafson Y 2001 Delirium before and after operation for femoral neck fracture. *Journal of the American Geriatrics Society* 49 (10) 1335-1340.

Egol KA, Strauss EJ 2009 Perioperative considerations in geriatric patients with hip fracture: what is the evidence? *Journal of Orthopaedic* Trauma 23 (6) 386-394.

Ennis RS 2003 Postoperative deep vein thrombosis prophylaxis: a retrospective analysis in 1000 consecutive hip fracture patients treated in a community hospital setting. *Journal of the Southern Orthopaedic Association* 12 (1) 10-17.

Eriksson BI, Lassen MR 2003 Duration of prophylaxis against venous thromboembolism with fondaparinux after hip fracture surgery: a multi-center, randomized, placebo-controlled, double-blind study. *Archives of Internal Medicine* 163 (11) 1337-1342.

Foss NB, Kristensen MT, Kristensen BB, Jensen PS, Kehlet H 2005 Effect of postoperative analgesia on rehabilitation and pain after hip fracture surgery: a randomised, double-blind, placebo-controlled trial. *Anaesthesiology* 102 (6) 1197-1204.

Gagliese L, Jackson M, Ritvo P, Wowk A, Katz J 2000 Age is not an impediment to effective use of patient-controlled analgesia by surgical patients. *Anaesthesiology* 93 (3) 601-610.

Geerts WH, Bergqvist D, Pineo GF, Heit JA, Samama CM, Lassen MR, Colwell CW; American College of Chest Physicians 2008 Prevention of venous thromboembolism: American College of Chest Physicians Evidence-Based Clinical Practice Guidelines (8th Edition). *Chest* 133 (6 suppl) 381S-453S.

Gunningsberg L, Lindholm C, Carlsson M, Sjoden PO 2000 The development of pressure ulcers in patients with hip fractures: inadequate nursing documentation is still a problem. *Journal of Advanced Nursing* 31 (5) 1155-1164.

Gustafson Y, Berggren D, Brannstrom B, Bucht G, Norberg A, Hansson LI, Winblad B 1988 Acute confusional states in elderly patients treated for femoral neck fracture. *Journal of the American Geriatrics Society* 36 (6) 525-530.

Hall C, Khan WS, Ahmed SI, Sochart DH (2009). A rare case of arterial avulsion presenting with occult blood loss in a patient following total hip arthroplasty: A case report. *J. Med. Case Rep*. 3: 9320.

Handoll HH, FTytherleigh-Strong G, Milne AA, Gillespie WJ 2002 Heparin, low molecular weight heparin and physical methods for preventing deep vein thrombosis and pulmonary embolism following surgery for hip fractures. *Cochrane Database of Systematic Reviews* (4):CD000305.

Hofman A, Geelkerken RH, Willie J, Hamming JJ, Hermans J, Breslau PJ 1994 Pressure sores and pressure-decreasing mattresses: controlled clinical trial. *Lancet* 343 (8897) 568-571.

Horgas AL, Elliott AF, Marsiske M 2009 Pain assessment in persons with dementia: relationship between self-report and behavioral observation *Journal of the American Geriatrics Society* 57 (1) 126-132.

Jaul E 2010 Assessment and management of pressure ulcers in the elderly: current strategies. *Drugs Aging* 27 (4) 311-325.

Juliebo V, Bjoro K, Krogseth M, Skovlund E, Ranhoff AH, Wyller TB 2009 Risk factors for preoperative and postoperative delirium in elderly patients with hip fracture. *Journal of the American Geriatrics Association* 57 (8) 1354-1361.

Kwong LM 2004 Hip fracture and venous thromboembolism in the elderly *Journal of Surgical Orthopaedic Advances* 13 (3) 139-148.

Lawrence VA, Hilsenbeck SG, Noveck H, Poses RM, Carson JL 2002 Medical complications and outcomes after hip fracture surgery. *Archives of Internal Medicine* 162 (18) 2053-2057.

Lowe JA, Crist BD, Bhandari M, Ferguson TA 2010 Optimal treatment of femoral neck fractures according to patient's physiologic age: an evidence-based review. *Orthopaedic Clinics of North America* 41 (2) 157-166.

Lundstrom M, Olofsson B, Stenvall M, Nyberg L, Englund U, Borssen B, Svensson O, Gustafson Y 2007 Postoperative delirium in old patients with femoral neck fracture: a randomised intervention study. *Ageing Clinical and Experimental Research* 19 (3) 178-186.

Malik AA, Kell P, Khan WS, Ihsan KM, Dunkow P 2009 Surgical management of fractured neck of femur. Journal of Perioperative Practice 19 (3) 100-104.

Marks R 2010 Hip fracture epidemiological trends, outcomes, and risk factors, 1970-2009. International Journal of General Medicine 8 (3) 1-17.

Mercantonio ER, Goldman L, Orav EJ, Cook EF, Lee TH 1998 The association of intraoperative factors with the development of postoperative delirium. *The American Journal of Medicine* 105 (5) 380-384.

Mercantonio ER, Flacker JM, Wright RJ, Resnick NM 2001 Reducing delirium after hip fracture: a randomised trial. *Journal of the American Geriatrics Society* 49 (5) 516-522.

Michel J, Klopfenstein C, Hoffmeyer P, Stern R, Grab B 2002 Hip fracture surgery: is the pre-operative American Society of Anaesthesiologists (ASA) score a predictor of functional outcome? *Ageing Clinical and Experimental Research* 14 (5) 389-394.

Morrison RS, Magaziner J, McLaughlin MA, Orosz G, Silberzweig SB, Koval KJ, Siu AL 2003 The impact of post-operative pain on outcomes following hip fracture. *Pain* 103 (3) 303-311.

Muravchick S 2000 Preoperative assessment of the elderly patient. *Anesthesiology Clinics of North America* 18 (1) 71-89.

The National Hip Fracture Database National Report 2010 [online] Available from: http://www.ccad.org.uk/nhfd.nsf/NHFD%20National%20Report%202010.pdf [Accessed September 2010]

Nettleman MD, Alsip J, Schrader M, Schulte M 1996 Predictors of mortality after acute hip fracture. *Journal of General Internal Medicine* 11 (2) 765-777.

Paqueron X, Lumbroso A, Mergoni P, Aubrun F, Langeron O, Coriat P, Riou B 2002 Is morphine-induced sedation synonymous with analgesia during intravenous morphine titration? *British Journal of Anaesthesia* 89 (5) 697-701.

Parker MJ, Handoll HHG, Bhargara A 2000 Conservative versus operative treatment for hip fractures. *Cochrane Database Systematic* Reviews Issue 4.

Penrod JD, Litke A, Hawke WG, Magaziner J, Doucette JT, Koval KJ, Silberzweig SB, Egol KA, Siu AL 2008 The association of race, gender, and co-morbidity with mortality and function after hip fracture. *The Journals of Gerontology* 63 (8) 867-872.

Prevention of pulmonary embolism and deep vein thrombosis with low dose aspirin: Pulmonary Embolism Prevention (PEP) trial 2000. *Lancet* 355 (9212) 1295-1302.

Ranhoff AH, Holvik K, Martinsen MI, Domaas K, Solheim LF 2010 Older hip fracture patients: three groups with different needs. *BMC Geriatrics* 10 (1) 65.

Richmond J, Aharonoff GB, Zuckerman JD, Koval KJ 2003 Mortality risk after hip fracture. *Journal of Orthopaedic Trauma* 17 (1) 53-56.

Roche JJ, Wenn RT, Sahota O, Moran CG 2005 Effect of comorbidities and postoperative complications on mortality after hip fracture in elderly people: prospective observational cohort study *British Medical Journal* 331 (7529) 1374-1379.

Schmidt AH, Asnis SE, Haidukewych G, Koval KJ, Thorngren KG 2005 Femoral neck fractures. *Instructional Course Lectures* 54 417-445.

Shorr AF, Kwong LM, Sarnes M, Happe L, Farelly E, Mody-Patel N 2007 Venous thromboembolism after orthopaedic surgery: implications of the choice for prophylaxis. *Thrombosis Research* 121 (1) 17-24.

Sieber FE 2009 Postoperative delirium in the elderly surgical patient. *Anaesthesiology Clinics* 27 (3) 451-464.

Soderqvist A, Ekstrom W, Ponzer S, Petterson H, Cederholm T, Dalen N, Hedstrom M, Tidermark J 2009 Prediction of mortality in elderly patients with hip fractures: a two-year prospective study of 1944 patients. *Gerontology* 55 (5) 496-504.

Turpie AG, Eriksson BI, Lassen MR, Bauer KA 2002 A meta-analysis of fondaparinux versus enoxaparin in the prevention of venous thromboembolism after major orthopaedic surgery. *Journal of the Southern Orthopaedic Association* 11 (4) 182-188.

In: Perioperative Practice in Trauma and Orthopaedic Surgery ISBN: 978-1-63483-325-7
Editor: Wasim S. Khan

Chapter 21

THE PERIOPERATIVE MANAGEMENT OF SKELETAL METASTASES

***Jagmeet S. Bhamra*[1], *Atif Malik*[2], *Wasim S. Khan*[3,*] *and Rob Pollock*[1]**

[1]Bone Tumour Unit, Royal National Orthopaedic Hospital, Stanmore, London, UK
[2]Department of Trauma and Orthopaedics, Queens Hospital, Barking Havering and Redbridge NHS Trust, Romford, Essex, UK
[3]University College London Institute of Orthopaedics and Musculoskeletal Sciences, Royal National Orthopaedic Hospital, Stanmore, London, UK

ABSTRACT

Bone metastasis is a common problem affecting a significant proportion of patients with metastatic cancer. Bone metastasis can present in a number of ways and the patients may need surgical stabilisation of their lesions. There are many important considerations in the care of these patients that need to be borne in mind including their increased anesthetic risks and potential risk of complications. There are continuous developments in the prevention, diagnosis and treatment with advances in imaging, orthopaedic technique and medication, particularly radiopharmaceuticals and cytotoxic, endocrine treatments with newer treatments based around the tumour cell-osteoclast interaction. Having a better understanding of these considerations and developments is important in allowing the optimisation of the care of the patient with bone metastasis.

Keywords: Perioperative management, metastases, bone lesions, cancer, surgery

* Corresponding Author: Mr Wasim S Khan, Clinical Lecturer, University College London Institute of Orthopaedic and Musculoskeletal Research, Royal National Orthopaedic Hospital, Stanmore, London, HA7 4LP, UK. Telephone number: +44 (0) 77791 025554. Fax number: +44 (0) 1707 655059. E-mail address: wasimkhan@doctors.org.uk.

Cancer of the bone may be either primary, arising from the bone itself, or secondary, metastasising from a different source. It is widely accepted that secondary cancers are more common than their primary counterparts; however the true incidence is the subject of much debate. This chapter discusses the perioperative management of skeletal metastases (Bhamra et al. 2012). Calculating incidence of metastatic bone disease is dependent on the sources methods; i.e. pathological presentation, incidental imaging findings, autopsy, etc. (table 1). The probability of disease can however be estimated by determining the prevalence of the primary cancer and its predilection for bone (Coleman et al. 2001).

Table 1. Incidence of new cancers diagnosed and sources of metastatic disease. ***Office for National Statistics (ONS), Annual, Online edition***

Type of cancer	New cases of cancer diagnosed in England, 2007*	Incidence of Bone Metastases in Cancer**
Multiple myeloma	3,357	70%-95%
Breast	38,291	65%-75%
Prostate	30,201	65%-75%
Renal	5,756	20%-25%
Lung	31,522	30%-40%
Malignant melanoma of skin	8,809	14%-45%

PATHOLOGY

Skeletal metastases to bone may occur through one of three mechanisms:

1. Seeding of embolic tumour cells via the systemic circulation
2. Direct extension
3. Retrograde venous flow

The bone matrix provides a favourable microenvironment for the adherence and extravasation of tumour cells. Once there, they stimulate osteoclasts to reabsorb bone, which in turn triggers the release of growth factors, stimulating tumour cell growth. The surrounding bone is characterised by a deranged metabolism and re-models around the destruction of the tumour cells, with either osteoclastic or osteoblastic cells predominating (Clines et al., 2008, Coleman et al., 2001, Mundy et al., 2002, Salmon et al. 2000).

The degree of bone reabsorption and turnover is highly dependant on the bone affected and the origin of the metastatic tumour cell. The relationship between the predominating cell type and remodelling process determines whether a sclerotic, lytic or mixed lesion is seen on radiographs. Disruption of the bone remodelling process results in significant bone loss and therefore a reduced skeletal integrity, which underlies skeletal complications of metastatic cancers (Coleman et al. 1997).

EFFECTS OF METASTATIC BONE DISEASE

Different primary cancers cause different rates of events in skeletal metastases (table 2). Breast cancers tend to cause the most skeletal events (68% over 24 months) (Figure 1), closely followed by myelomas (51% over 21 months) and prostatic cancers (49% over 24 months) (Coleman et al. 2004).

Table 2. Rates of skeletal metastases from primary cancers *(Coleman 2004)*

Primary tumour	Rate of spread
Breast	68% (24 months)
Prostate	49% (24 months)
Myeloma	51% (21 months)

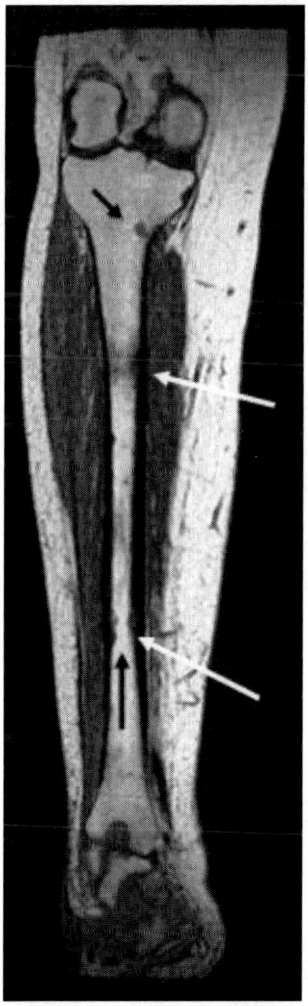

Figure 1. MRI demonstrating right tibial metastases in a 70 year old woman from breast carcinoma.

1. Pain

Bone pain in patients with a known primary cancer is highly suspicious of metastatic disease and should be investigated thoroughly. Pain may be caused by direct invasion of the bone causing micro-fractures, increased pressure of the endosteum or distortion of the periosteum. Vertebral collapse can lead to nerve root compression and muscles in the affected have a tendency to spasm (Roger von Moos et al. 2008). Pain can be treated by adhering to the WHO analgesic pyramid, initially with non steroidal anti-inflammatories and then opioids. In severe cases radiotherapy or radionuclide therapy can be used and although surgery is generally used to treat or prevent fractures, it is also successful in treating pain (Dalton et al. 2000).

2. Hypercalcaemia

Hypercalcaemia of malignancy results from the up-regulation of osteoclastic activity, resulting in increased bone re-absorption and reduced renal clearance of calcium and phosphate. The hypercalcaemic state can cause a variety of symptoms including thirst, drowsiness, vomiting and ultimately death. Furthermore, it has been demonstrated that hypercalcaemia can precipitate or exacerbate pain threshold (Fleisch et al. 1991). Patients with breast cancer are most susceptible to hypercalcaemia (13% over 24 months). The mainstay of treatment for hypercalcaemia of malignancy is Bisphosphonates, both prophylactically and therapeutically (Coleman et al. 2004).

3. Bone Marrow Depletion and Anaemia

Metastases to bone generally affect areas that contain red marrow. The marrow which cancerous cells adhere to contains haematopoietic stem cells, stromal cells and immune cells that release inflammatory mediators such as cytokines and growth factors. This provides a fertile microenvironment for tumour cells to grow, which disrupts the normal physiology of bone marrow (Lipton et al. 2004). This leads to a leukoerythroblastic anaemia which is most commonly seen in association with metastasis of cancers from the breast, lung, stomach and prostate (Rubins et al. 1983).

4. Spinal Cord Compression

Spinal column metastases occur in 3–5% of cancer patients (Figure 2). The most commonly affecting cancers are breast, prostate and lung cancers, in which the incidence may be as high as 19%. Spinal metastases cause pain, vertebral collapse and metastatic spinal cord compression (MSCC). The pathology is caused by compression of the dural sac and its contents (the spinal cord and cauda equina), by an extradural mass.

In an ageing population, patients are more frequently presenting with oncological emergencies. MSCC is one of the most common, currently affecting 5-10% of patients

(Loblaw et al., 2003, Levack et al. 2001). Once the spinal cord or cauda equina are compressed, irreversible neurological damage ensues, with resulting paraplegia.

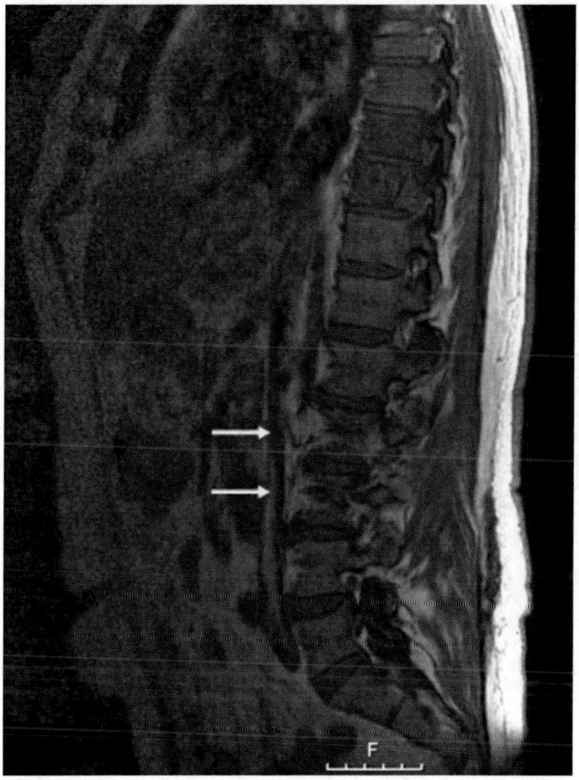

Figure 2. 66 year old male with known renal cell carcinoma, presenting with back pain. MRI spine reveals metastatic lesions T9-T10 vertebral bodies.

The gold standard for diagnosis is MRI of the whole spine (Levack et al., 2001, Cook et al. 1998) and once a diagnosis is made, the treatment goals are the restoration of neurology and prevention of further neurological decline, stabilisation of the spine and analgesia (Husband et al., 1998, Held et al. 1993).

5. Pathological Fractures

A pathological fracture occurs when an area of bone which has already been weakened by a pre-existing abnormality, i.e. a cancer, is fractured following a low velocity injury (Figure 3).

Tumour extension and growth cause a local destructive effect in the bone cortex and matrix and this initially leads to micro-fractures causing pain and pathological fractures. Large, predominantly lytic lesions which affect the cortex of the bone are most likely to cause fractures, particularly in weight baring bones. The fracture of long bones or the spine cause the biggest disability and detriment to patients' health and so efforts are made to predict and prevent such fractures.

Pathological fractures are not a sign of terminal disease and so prophylactic fixation with internal stabilisation and radiotherapy to prevent progression are viable options (Haberman et al. 1989) (Figure 4).

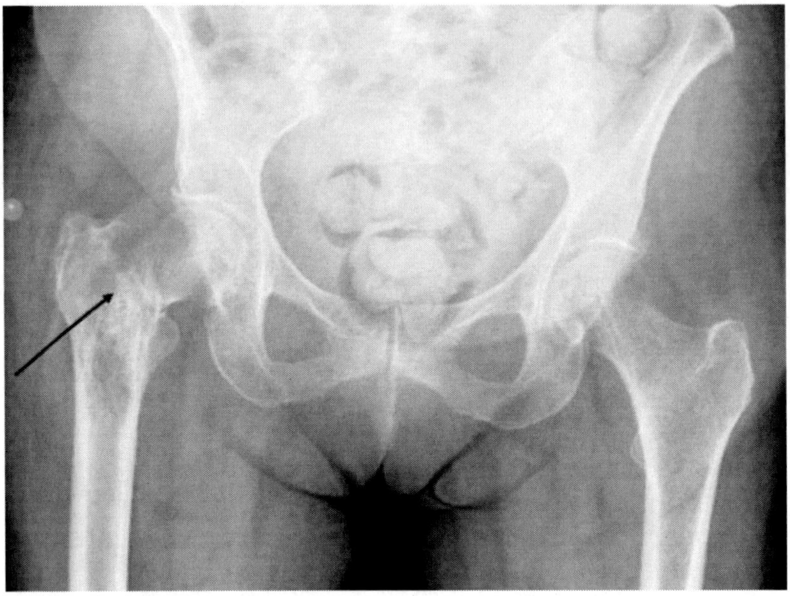

Figure 3. Pathological right neck of femur fracture (metastases from breast primary to right femur and acetabulum) in a 76 year old female. Surgically treated with a total hip arthroplasty for pain management and to restore mobility.

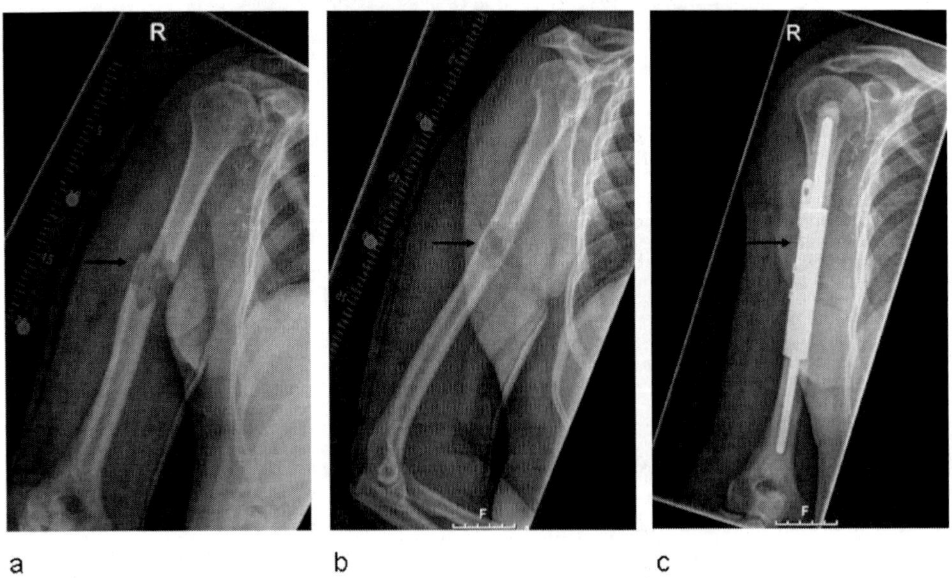

Figure 4. Pathological fracture (b) following metastases (a) from malignant melanoma to right humerus that was subsequently treated with fixation with humeral diaphyseal replacement (c).

Assessment of the Patient

It is imperative to take a thorough history and examination of the patient as bone metastases are often multiple at time of presentation. “Red flag” signs, such as pain (particularly at night); weight loss; loss of appetite; malaise and lethargy; fevers and temperatures, fractures and neurological signs (e.g., malignant cord compression) should be sought in the history taking. It is also important to include a systems review highlighting any areas of concern which may need investigating; such as shortness of breath suggesting a lung primary, or history of a breast lump which may be indicative of breast carcinoma. A complete laboratory blood work-up is completed; full blood count, urea & electrolytes, clotting, ESR, CRP, liver function tests and if relevant tumour markers requested (Weber 2010).

In the majority of cases, patients are initial complaints are dealt with by their family doctor. An urgent cancer referral (within two weeks), is then made to specialist tertiary referral centres for definitive management. These specialist units consist of a large multidisciplinary team; constituting surgeons, radiologists, specialist cancer nurses, pathologists, dieticians, physiotherapists and occupational therapists. All referred cases are discussed at meetings and specialist opinions are sought and management plans established.

Patients are then investigated with relevant radiological imaging, biopsy of the lesion and further clinical assessment in an outpatient setting with histological results and relevant imaging available.

All patients with metastatic bone disease undergo a Technetium-99 (^{99m}Tc) radionuclide scintiscanning bone scan. This modality is the most cost-effective and sensitive whole body imaging for assessing skeletal metastases, but is non-specific. Other screening radiology includes whole body MRI and flourodeoxyglucose (FDG) positive emission tomography. Both are more expensive, but more accurate than nuclear bone scanning (Aoki et al. 2001, Cook et al. 2000). Conventional imaging is reserved for investigating lesions identified on the bone scan (plain radiographic films, MR and Ultrasound imaging (Peh 2000, Merrick et al., 1992, Traill et al. 1999). Patients are further assessed for surgery using a staging CT (chest, abdomen and pelvis) which helps in deciding management options. Histological diagnosis is usually obtained by needle biopsy (under radiological guidance, CT) and in difficult (eg. anatomical) or painful cases; open biopsy is an option which is performed under general anaesthesia. Confirmed histological diagnosis, together with the extent of disease spread is then considered and finally, depending on patient prognosis a treatment plan is made after re-discussion at the multi-disciplinary meeting.

Treatment Options

Depending on the outcome of the investigations above, fitness for surgery is assessed. If surgery is not an option; (such as extensive spread of disease, frailty of patient, presence of multiple co-morbidities) then referral to the palliative team is made. Symptomatic treatment is the mainstay is such cases. Patients fit for surgery may undergo radiotherapy prior to surgery and in palliative patients; radiotherapy may be an option in treating ‘bony pain.’

The changes to the metabolic and bone remodelling processes underlies the manifestation of skeletal complications. Better understanding of these processes has meant that there are better treatment options for skeletal metastases, preventing the aforementioned complications. Orthopaedic surgery is used to repair pathological fractures and stabilise impending fractures. Radiotherapy is used to treat bone pain and to stabilise bony lesions.

1. Bisphosphonates

Bisphosphonates are currently the standard of care for preventing skeletal complications of metastatic disease and are used to treat bone pain. They preferentially bind to bone surfaces which are undergoing remodelling and are released by the bone matrix during reabsorption, inhibiting osteoclastic activity. This mechanism may reduce osteoclast-mediated bone reabsorption (Fleisch 2002). Various clinical trials have compared the various bisphosphonates to each other and to placebos using "end points" or "skeletal related events" (SRE) which generally include pathological fractures, cord compression, hypercalcaemia, radiation to bone or surgery.

Zoledronic acid, a bisphosphonate, is the current standard treatment for patients with osteolytic or mixed bone metastases or lesions. Studies have shown this drug to be more potent than bisphosphonates (eg. Pamidronate) and is administered by intravenous infusion. Furthermore, it has been shown to significantly reduce rates of SREs in patients with breast, prostate cancer as well as other solid tumours and multiple myelomas (Rosen et al., 2001, Kohno et al., 2004, Small et al., 2003, Major et al. 2004).

It is widely accepted that the release of growth factors and cytokines during the normal bone reabsorption process attracts malignant cells to the bone surface and facilitates its growth and proliferation (Yomeda et al., 1999, Van Der Pluijim et al. 2000).

Several animal models have demonstrated a reduction in metastatic bone disease, but these results have not been easily transferred to human trials, although there some evidence does suggest that clodronate may be of benefit. For example, Diel et al., (2008), looked at 302 patients with breast cancer who had cancer cells in the bone marrow identified by immunocytochemistry. There was a reduction in bone metastases at 36 months by using clodronate (11 versus 25, $p<0.002$). Interestingly, there was also a reduction in extra skeletal metastases (19 versus 42 $p<0.001$). However a Scandinavian trial of 299 breast cancer patients receiving adjuvant systemic treatment showed an increase in frequency of skeletal metastases (26% versus 18%, $p = 0.09$) and extra skeletal metastases (45% versus 27%, $p = 0.001$) in patients randomised to receive 3 years of clodronate, at a minimum of 5 year follow up. It is therefore clear to conclude that bisphosphonates have an established role in preventing SREs in patients with metastatic bone cancer; there does however require more work identify the role of Bisphosphonates in the prevention of skeletal metastases (Fleisch 2002).

2. Orthopaedic Surgery

The roles of the orthopaedic surgery in the management of skeletal metastases are (BASO 1999):

1. Prophylactic fixation of bone where there is a significant risk of fracture.

2. Fixation and stabilisation following a fracture (Figure 5).
3. Decompression of spinal nerve roots and stabilisation of the affected vertebrae.

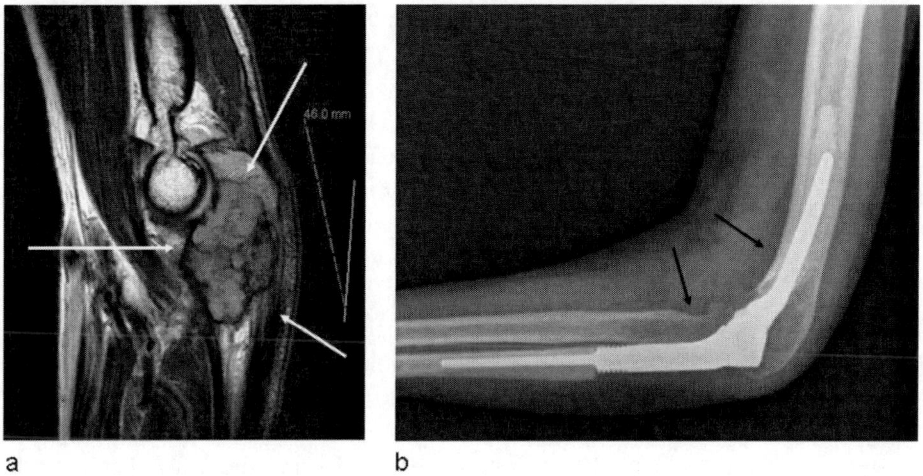

Figure 5. 60 year old male presenting with lytic lesion of the left elbow (olecranon) (a) that was treated with an elbow replacement (b).

Mirels (1989) suggested a scoring system (table 3) to evaluate the risk of a pathological fracture, which is widely used in the USA. A high score would mean a high risk of fracture and so prophylactic fixation could be considered. This study found that scores of 7 or less carry a less than 5% risk of fracture and so conservative management and primary radiotherapy is indicated. Scores of 9 or more carry a high risk of fracture and so prophylactic surgery is indicated, whereas scores of 8 carry an intermediate (≈15%) and therefore a decision should be made based on the clinical picture.

Table 3. Mirels' scoring system for evaluation of risk of pathological fracture *(1989)*

Variable	Score 1	Score 2	Score 3
Site	*Upper limb*	*Lower limb*	*Peri-trochanter*
Pain	*Mild*	*Moderate*	*Functional*
Lesion	*Blastic*	*Mixed*	*Lytic*
Size	*<1/3**	*1/3–2/3**	*>2/3**

*Refers to the proportion (on radiograph) of a single cortical layer destroyed.

An anaesthetic review is performed in all patients prior to surgery and specialist opinions sought with relevant investigations completed (RCoA Guidelines). Anaesthetic risk is assessed based on The American Society of Anaesthesiologists classification system, consisting of four grades (ASA I-IV). A patient with a higher ASA class has a higher risk of postoperative complications (RCS).

Systemic disease presents with a multitude of symptoms. Symptomatic control is paramount in managing patients with skeletal metastases. At least 60% of surgical patients suffer from coexisting medical issues (Nierman et al. 1999) Haematological, electrolyte and metabolic disturbance, respiratory support, analgesia, bowel and urinary management in particular, need to be addressed urgently prior to surgical treatment. The burden of malignancy also increases the risk of thromboembolic events (deep vein thrombosis and pulmonary embolus) and therefore advice from haematologists should be sought or local guidelines strictly adhered to. A vena cava filter may also be required in patients with coexisting DVT's before to surgery.

Meticulous preoperative planning and a multidisciplinary approach are vital prior to proceeding with surgery. An alternative strategy must be made by the surgeon if the primary surgical plan fails. All surgical equipment must be sterilised, checked and be available prior to surgery (endoprostheses, cement, internal fixation instruments). In certain cases, the availability of general and vascular surgeon teams should be checked.

It is mandatory for the operating room to be well prepared (monitoring equipment, sterility) before surgery. Extra care must be given to patient positioning to pervent decubiti and nerve palsies. The use of extra padding is often helpful. Patient warming prevents risk of hypothermia in lengthy cases. Sequential compression devices, arterial and central venous lines, urethral catheters are all placed for monitoring and continuous blood sampling. End tidal Co_2 is monitored during cementation as this can evoke a cardiopulmonary event. Spinal monitoring may also be required. Broad spectrum antibiotics are administered on induction of anaesthesia, followed by two postoperative doses in routine cases. Finally, the World Health Organisation (WHO) checklist should be performed in the operating room before surgery commences to minimise errors (Haynes et al. 2009).

Postoperatively, patients are managed on the surgical unit. Unstable patients are transferred to high dependency or intensive care unit, where closer monitoring and higher nurse to patient ratio is provided. Cardiopulmonary and haemodynamic monitoring provides a good indication of fluid balance, electrolyte and oxygenation. Drains which are placed intraoperatively also need requiring strict monitoring (ongoing blood loss) and play a role in the fluid replacement regime (Bibbo et al. 2000).

3. Radiotherapy

Radiotherapy has for a number of years been used to successfully treat bone pain, to great effect. It also induces remineralisation of bones which helps stability and can further be used to treat neurological symptoms due to nerve or spinal damage (Kardamakis et al. 2009).

This is generally achieved through a short regime of one to five fractions, although several randomised control trials have shown that a singly fraction of 8 Gy is sufficient to alleviate bone pain (Janjan et al. 1997).

Conclusion

Bone metastasis is a common problem affecting a significant proportion of patients with metastatic cancer. There are continuous developments in the prevention, diagnosis and treatment with advances in imaging, orthopaedic technique and medication, particularly radiopharmaceuticals and cytotoxic, endocrine treatments with newer treatments based around the tumour cell-osteoclast interaction.

REFERENCES

Aoki J, Inoue T, Tomiyoshi K, Shinozaki T, Watanabe H, Takagishi K, Endo K 2001. Nuclear imaging of bone tumors: FDG-PET. Semin Musculoskelet Radiol 5 (2) 183-7.

Bhamra J, Malik AA, Khan WS, Pollock R (2012). The perioperative management of skeletal metastases. *J Periop Pract*. 22(1): 24-9.

Bibbo C, Patel D, Benevenia J. Perioperative considerations in patients with metastatic disease 1999 Orthop Clin North Am 31 (4) 577-595.

Clines GA, Guise TA 2008 Molecular mechanisms and treatment of bone metastasis. *Expert Rev Mol Med* 6 (10) e7.

Coleman RE 2001 Metastatic bone disease: clinical features, pathophysiology and treatment strategies. *Cancer Treat Rev* 27 165–176.

Coleman RE 2004 Bisphosphonates: Clinical Experience. *The Oncologist* 9 (S4)14-27.

Coleman RE 1997 Skeletal complications of malignancy. *Cancer* 80 (S)1588–1594

Cook AM, Lau TN, Tomlinson MJ, Vaidya M, Wakeley CJ, Goddard P 1998 Magnetic resonance imaging of the whole spine in suspected malignant spinal cord compression: Impact on management. *Clinical Oncology* 10 (1) 39-43.

Cook GJ, Fogelman I 2000 The role of positron emission tomography in the management of bone metastases. Cancer 88 (S12) 2927-33.

Dalton JA, Youngblood R 2000 Clinical application of the World Health Organization analgesic ladder. *J Intraven Nurs* 23 (2) 118–124.

Diel IJ, Jaschke A, Solomayer EF, Gollan C, Bastert G, Sohn C, Schuetz F 2008 Adjuvant oral clodronate improves the overall survival of primary breast cancer patients with micrometastases to the bone marrow—a long-term follow-up. *Ann Oncol* 19 (12) 2007–2011.

Fleisch H. Bisphosphonates 1991 Pharmacology and use in the treatment of tumour-induced hypercalcaemic and metastatic bone disease. *Drugs* 42 (6) 919-44.

Fleisch H 2002 Development of bisphosphonates. *Breast Cancer Res* 4 (1) 30-4.

Habermann ET, Lopez RA 1989 Metastatic disease of bone and treatment of pathological fractures. *Orthop Clin North Am* 20 (3) 469-86.

Haynes AB, Weiser TG, Berry WR, Lipsitz SR, Breizat AH S, Dellinger EP, Herbosa T, Joseph S, Kibatala PL, Lapitan MCM, Merry AF, Moorthy K, Reznick RK, Taylor B, Gawande AA 2009 A Surgical Safety Checklist to Reduce Morbidity and Mortality in a Global Population. *N Engl J Med* 360: 491-499.

Held JL, Peahota A 1993 Nursing care of the patient with spinal cord compression. *Oncol Nurs Forum* 20 (10)1507–1516.

Husband DJ 1998 Malignant spinal cord compression: prospective study of delays in referral and treatment. *BMJ* 317 (7150) 18–21.

Kardamakis D, Vassiliou V, Chow E 2009 Bone Metastases: A translational and clinical approach Cancer Metastasis - *Biology and Treatment* 12, DOI: 10.1007/978-1-4020-9819-2.

Kohno N, Aogi K, Minami H, Nakamura S, Asaga T, Yuichi 2005 Zoledronic Acid Significantly Reduces Skeletal Complications Compared With Placebo in Japanese Women With Bone Metastases From Breast Cancer:A Randomized, Placebo-Controlled. *Trial* Journal of Clinical Oncology 23 (15) 3314-3321.

Janjan NA 1997 Radiation for bone metastases: conventional techniques and the role of systemic radiopharmaceuticals. *Cancer* 80 (S8):1628-1645.

Levack P, Graham J, Collie D, Grant R, Kidd J, Kunkler I, Gibson A, Hurman D, McMillan N, Rampling R, Slider L, Statham P, Summers D 2001 A prospective audit of the diagnosis, management and outcome of malignant spinal cord compression. *Clinical Resource and Audit Group* (CRAG) 97/08.

Lipton A 2004 Pathophysiology of bone metastases: how this knowledge may lead to therapeutic intervention. *Support Oncol* 2 205-220.

Loblaw DA, Laperriere NJ, Mackillop WJ 2003 A population-based study of malignant spinal cord compression in Ontario. *Clin Oncol* (R Coll Radiol) 15 (4) 211-7.

Major PP, Cook RJ 2004 Clinical Endpoints forAssessing Bisphosphonate Efficacy in the Prevention of Skeletal Complicationsof Bone Metastases *European Urology* S3 34–39.

Mirels H 1989 Metastatic disease in long bones: A proposed scoring system for diagnosing impending pathologic fracture. *Clin Orthop Rel Res* 249 256.

Merrick MV, Beales JS, Garvie N, Leonard RC 1992 Evaluation and skeletal metastases. Br J Radiol 65 (777) 803-6.

Moos RV, Strasser F, Gillessen S, Zaugg K 2008 Metastatic bone pain: treatment options with an emphasis on bisphosphonates Support Care *Cancer* 16:1105–1115.

Mundy GR 2002 Metastasis to bone: causes, consequences and therapeutic opportunities. *Nature Rev Cancer* 2 584–593.

Nierman E, Zakrzewski K 1999 Recognition and management of preoperative risk Rheum. *Dis Clin North Am* 25 585-622.

Peh WC 2000 Screening for bone metastases. *Am J Orthop* 2 (5) 405.

Rosen LS, Gordon D, Kaminski M, Howell A, Belch A, Mackey J, Apffelstaedt J, Hussein M, Coleman RE, Reitsma DJ, Seaman JJ, Chen BL, Ambros Y 2003 Zoledronic acid versus pamidronate in the treatment of skeletal metastases in patients with breast cancer or osteolytic lesions of multiple myeloma: a phase III, double-blind, comparative trial. Journal of Clinical Oncology 21 (16) 3150-3157.

Rubins JR 1983 The role of myelofibrosis in malignant myelosclerosis. *Cancer* 51 308–11.

Saarto T, Blomqvist C, Virkkunen P 1999 No reduction of bone metastases with adjuvant clodronate treatment in node-positive breast cancer patients *Proc Am Soc Clin Oncol* 18 128a.

Salmon JM, Kilpatrick SE. Pathology of skeletal metastases 2000. *Orthop Clin North Am* 31 (4) 537-44 vii-viii.

Small EJ, Smith MR, Seaman JJ, Petrone S, Kowalski MO 2003 Combined analysis of two multicenter, randomized, placebo-controlled studies of pamidronate disodium for the palliation of bone pain in men with metastatic prostate cancer. *J Clin Oncol* 21 (23) 4277-84.

The management of metastatic bone disease in the UK 1999 The Breast Specialty Group of the British Association of Surgical Oncology (BASO) *European Journal of Surgical Oncology* 25 3–23.

The Royal College of Anaesthetists http://www.rcoa.ac.uk

The Royal College of Surgeons. Preoperative Tests - the use of routine preoperative tests for elective surgery. *Appendices, Guidelines & Information* www.rcseng.ac.uk

Traill ZC, Talbot D, Golding S, Gleeson FV 1999 Magnetic resonance imaging versus radionuclide scintigraphy in screening for bone metastases. *Clin Radiol* 54 (7) 448-51.

Van der Pluijm G, Lowik C, Papapoulos S 2000 Tumour progression and angiogenesis in bone metastases from breast cancer: new approaches to an old problem. *Cancer Treat Rev* 26 11-27.

Weber K L 2010 Evaluation of the Adult Patient (Aged >40 Years) With a Destructive Bone Lesion. *J Am Acad Orthop Surg* 18 (3) 169-179.

Yoneda T, Michigami T, Yi B 1999 Use of Bisphosphonates for the treatment of bone metastasis in experimental animal models. *Cancer Treat Rev* 25 293-299.

In: Perioperative Practice in Trauma and Orthopaedic Surgery ISBN: 978-1-63483-325-7
Editor: Wasim S. Khan

Chapter 22

Arthroscopic Knee Surgery: An Evidence-Based Practice

Christopher Onyema, Emeka Oragui, Jonathan White and Wasim S. Khan*

University College London Institute of Orthopaedics and Musculoskeletal Sciences,
Royal National Orthopaedic Hospital, Stanmore, London, UK

Abstract

Knee arthroscopy is a minimally-invasive technique that allows intra-articular assessment and treatment of knee joint pathology. It has proven benefits of reduced patient morbidity, earlier recovery and mobilisation, and it is cost-effective. In this chapter we review the anatomy of the knee joint, indications and contra-indications to knee arthroscopic use, and consider the main techniques of knee arthroscopy including types of anaesthetic, prophylactic antibiotics, theatre setup and arthroscopic portals, and post-operative care.

Keywords: Knee, arthroscopy, evidence-based practice, Minimally Invasive Surgery (MIS)

In this chapter we review the evidence base behind arthroscopic knee surgery (Onyema et al. 2011). Arthroscopy of the knee is the most common operative procedure in orthopaedic surgery today. Like all arthroscopic procedures, it delivers a minimally invasive approach to orthopaedic operations that previously necessitated open surgery. The basic principle involves the insertion of a camera and associated equipment through small portals in the skin to allow intra-articular evaluation and treatment of pathology. Professor Kenji Takagi of Tokyo has

* Corresponding Author: Mr Wasim S Khan, Clinical Lecturer, University College London Institute of Orthopaedic and Musculoskeletal Research, Royal National Orthopaedic Hospital, Stanmore, London, HA7 4LP, UK. Telephone number: +44 (0) 77791 025554. Fax number: +44 (0) 1707 655059. E-mail address: wasimkhan@doctors.org.uk.

traditionally been cited as having performed the first arthroscopic assessment of the knee in 1919 although it may be that the Danish physician Severin Nordentoft actually pioneered the technique seven years earlier. The technique became an established feature of orthopaedic practice during the 1970s, and today surgeons can perform an array of complex intra-articular operations through small incisions (Katz & Gomoll 2007). Knee arthroscopy is used to perform many procedures that previously necessitated an open procedure such as simple meniscectomies, ligament reconstruction and cartilage restoration.

There are many advantages of arthroscopic surgery over traditional open surgery. The minimally invasive technique results in less trauma to the patient, less post-operative pain and less blood loss. Patients recover faster and can quickly return to their normal daily activities. A day surgery arthroscopic procedure is more readily accepted by patients than an in-patient arthrotomy and may facilitate earlier intervention. Cosmetically-speaking, smaller skin scars are more appealing. An economic benefit is provided as patients spend less time in hospital, can quickly return to work, and overall, the procedure is less expensive compared to open operations.

Arthroscopic Knee Anatomy

The knee joint comprises articulations between the medial and lateral compartments of the distal femur and proximal tibia as well as an articulation between the patella and the anterior aspect of the distal femur, which forms the third, patellofemoral compartment. The surfaces of these bones are lined with articular cartilage and in addition two crescent-shaped fibro-cartilaginous pads called menisci lie between the femoral and tibial compartments and are joined by a transverse inter-meniscal ligament that connects them anteriorly. These menisci protect articular surfaces by providing lubrication and reducing friction. They may also have a role in providing nutrition to tissues (Katz 2007).

The peripheral part of the meniscus is vascular and DeHaven (1990) suggested that tears in the peripheral 3 mm are amenable to repair (Koval & Zuckerman 2004), whereas tears more than 5 mm from the menisco-capsular aspect are avascular with little or no potential for healing or repair.

The knee joint is stabilised by ligaments around the knee. These include the medial and lateral collateral ligaments which can be palpated at the joint line and resist varus and valgus strain respectively. The anterior cruciate ligaments (ACL) and posterior cruciate ligaments (PCL) lie within the joint and resist displacement of the tibia on the femur in an anterior or posterior direction respectively. The fibrous capsule contributes to the stability of the joint. The knee is also supported by several muscles that include the quadriceps and the hamstrings (Koval & Zuckerman 2004).

Indications and Contra-Indications to Knee Arthroscopy

Knee arthroscopy may be diagnostic or therapeutic, and is indicated when there is no other way to confirm the diagnosis, or the lesion is amenable to arthroscopic surgery and no easier technique to treat the pathology exists. The final decision on whether to perform an elective knee arthroscopy or not usually relies upon symptoms and disabilities that negatively impact on the quality of a patient's life but may be hard to quantify (DeHaven 1990). The use of knee arthroscopy has been demonstrated for diagnosis and treatment of intra-articular lesions, loose bodies, meniscal tears, osteoarthritis, cartilage repair, ACL reconstruction, synovectomy and plicectomy, unexplained knee pain, intra-articular tumours, painful knee after total knee replacement, pyogenic arthritis, and arthro-fibrosis (Marx 2008).

Only a few contraindications for knee arthroscopy exist. These include localised soft tissue infection where the insertion of the equipment into the knee joint may introduce infection into the joint and cause overt sepsis. Infection in the joint itself is not a contraindication, and in such cases arthroscopic techniques may be employed for debridement and drainage.

Severe degenerative joint diseases resulting in stiffness or ankylosis of the knee may prohibit manoeuvring of the arthroscope within the various compartments and access may be difficult. It may also be difficult to operate on any patient with a recent haemarthrosis as visualisation may be compromised. Training and technical ability also limits the procedures that may be performed by any knee surgeon (Noble 1992).

A thorough evaluation of the patient before the procedure is mandatory and should include a relevant history, examination and appropriate imaging. Magnetic resonance imaging (MRI) is useful as it has been shown to be reliable for the exclusion of intraarticular lesions, thus reducing the number of unnecessary arthroscopies (Friemert 2004). During the operation, all necessary imaging should be made available (Jackson 1972).

Anaesthesia

Arthroscopic knee surgery can be performed with general, regional or local anaesthesia, each having its own advantages and disadvantages. The anaesthetic technique(s) used will depend on the preferences of the anaesthetist, patient and operating surgeon, as well as local guidelines.

1. General Anaesthetic

General anaesthesia has remained the most common modality for knee arthroscopy. This technique puts the patient to sleep, allowing complete muscle relaxation for the entire procedure and is a good choice for very young or anxious patients. However, there are associated risks of allergic/ anaphylactic reactions to the anaesthetic agents and the risk associated with intubation and ventilation during general anaesthesia (Dandy 1997). In the anaesthetic room, a laryngeal mask airway is commonly used. Before starting the procedure the portal sites may be injected with a local anaesthetic as this has been shown to reduce post-operative pain and opioid requirements (Buckenmaier 2002).

2. Spinal Anaesthetic

Spinal anaesthesia provides good single-injection anaesthesia for knee arthroscopy. It is preferred for lower limb orthopaedic surgery because of its reliability and simplicity. It permits the patient to be awake during the procedure if desired. Other advantages include a rapid onset, high reliability, and a reduction in the time that the patient spends in post-anaesthesia recovery and facilitates early hospital discharge. Low dose, short-acting agents such as lidocaine have considerable benefits over long-acting agents in terms of recovery and home discharge. Disadvantages include the small risk of spinal headache despite using newer spinal needles, and the possibility of a difficult spinal puncture (McKeon et al., 2009).

3. Local Anaesthetic

Although not commonly practiced in the UK or US, knee arthroscopy under local anaesthesia has been shown to be reliable and safe with appropriate case selection by an experienced anaesthetist. Evidence for its efficacy has been demonstrated in Hong Kong, Japan and Sweden (Law et al., 2009, Jacobsen et al., 2000, Yoshiya et al., 1988). The disadvantages are that this method of anaesthesia may limit tourniquet use, and the patient's tolerance to movement of the limb may limit the amount of forceful manipulation that can be achieved.

In some cases, conversion to general anaesthesia is required. Local anaesthesia is cost-effective, allows for a quicker recovery and shorter hospital stay (O'Donnell BD & Iohom, 2008). Nevertheless, the use of arthroscopy under local anaesthesia will depend on surgeon preference and local practice.

The local anaesthetic should be injected into the portal sites and joint itself, with most of the agent being injected into the subcutaneous layer. Successful intra-articular injection can be confirmed by a positive patellar tap and bulging from the medial gutter. Introduction of the agent into the subcapsular layer should be avoided as this will push the fat pad into the joint, hindering visualisation in the initial stages. A twenty minute waiting interval should be given after the injection to allow for onset of action of the agent. Sedatives can also be given for anxious or apprehensive patients.

Prophylactic Antibiotics

Prophylactic antibiotics are not routinely used for knee arthroscopy because the procedure is considered clean. This is supported by the low rate of post-operative infection reported in the literature. The use of antibiotics also increases costs and introduces a risk of allergic reactions and the development of antibiotic resistant organisms (Law et al., 2009, Allum, 2002). In a study of 2,780 arthroscopic meniscectomies Bert et al., (2007) showed that there was no value in administering antibiotics. They reported infection rates of 0.15% when prophylactic antibiotics were administered compared to 0.16% in patients who received no antibiotics ($P = 0.59$).

Complex procedures of long duration or those that involve the use of implants may require antibiotics. Patients who have a high risk of infection and those with conditions such as diabetes, skin and immunological disorders should also be considered for prophylactic antibiotics (Allum, 2002).

THEATRE SETUP

1. Skin Preparation

Full aseptic precautions must be taken and the skin should be prepped and draped. A standard antiseptic solution such as a chlorhexidine-based one should be used to prepare the skin from ankle to groin. Special precautions should be taken when dealing with the skin around the foot as the bacterial load is high and the risk of cross contamination of the operative site greater (Bert et al., 2007).

2. Tourniquet

A tourniquet may be used to produce a bloodless field during the procedure although some surgeons may prefer not to. It may be sensible to apply the tourniquet before the operation, reserving inflation for cases where unexpected bleeding has occurred and sufficient visibility cannot be maintained. Tourniquet pressure is determined by the anaesthetist based on the patient's blood pressure; a pressure of 300 mm Hg has been shown to be safe in the lower limb (Wu and Richmond 2003). Using a wide and padded tourniquet minimises the incidence of complications such as compression neurapraxia and temporary paresis (Dandy 1986, Wakai et al., 2001, Oragui et al., in press).

3. Equipment Setup

In the operating room careful planning and communication is essential in setting up the operating room to allow the anaesthetist to provide a safe anaesthetic and the surgeon to make best use of all the necessary equipment. Special consideration should be placed upon the position of video equipment, the arthroscope, light source, shaving and cauterising systems, the irrigation pump, and an array of arthroscopic hand instruments.

4. Patient Positioning

The patient is positioned supine on the operating table. The operative limb may be placed in a leg holder, so that the joint can be adequately manipulated and opened. If a leg holder is used it should be well-padded and placed high on the thigh and snug. Some surgeons prefer to use a lateral side post and choose to leave the limb on the table, adjusting the patient's knee during the procedure. A lateral side post should be carefully set up to ensure that it will be at the correct level. Incorrect use of the leg holder or unpadded leg holders will increase the risk of pressure injury (Buckenmaier 2002, Malik et al., 2009). Adequate light source is essential for placement of the portals (Marx 2000).

ARTHROSCOPIC PORTALS

Accurate placement of portals is essential to optimise visualisation and manipulation of the joint. Palpating and drawing bony landmarks, joint lines and soft tissue structures can help to identify correct sites of entry. The inflow cannula is usually inserted into the supero-medial supra-patella pouch once landmarks have been marked out. The irrigation fluid bag should be raised 1.5 metres higher than the patient and the fluid outflow regulated to ensure distension of the knee joint. This will remove soft tissue such as the synovium and fat pad from view (Aiello 1986). Most procedures require only two portals, however a third portal may be needed for fluid flow with certain irrigation systems.

1. Antero-Lateral Portal

The antero-lateral portal is most commonly employed for diagnostic arthroscopy as it offers superior visualisation of most parts of the knee joint. A 4 mm incision is made approximately 1 cm lateral to the border of the patellar tendon and about 1 cm above the lateral joint line (Aiello, 1986). To avoid damaging the meniscus, the cutting edge of the blade should be pointing up when extended through the capsule and synovium, and the scalpel should not plunge too deep as to damage the articular cartilage. A blunt trocar in an arthroscope sheath is then introduced through the portal, directed toward the medial wall of the intercondylar notch, with the knee in approximately 30 degrees of flexion. The arthroscope is then inserted into the sheath, replacing the blunt trocar (Katx & Gomoll 2007, Aiello, 1986).

2. Antero-Medial Portal

The antero-medial portal is used for additional visualisation of the lateral compartment, and instrumentation of the medial or lateral compartment structures. It is created with the knee in 30 degrees of flexion, where the soft spot is palpated, 1 cm medial to the border of the patellar tendon and about 1 cm above the medial joint line (Aiello, 1986).

3. Postero-Medial Portal

The postero-medial portal is placed in a small triangular soft spot about 1 cm posterior to the postero-medial edge of the femoral condyle, and about 1 cm above the postero-medial joint line. For best results with creating this portal, the knee should be fully distended, with 90 degrees of flexion, external rotation, and abduction. With the arthroscope angled at 30 degrees, it should be possible to view and inspect all the structures in the postero-medial compartment including the PCL, posterior horn of the medial meniscus, and the postero-medial aspect of the femoral condyle and synovial lining (Katx & Gomoll 2007, Buckenmaier, 2002).

4. Supero-Lateral Portal

The supero-lateral portal is the best approach for viewing the articulation between the patella and femur diagnostically, with a 70 degree arthroscope. The surgeon should be able to track the patella and assess congruity. The portal should be established as close to the lateral margin of the quadriceps tendon as possible, and about 2.5 cm superior to the supero-lateral edge of the patella (Katx & Gomoll 2007, Aiello, 1986).

5. Additional Portals

Other portals exist, and their placement depends on the pathology that is expected or encountered. These include postero-lateral, medial and lateral proximal mid-patellar, and the central trans-patellar tendon portals (Buckenmaier 2002, Aiello, 1986).

Some Common Arthroscopic Procedures

1. Diagnostic Arthroscopy

The most common use for knee arthroscopy has been that of a diagnostic tool and includes staging osteoarthritic degenerative disease, assessing osteochondritis dessicans defects, obtaining biopsies for diagnosis confirmation e.g., rheumatoid arthritis, managing septic arthritis and haemoarthrosis, and assessing tibial plateau fractures. The method should be conducted in the same sequence each time, dividing the knee into individual compartments (suprapatellar pouch and patellofemoral joint; medial gutter; medial compartment; intercondylar notch; posteromedial compartment; lateral compartment; and lateral gutter). This allows for a thorough evaluation and diagnosis of knee joint pathology with the option of intervention if required.

In the current economic climate, the role of diagnostic knee arthroscopy is under review. Although arthroscopy remains the gold standard for the investigation of intra-articular abnormalities, MRI provides a less invasive and more cost-effective alternative (Vincken et al. 2007). It is a highly accurate modality for diagnosing meniscal and ACL lesions, although for PCL lesions the sensitivity and accuracy is low (Crawford et al. 2007). Its high specificity and negative predictive value confirm its use as the most accurate screening tool prior to therapeutic arthroscopy. In the non-acute setting, when used in combination with a full history and clinical examination, MRI can obviate the need for arthroscopy, saving costs and preventing unnecessary risk.

2. Meniscal lesions

Meniscal injury is the most common indication for the therapeutic application of knee arthroscopy. Meniscal tears are classified intra-operatively according to macroscopic appearance. They may be classified as longitudinal, horizontal, oblique and radial tears, as well as flap, basket handle, complex and degenerative tears (Aiello 1986). When the meniscus is torn the site will determine whether the lesion is amenable to healing and whether arthroscopic surgery is required to either repair or to excise a portion of the meniscus (Koval & Zuckerman 2004). Excisions can be performed with a basket-punch or a motorised shaver, although the use of radiofrequency ablation has also been demonstrated. It is always preferable to save as much of the meniscus as possible by performing a partial meniscectomy, where only loose fragments are excised (Marx 2000, Pasa & Visna 2005).

3. Loose Body Extraction

Removing loose bodies from the knee arthroscopically is a relatively common procedure and surgeons should select the correct portal depending on the site of the lesion (Gold et al. 1995). Due to gravity, intra-articular loose bodies are often found in the posterior compartment and an appropriate portal should be selected (Dandy & O'Carroll 1982). The loose body should then be immobilised, grasped and removed. The smallest should be removed first and then the knee re-examined before closure.

4. Focal Articular Cartilage Lesions

A number of options for the repair or replacement of focal cartilaginous lesions have been used arthrosopically including abrasive chondroplasty, subchondral drilling, micro-fracture, cartilage transplantation and Autologous Chondrocyte Implantation (ACI) (Spahn et al., 2008, Jaiswal et al., 2010, 2011). A promising new approach is the use of tissue engineering applications for the arthroscopic replacement of articular cartilage defects using stem cells (Khan et al., 2010, Ong et al. 2013).

5. ACL Reconstruction

Ligament reconstruction of both the ACL and PCL can be achieved using arthroscopic techniques. A minimally invasive, arthroscopic approach has several advantages: smaller incisions, fewer adhesions, less disruption to the extensor mechanism, less pain, faster rehabilitation and enhanced visualisation of the ligament insertion points. Graft selection is surgeon and patient-dependent and options include autograft (patellar tendon or hamstrings) or allograft (patellar tendon or Achilles' tendon).

6. Osteoarthritis

Techniques such as joint lavage and debridement, loose body extraction, partial synovectomy, and meniscectomy are currently being utilised for treatment of osteoarthritis of the knee (Khan & Hardingham 2010). Arthroscopy may not be beneficial to all patients with knee osteoarthritis and controversy exists as to whether it provides any additional benefit over conventional treatment (Siparsky et al., 2007, Minocha & Khan 2014).

During arthroscopy the severity of osteoarthritis can be graded using the Outerbridge scale grading system. This may help determine the specific arthroscopic technique to be use when treating osteoarthritis. Grade I refers to softening of articular cartilage; grades II and III refer to fragmentation of an area of articular cartilage less than 1 cm and greater than 1 cm respectively; in grade IV there is erosion of articular cartilage through to the underlying bone (Nutton 2009).

Dressings and Post-Operative Care

Once the case is finished, excess irrigation fluid is removed and long acting local anaesthetic may be injected into the joint to help reduce post-operative pain. The wound may be closed with appropriate sutures or steri-strips. Before a compressive wrap is applied, the wound should ideally be covered with absorbable pads and sterile dressing (Buckenmaier 2002, Stuart & Lubowitz 2006). The regime will vary depending on the surgeon's preference and local practice.

Specific post operative rehabilitation will depend upon findings and procedures undertaken. For basic arthroscopy the patient should be instructed in the use of crutches and exercises, and should continue to use crutches for one to three days. Early exercise is usually allowed however the weight bearing status varies with the procedure performed. Patients may remove dressings for simple arthroscopy after forty-eight hours and maintain hygienic wound care (Buckenmaier 2002, Stuart & Lubowitz 2006). The patient may have a brace applied for up to six weeks if they have undergone a focal cartilage repair procedure (Burkhart 2003).

Complications

Although knee arthroscopy is a relatively safe procedure, complications can and do occur and may depend upon the exact procedure being carried out. Intra-operative complications such as nerve compression injury may result from leg holders or prolonged tourniquet use (Khan et al. 2007). Other operative complications include compartment syndrome and vascular injury (Kim et al. 2002). Penetrating injuries to the popliteal artery have also been reported (Law et al. 2009).

Post-operative complications include pain, haemarthrosis, complex regional pain syndrome, synovial fistula, infection and thrombo-embolism. Most arthroscopic procedures are of short duration and early post-operative mobilisation reduces the risk of thrombo-embolism. For this reason thrombo-prophylaxis is not routinely given in arthroscopic surgery. However, thrombo-prophylaxis is indicated for high risk patients such as those with a previous history of thrombo-embolic disease, morbidly obese patients and procedures that have involved prolonged tourniquet use (Ramos et al. 2007).

Conclusion

The advantages of arthroscopic surgery are clear when compared to traditional open surgery. Patients recover faster and can quickly resume their normal daily activities. Procedures can be done on a day case basis, and in general are more readily accepted by patients than an in-patient arthrotomy, thus facilitating earlier intervention. Day surgery is also more economical as patients spend less time in hospital and return to work sooner.

In the current economic climate, the role of diagnostic knee arthroscopy is under review. Although arthroscopy remains the gold standard for the investigation of intra-articular abnormalities with the potential benefit of intervention, MRI provides a less invasive, highly accurate and more cost-effective alternative and has a role as a screening tool prior to therapeutic arthroscopy. In the non-acute setting, when used in combination with a full history and clinical examination, MRI can obviate the need for arthroscopy, saving costs and preventing unnecessary risk.

Knee arthroscopy is indicated in the diagnosis and treatment of a variety of knee pathology. A thorough understanding of the principles and techniques of knee arthroscopy and evidence-base is crucial to a successful outcome and low complication rate.

References

Ahn JH, Yoo JC, Lee SH 2007 Arthroscopic loose-body removal in posterior compartment of the knee joint: a technical note. Knee Surgery, Sports Traumatology, *Arthroscopy* 15 (1) 100-106.

Aiello D 1986 Arthroscopy of the knee. A perioperative nursing challenge AORN Journal 43 (4) 824-827

Allum R 2002 Complications of arthroscopy of the knee Journal of Bone and Joint Surgery. *British Volume* 84 (7) 937-945.

Bert J, Giannini D, Nace L 2007 Antibiotic prophylaxis for arthroscopy of the knee: is it necessary? *Arthroscopy* 23 (1) 4-6.

Buckenmaier C 3rd 2002 Anaesthesia for outpatient knee surgery Best Practice & Research. *Clinical Anaesthesiology* 16 (2) 255-270.

Burkhart SS 2003 *Operative arthroscopy 3rd ed.* Philadelphia, Lippincott Williams & Wilkins.

Campbell W, Canale S 2003 *Campbell's operative orthopaedics 10th ed.* St Louis, Mosby.

Crawford R, Walley G, Bridgman S, Maffulli N 2007 Magnetic resonance imaging versus arthroscopy in the diagnosis of knee pathology, concentrating on meniscal lesions and ACL tears: systematic review *British Medical Bulletin* 84 5-23.

Dandy D, O'Carroll P 1982 The removal of loose bodies from the knee under arthroscopic control. Journal of Bone and Joint Surgery. *British Volume* 64 (4)473-474.

Dandy D 1986 Arthroscopy: the endoscopy of joints. *British Medical Bulletin* 42 (3) 301-306.

Dandy D 1997 Arthroscopy and MRI for the knee Journal of Bone and Joint Surgery. *British Volume* 79 (4) 520.

DeHaven K 1990 Decision-making factors in the treatment of meniscus lesions. *Clinical Orthopaedics and Related Research* 252 49-54.

Friemert B, Oberlander Y, Schwarz W, Haberle HJ, Bahren W, Gerngross H, Danz B 2004 Diagnosis of chondral lesions of the knee joint: can MRI replace arthroscopy? A prospective study Knee Surgery, Sports Traumatology, *Arthroscopy* 12 (1) 58-64.

Gold D, Schaner P, Sapega A 1995 The posteromedial portal in knee arthroscopy: an analysis of diagnostic and surgical utility. *Arthroscopy* 11 (2) 139-145.

Jackson R, Abe I 1972 The role of arthroscopy in the management of disorders of the knee. An analysis of 200 consecutive examinations Journal of Bone and Joint Surgery. *British Volume* 54 (2) 310-322.

Jacobsen E, Forssblad M, Rosenberg J, Westman L, Weidenhielm L 2000 Can local anaesthesia be recommended for routine use in elective knee arthroscopy? A comparison between local, spinal, and general anaesthesia *Arthroscopy* 16 (2) 183-190.

Jaiswal PK, Wong K, Khan WS (2010). Current cell based strategies for knee cartilage injuries. *J Stem Cells*. 5(4):177-85.

Jaiswal PK, Wong K, Khan WS (2011). Operative Treatment of Knee Cartilage Injuries: A Review of the Current Literature on Non-Cell-Based and Cell-Based Therapies. *Br J Med Med Res*. 1(4): 516-537.

Katz J, Gomoll A 2007 Advances in arthroscopic surgery: indications and outcomes. *Current Opinion in Rheumatology* 19 (2) 106-110.

Khan WS, Jones RK, Nokes L, Johnson DS 2007 How accurate are lockable orthotic knee braces? An objective study with the use of gait analysis. *The Knee* 14 (6) 497-499.

Khan WS, Hardingham TE 2010 Stem Cell Applications and Cartilage Tissue Engineering Approaches in Orthopaedic Surgery New York, Nova Science Publishers.

Khan WS, Johnson DS, Hardingham TE 2010 The potential use of stem cells for knee articular cartilage repair. *The Knee* 17 (6) 369-374

Kim TK, Savino RM, McFarland EG, Cosgarea HJ 2002 Neurovascular complications of knee arthroscopy. *The American Journal of Sports Medicine* 30 (4) 619-629.

Koval K, Zuckerman J 2004 Atlas of orthopaedic surgery: a multimedia reference Philadelphia, Lippincott Williams & Wilkins.

Kurzweil P 2006 *Antibiotic prophylaxis for arthroscopic surgery Arthroscopy* 22 (4) 452-454.

Law BK, Yung PS, Ho EP, Chang JJ, Kwok GK, Fung KY, Chan KM 2009 Review of knee arthroscopy performed under local anesthesia. *Sports Medicine, Arthroscopy, Rehabilitation, Therapy & Technology* 1 (1) 3.

Malik AA, Khan WS, Chaudhry A, Ihsan M, Cullen NP 2009 Acute Compartment Syndrome- A Life and Limb Threatening Surgical Emergency. *Journal of Perioperative Practice* 19 (5) 137-142.

Marx RG 2000 Tourniquet use during arthroscopy did not adversely affect patient outcomes Journal of Bone and Joint Surgery. *American Volume* 82 (9) 1325.

Marx RG 2008 Arthroscopic surgery for osteoarthritis of the knee? *The New England Journal of Medicine* 359 (11) 1169-1170.

McKeon B, Bono JV, Richmond JC 2009 Knee Arthroscopy New York, Springer Noble J 1992 Unnecessary arthroscopy. *Journal of Bone and Joint Surgery. British Volume* 74 (6) 797-798.

Minocha A, Khan WS (2014). *Knee osteoarthritis: review of treatment options*. GM: Midlife & Beyond. 44(9): 88-91.

Nutton RW 2009 Is arthroscopic surgery a beneficial treatment for knee osteoarthritis? Nature Clinical Practice. *Rheumatology* 5 (3) 122-123.

O'Donnell B, Iohom G 2008 Regional anesthesia techniques for ambulatory orthopedic surgery. *Current Opinion in Anaesthesiology* 21 (6) 723-728.

Ong E, Chimutengwende-Gordon M, Khan W (2013). Stem cell therapy for knee ligament, articular cartilage and meniscal injuries. *Curr Stem Cell Res Ther*. 8(6): 422-8.

Onyema C, Oragui E, White J, Khan WS (2011). Evidence-based practice in arthroscopic knee surgery. *J Perioper Pract*. 21(4): 128-134.

Oragui E, Parsons A, White T, Khan WS, Longo UG. Tourniquet Use in Upper Limb Surgery. *Hand* (NY) (in press).

Pasa L, Visna P 2005 Suture of meniscus. *Scripta Medica* 78 (3) 135-150.

Ramos J, Perrotta C, Badariotti G, Berenstein G 2007 Interventions for preventing venous thromboembolism in adults undergoing knee arthroscopy. *Cochrane Database of Systematic Reviews* (online) 18 (2):CD005259.

Siparsky P, Ryzewicz M, Peterson B, Bartz R 2007 Arthroscopic treatment of osteoarthritis of the knee: are there any evidence-based indications? *Clinical Orthopaedics and Related Research* 455 107-112.

Spahn G, Kahl E, Mückley T, Hoffman GO, Klinger HM 2008 Arthroscopic knee chondroplasty using a bipolar radiofrequency-based device compared to mechanical shaver: results of a prospective, randomized, controlled study. *Knee Surgery, Sports Traumatology, Arthroscopy* 16 (6) 565-573.

Stuart MJ, Lubowitz JH 2006 What, if any, are the indications for arthroscopic debridement of the osteoarthritic knee? *Arthroscopy* 22 (3) 238-239.

Vincken PW, ter Braak AP, van Erkel AR et al., 2007 MR imaging: effectiveness and costs at triage of patients with nonacute knee symptoms *Radiology* 242 (1) 85-93.

Wakai A, Winter DC, Street JT, Redmond PH 2001 Pneumatic tourniquets in extremity surgery. *The Journal of the American Academy of Orthopaedic Surgeons* 9 (5) 345-351.

In: Perioperative Practice in Trauma and Orthopaedic Surgery ISBN: 978-1-63483-325-7
Editor: Wasim S. Khan

Chapter 23

TOTAL KNEE REPLACEMENT: RECENT ADVANCES IN DESIGNS, APPROACHES AND MATERIALS

James M. Wong, Wasim S. Khan**, Mukai Chimutengwende-Gordon, Ernest Chew and George S. E. Dowd

Department of Trauma and Orthopaedics,
Royal Free Hampstead NHS Trust, London, UK

ABSTRACT

Ever since Themistocles Gluck described the use of an ivory cup as a tibial hemiarthroplasty in 1894, knee arthoplasty has continued to evolve. Both human ingenuity and intensive clinical research has led to an improved understanding of biomaterials and knee kinematics, resulting in the modern total knee replacement which has enjoyed such a clinical and commercial success. As it increases in popularity, attempts to improve knee arthroplasty have been driven by demands for improved function and implant survival, particularly in younger, more demanding patients. Research continues to see if advances in implant instrumentation, materials and design will translate into improved clinical outcomes and longevity.

Keywords: Knee, arthroplasty, advances, design, materials

INTRODUCTION

Knee replacement surgery is an increasingly popular procedure with good long-term results (Minocha & Khan 2014). In this chapter we discuss recent advances in designs,

* Corresponding Author: Mr Wasim S Khan, Clinical Lecturer, University College London Institute of Orthopaedics and Musculoskeletal Science, Royal National Orthopaedic Hospital, Stanmore, Middlesex, London, HA7 4LP, UK, Telephone number: +44 (0) 7791 025554, Fax number: +44 (0) 20 8570 3864, E-mail address: wasimkhan@doctors.org.uk.

approaches and materials in total knee replacement. We present a review of the literature and provide current evidence (Wong et al. 2011).

Since the development of modern total knee arthroplasty implants in the 1970's, total knee replacements have been overwhelmingly successful in their primary function of abolishing pain in degenerative joints (Ritter et al. 2001). Modern implants enjoy a high satisfaction rate and an acceptably low revision rate (Noble et al. 2006, Bourne et al. 2010). This success can account for their popularity, with the 7th National Joint Registry (NJR) Report documenting 79,263 primary total knee arthroplasties performed in the England and Wales alone in 2009-2010 (NJR 2010). This demand is expected to expand, with some estimates from the United States predicting a 673% increase by the year 2030 (Kurtz et al. 2007). With an increasing incidence of early onset degenerative, disabling rheumatoid and post traumatic arthritis total knee replacements are now being offered to patients at a younger age. The continued evolution of knee arthroplasty has been driven by the need for longer lasting implants for these patients, with both the latest NJR report (NJR 2010) and the Swedish Knee Arthroplasty Register (SKAR 2010) documenting higher revision rates in younger patients. However, some of these changes are undoubtedly market driven, with a specific procedure often marketed directly at patients. Developments in knee arthroplasty have explored the possibilities of new implant designs, new surgical techniques and new implant materials and these are discussed below.

New Total Knee Replacement Designs

The vast majority of total knee arthroplasty implants in use today are versions of the 'condylar' knee replacements developed in the 1970's, widely credited to work by Freeman and Swanson of the London Hospital and Imperial College, and Insall, Burstein and Walker of the Hospital for Special Surgery in New York (Shetty et al. 2003). These advances in design have resulted in a marked improvement in results and longevity. Condylar knee replacements incorporate an anatomically shaped femoral component, usually made from a cobalt-chrome alloy, with an anterior flange to articulate with the patella. The femoral component articulates with a polyethylene tibial tray, which is usually attached to a titanium tibial component (Figure 1). Inserting these implants involves resection of the bone ends to create parallel and equal spaces in flexion and extension, and then balancing the soft tissues to convey stability. These implants are normally cemented in place using acrylic polymethylmethacrylate cement. Alterations to this design in recent years include modifications to improve flexion and altering the implant's dimensions based on the patient's gender.

1. The High Flexion Knee

Postoperative flexion is one of the parameters that surgeons and patients use to evaluate the success of total knee arthroplasty. Whilst the human knee is capable of 150 degrees of flexion, patients after total knee arthroplasty rarely achieve more than 110 degrees. Attempts have therefore been made to modify prostheses to allow more flexion, particularly in the younger patient. This can be achieved by increased 'wraparound' of the femoral component around the posterior femoral condyles. This theoretically enables flexion of the prosthetic knee in excess of 130 degrees, whilst maintaining the same performance at normal ranges of flexion.

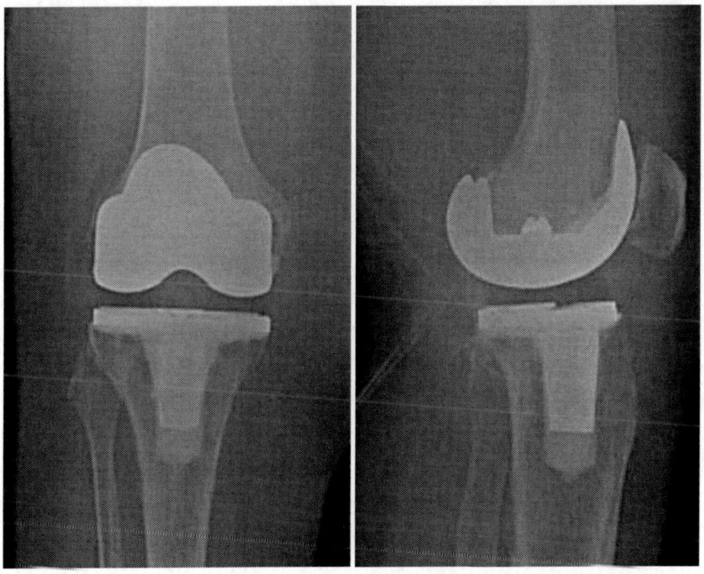

Figure 1. Postoperative radiographs of a modern total knee replacement prosthesis.

Several high-flexion prostheses are now available, with varied results in the published literature. Although some randomised, prospective studies have shown high flexion designs achieve 10-13 degrees more flexion than standard knee arthroplasties (Huang et al. 2005, Weeden and Schmidt 2007), others have shown no difference in eventual flexion (Kim et al. 2005, Mehin et al. 2010). Some have questioned the need for these implants, with one study investigating knee movements after high flex TKR showing flexion greater than 90 degrees was needed 0.5% of the time, and 120 degrees less than 0.1% of the time during activities of daily living (Huddleston et al. 2009). Of some concern is the finding that high flexion activities induce higher implant stress levels, raising the possibility that implant longevity may be compromised (Barink et al. 2008). Clearly, long term results regarding flexion and implant survival are needed.

2. Gender Specific Designs

Small but significant anatomical variations in male and female knees have long been recognised. Measurements taken intraoperatively suggest women have narrower femoral condyles than men (Chin et al. 2002). This can make sizing of femoral components, which is typically based on the anteroposterior dimensions of the femur, awkward. An appropriately sized femoral component may be too wide, altering collateral ligament balancing. This may have to be accepted, or alternatively a smaller femoral component may be used, resulting in laxity in flexion. Women also differ from men in that they have a different orientation of the articulation between the femur and the patella.

Manufacturers have now introduced gender specific total knee arthroplasty designs with modified dimensions to accommodate the anatomical differences between sexes. Clinical results are starting to appear in the medical literature. In a prospective randomised trial comparing gender specific with standard implants, Kim et al. (2010a) found no significant differences between the two groups in terms of satisfaction, clinical or radiological outcome.

3. The Medial Pivot Knee

Attempts have also been made to adapt knee arthroplasty designs as our understanding of knee kinematics changes. Work by Freeman using MRI studies of cadaveric knees have demonstrated that whilst the lateral femoral condyle moves posteriorly on the tibia up to 2 cm when the knee flexes, the position of the medial femoral condyle hardly moves, pivoting like a ball and socket joint (Freeman 2001). The Medial Rotation Knee (Wright Medical Technology, Arlington, Tennessee, USA) was designed to reproduce this movement. This design has a spherically shaped medial femoral condyle which articulates with a matched, conforming tibial component. Although this represents an increase in constraint, and potentially increases the forces being transmitted through the tibial component, early results have not shown an increase in loosening (Amin et al. 2008). Results after five years have shown 99% survival of the implant (Karachalios et al. 2009), and longer term results are now awaited.

New Surgical Approaches

1. Minimally Invasive Surgery

Minimally Invasive Surgery (MIS) represents an alteration to the standard medial parapatellar approach to the knee used in 92% of knee arthroplasties (NJR 2010). It is defined as a minimally invasive technique in which the incision and surgical dissection have been modified to reduce surgical morbidity (Malik and Dorr 2007). Several approaches have been described, all aiming to reduce size of the skin incision, but also reducing the amount of soft tissue dissection, conserving the subvastus insertion and not everting the patella. New instrumentation has been introduced to allow joint arthroplasty through this more limited exposure, without causing trauma to tissue due to excessive traction. A worrying development is that MIS appears to have been marketed directly at patients eager for a better cosmetic result.

Advocates of MIS feel that it represents a natural evolution in the approach to knee arthroplasty, limiting soft-tissue disruption, and therefore some of the pain and functional delays in recovery observed postoperatively. Detractors feel that the more limited exposure may result in component malposition (Dalury et al. 2008) and hence increased complication rates. The debate regarding the role of MIS has not been settled by the medical literature, with studies for total knee arthroplasty reporting a wide range of clinical results. Some have shown early benefits, such as decreased pain, shorter functional recovery, and improved range of knee flexion (Haas et al. 2004, Laskin 2005, Varela-Egocheaga et al. 2010). Others, however, have failed to demonstrate any substantial difference between MIS and conventional approaches in the postoperative period (Seon and Song 2006, Kolisek et al. 2007, Wulker et al. 2010).

2. Navigation

Although excellent results have been reported with modern implant designs, malpositioning of implants can contribute significantly to early failure (Ritter et al. 1994). Most knee systems utilise a combination of intramedullary and extramedullary instrumentation together with extensive visual referencing to guide appropriate resection of bone. Variations in anatomy, difficulty with exposure, and bone loss can affect the accuracy of conventional instrumentation and compromise postoperative limb and component alignment. Some studies have suggested that component malposition greater than 3 degrees can occur in up to 10% of knee replacements using conventional jigs (Stulberg et al. 2002). Rotational malalignment in particular is a significant problem, and often difficult to identify postoperatively. Computer assisted surgery, or navigation, has been introduced in an attempt to improve the accuracy of bone cuts and implant placement.

Several navigation systems are now available (Wong et al. 2013). These systems utilise preoperative CT scans, intraoperative fluoroscopy or intraoperative digital registration to determine the location and orientation of multiple anatomical landmarks. Many systems utilise pins with reflective trackers drilled into the femur and tibia. The positions of these trackers are monitored by infrared cameras.

This data is used to calculate the mechanical and anatomical axes of the limb, and then guide the appropriate position and orientation of bone cuts. Many of these systems are designed to coincide with MIS approaches. Despite improvements, many find these systems cumbersome, and time consuming to use (Dutton et al. 2008). There are also concerns regarding cost.

Multiple prospective randomised controlled trials (Dutton et al. 2008, Matziolis et al. 2007, Mullaji et al. 2007), and more recently meta-analyses (Mason et al. 2007) have shown increased accuracy in bone cuts when compared to conventional jigs, achieving accuracy to within 1 degree in the coronal and sagittal planes, and showing improved accuracy in rotational alignment (Chauhan et al. 2004). Whether or not this increased accuracy will translate into improved function and implant survival, however, remains to be seen (Bauwens et al. 2007).

One study has already pointed out that accurate bone cuts do not guarantee reproducible implant positioning, recording inaccuracies related to implant insertion after accurate bone cuts (Catani et al. 2008).

Many feel that navigated systems already have a place in knee replacement surgery, particularly in the difficult patient where tibial or femoral deformities prevent the accurate use of conventional jigs. Whether or not these systems will gain widespread acceptance for more straightforward procedures depends on their ongoing evolution, especially regarding their expense as well as their speed and ease of use (Lau & Khan 2012).

NEW ARTHROPLASTY MATERIALS

In the early 1900's, surgeons experimented with interposition arthroplasty in the knee as a means of treating arthritis whilst preserving movement. Materials used were initially biological, including pieces of pig bladder, fascia lata and skin flaps. Non-biological implants made of cellophane and nylon were also tried, eventually giving way to metallic implants in the 1940's. The composition of knee arthroplasty implants continued to evolve as knowledge of biomaterials and their properties improved. The vast majority of modern implants incorporate a cobalt-chrome alloy femoral implant articulating with a polyethylene tibial tray, usually attached to a titanium tibial component. The continued improvement of these materials remains the subject of intense research.

1. Improving Polyethylene

Ultra-high molecular weight polyethylene (UHWPE) was first introduced as a bearing surface for joint arthroplasty by Sir John Charnley over 40 years ago. Its strength, wear properties, low coefficient of friction and the ability to mould or machine it into a desired shape have contributed to its success. Knee replacements normally fail due to fatigue and delamination of polyethylene, but implant failure can also be caused by the generation of polyethylene wear particles. These particles are biologically active, and induce an inflammatory response when phagocytosed by macrophages. The degree of biological activity is dependent on the amount, size and shape of the wear particles generated. Inflammatory mediators released by macrophages stimulate osteoclasts to resorb bone, causing osteolysis, loosening and ultimately failure of the prosthesis. Polyethylene has therefore, despite its clinical success, been the subject of much research to improve its wear properties to reduce osteolysis. Attempts to improve performance by reinforcing UHWPE with carbon fibre, and the introduction of UHWPE with higher crystallinity (Ries et al. 1996) both failed clinically, despite considerable *in vitro* testing.

More promising in the evolution of polyethylene is the changes made to sterilisation via gamma irradiation, which increases the cross-linking between polyethylene polymer chains, producing Highly Cross-Linked Polyethylene (HXLPE). This improves the wear properties of the polyethylene, but at the cost of generating free radicals which induce an oxidative reaction, making the polyethylene brittle. Heating HXLPE stabilises it against oxidisation but alters its mechanical properties, notably reducing strength and fatigue resistance. Multiple manufacturers have produced HXLPE implants, all differing in their irradiation and thermal stabilisation regimes. This first generation of HXLPE implants have shown decreased wear rates when used in hip arthroplasty after 4-5 years (Dorr et al. 2005, Manning et al. 2005, Geerdink et al. 2006, Engh et al. 2006), with one study showing a 95% reduction in wear (Digas et al. 2007). Some failures have occurred, however, due to fractures of tibial polyethylene posts in knee arthroplasty (Sharkey et al. 2002). Further work is ongoing in the generation of so-called second generation HXLPE, aiming to further reduce oxidation through multiple cycles of irradiation and thermal stabilisation treatments. Thus far *in vitro* studies have suggested a further reduction in wear rates (Tsukamoto et al. 2008).

Another strategy to reduce HXLPE oxidation is adding the antioxidant alpha-tocopherol (vitamin E) to the polyethylene, avoiding thermal stabilisation treatments which can alter its mechanical properties. This has been shown to improve the fatigue crack propagation resistance of polyethylene (Oral et al. 2008) without compromising wear resistance *in vitro* (Wannomae et al. 2010). There are as yet no clinical trials published in the medical literature.

It should be noted that there are some concerns regarding the application of HXLPE to knee arthroplasty. Although joint simulator studies have shown decreased wear, the polyethylene wear particles generated are smaller than those produced from conventional polyethylene (Fisher et al. 2004) with evidence that these particles may be more biologically active (Illgen et al. 2008), with a greater potential to cause macrophage-mediated osteolysis and loosening.

2. Oxinium

Although numerous attempts have been made to decrease polyethylene wear, and thereby increasing the longevity of knee implants, most of these have centred on changes in polyethylene composition and implant design. A new approach has been to alter the composition of the surface articulating with the polyethylene (the femoral component). Ceramic components are much harder than metals with a lower coefficient of friction and better scratch profile. Ceramics have been used as bearing surfaces in hip replacements, with greatly reduced wear, but their brittleness makes them unsuitable for use in knee arthroplasty. A new metal alloy has been introduced for the manufacture of femoral components in knee arthroplasty as an alternative to the more conventional cobalt chrome. This oxidised zirconium, also called Oxinium (Smith and Nephew, Memphis, TN) is produced via a thermally driven oxygen diffusion process which converts the surface of the metallic zirconium alloy into a durable oxide with a low friction coefficient. This surface is essentially a ceramic, conveying excellent wear properties, but the remainder of the prosthesis remains a metal alloy, removing the fracture risk.

In vitro studies regarding oxinium knee components in wear simulators (Tsukamoto et al. 2006, Lee et al. 2009) have shown improved scratch resistance and decreased polyethylene wear when compared to standard implants. Clinical trials have shown good results at two years (Laskin 2003) and five years (Innocenti et al. 2010). Whether or not the theoretical advantage of using Oxinium implants is translated to improved long term clinical outcome remains to be seen. Studies comparing samples of synovial fluid from total knee replacements using oxinium and cobalt chrome have shown no difference in the weight, size or shape of generated polyethylene wear particles (Kim et al. 2010b), suggesting that rates of osteolysis and loosening may be unchanged.

3. Uncemented Knee Replacements

Fixation of implants with acrylic polymethylmethacrylate cement is currently the gold standard in total knee replacement, used in over 92% of total knee replacements (NJR 2010). In contrast, surgeons have been reluctant to utilise cementless fixation due to past failures in the early generations of cementless knee arthroplasty designs. With knee replacements being considered in younger patients, however, cementless fixation has enjoyed a renewal of interest as a potentially more durable mode of fixation. This has been aided by the availability of improved biomaterials, including highly porous tantalum and titanium biomaterials with morphologies and mechanical properties resembling native trabecular bone, encouraging new bone to grow into the implant. This may provide faster and better osseointegration than previous cementless fixation and are already popular in revision hip surgery. Early results have been encouraging, with clinical trials of a tantalum trabecular metal tibial tray reporting three year results equivalent to cemented prostheses (Dunbar et al. 2009, Helm et al. 2009). Although there have been numerous advances in the design of the knee replacement, it is nevertheless crucial to ensure patients are worked up adequately preoperatively, due consideration taken intraoperatively and rehabilitated well post-operatively to ensure optimal results (Sohail et al. in press)

CONCLUSION

Knee arthroplasty continues to evolve, with efforts to improve postoperative function and implant survival subjecting almost all aspects of the status quo to continued research and clinical trials. When reviewing these new developments it is worth considering that existing condylar knee replacement designs, utilising a cobalt chrome femoral component fixed with polymethylmethacrylate cement and articulating with a UHMWPE tibial tray, are already hugely successful, achieving excellent clinical results, high patient satisfaction and low revision rates. Caution must be exercised to ensure a theoretical advantage does not result in a poorer clinical outcome. Orthopaedics has seen many good implants ruined by 'improved' engineering.

REFERENCES

Amin A, Al-Taiar A, Sanghrajka AP, Kang N, Scott G 2008 The early radiological follow-up of a medial rotational design of total knee arthroplasty. *Knee* 15 222-6.

Barink M, De Waal Malefijt M, Celada P, Vena P, Van Kampen A, Verdonschot N 2008 A mechanical comparison of high-flexion and conventional total knee arthroplasty. *Proc. Inst. Mech. Eng. H* 222 297-307.

Bauwens K, Matthes G, Wich M et al. 2007 Navigated total knee replacement. A meta-analysis. *J. Bone Joint Surg.* 89A 261-9.

Bourne RB, Chesworth BM, Davis, AM, Mahed NN, Charon KDJ 2010 Patient Satisfaction after Total Knee Arthroplasty. *Clin. Orthop. Relat.* Res. 468 57-63.

Catani F, Biasca N, Ensini A et al. 2008 Alignment deviation between bone resection and final implant positioning in computer-navigated total knee arthroplasty. *J. Bone Joint Surg.* 90A 765-71.

Chauhan SK, Scott RG, Breidahl W, Beaver RJ 2004 Computer-assisted knee arthroplasty versus a conventional jig-based technique: a randomised, prospective trial. *J. Bone Joint Surg.* 86B 372–7.

Chin KR, Dalury DF, Zurakowski D et al. 2002 Intraoperative measurements of male and female distal femurs during primary total knee arthroplasty. *J. Knee Surg*. 15 213.

Dalury DF, Snow RG, Adams MJ 2008 Electromyographic evaluation of the midvastus approach. *J. Arthroplasty* 23 136-40.

Digas G, Karrholm J, Thanner J, Herberts P 2007 5-year experience of highly cross-linked polyethylene in cemented and uncemented sockets: Two randomized studies using radiostereometric analysis. *Acta. Orthop*. 78 746-54.

Dorr LD, Wan Z, Shahrdar C, Sirianni L, Boutary M, Yun A 2005 Clinical performance of a Durasul highly cross-linked polyethylene acetabular liner for total hip arthroplasty at five years. *J. Bone Joint Surg*. 87A 1816-21.

Dunbar MJ, Wilson DAJ, Hennigar AW, Amirault JD, Gross M, Reardon GP 2009 Fixation of a Trabecular Metal Knee Arthroplasty Component. *J. Bone Joint Surg*. 91A 1578-86.

Dutton AQ, Yeo S-J, Yang K-Y, Lo N-N, Chia K-U, Chong H-C 2008 Computer-Assisted Minimally Invasive Total Knee Arthroplasty Compared with Standard Total Knee Arthroplasty A Prospective, Randomized Study. *J. Bone Joint Surg*. 90A 2-9.

Engh CA Jr, Stepniewski AS, Ginn SD, Beykirch SE, Sychterz-Terefenko CJ, Hopper RH 2006 A randomized prospective evaluation of outcomes after total hip arthroplasty using cross-linked marathon and noncross-linked Enduron polyethylene liners. *J. Arthroplasty* 21 17-25.

Fisher J, McEwen HM, Tipper JL et al. 2004 Wear, debris, and biologic activity of cross-linked polyethylene in the knee: Benefits and potential concerns. *Clin. Orthop. Rel. Res*. 428 114–9.

Freeman MAR 2001 How the knee moves. *Curr. Orthop*. 15 444-50.

Geerdink CH, Grimm B, Ramakrishnan R, Rondhuis J, Verburg AJ, Tonino AJ 2006 Crosslinked polyethylene comparedto conventional polyethylene in total hip replacement: pre-clinical evaluation, in-vitro testing and prospective clinical follow-up study. *Acta. Orthop*. 77 719-25.

Haas SB, Cook S, Beksac B 2004 Minimally invasive total knee replacement through a mini midvastus approach: a comparative study. *Clin. Orthop. Rel. Res*. 428 68-73.

Huang HT, Su JY, Wang GJ 2005 The early results of high flex total knee arthroplasty: a minimum of two years of follow up. *J. Arthroplasty* 20 674-8.

Helm AT, Kerin C, Ghalayini SRA, Mclauchlan GJ 2009 Preliminary Results of an Uncemented Trabecular Metal Tibial Component in Total Knee Arthroplasty. *J. Arthroplasty* 24 941-4.

Huddleston JI, Scarborough DM, Goldvasser D, Freiberg AA, Malchau H 2009 How Often Do Patients with High-Flex Total Knee Arthroplasty Use High Flexion? *Clin. Orthop. Rel. Res*. 467 1898-906.

Illgen RL, Forsythe TM, Pike JW, Laurent M, Blanchard CR 2008 The Highly Crosslinked vs Conventional Polyethylene Particles—An In Vitro Comparison of Biologic Activities. *J. Arthroplasty* 23 721-31.

Innocenti M, Civinini R, Carulli C, Matassi F, Villano M 2010 The 5-year results of an oxidized zirconium femoral component for *TKA. Clin. Orthop. Rel. Res*. 468 1258-63.

Karachalios T, Roidis N, Goitikas D, Bargiotas K, Varitimidis S, Malizos K 2009 A mid-term clinical outcome study of the Advance Medial Pivot knee arthroplasty. *Knee* 16 484-8.

Wong J, Khan WS, Chimutengwende-Gordon M, Dowd GSE (2011). Recent advances in designs, approaches and materials in total knee replacement: Literature review and evidence today. *J. Perioper Pract.* 21(5): 165-171.

Kim YH, Sohn KS, Kim JS 2005 Range of motion of standard and high-flexion posterior stabilized total knee prostheses: a prospective randomized study. *J. Bone Joint Surg.* 87A 1470-5.

Kim YH, Choi,Y, Kim JS 2010a Comparison of standard and gender-specific posterior-cruciate-retaining high-flexion total knee replacements. A prospective, randomised study. *J. Bone Joint Surg.* 92B 639-45.

Kim YH, Kim JS, Huh W, Lee KH 2010b Weight of polyethylene wear particles is similar in TKAs with oxidized zirconium and cobalt-chrome prostheses. *Clin. Orthop. Rel. Res.* 468 1296-304.

Kolisek FR, Bonutti PM, Hozack WJ et al. 2007 Clinical experience using a minimally invasive surgical approach for total knee arthroplasty: early results of a prospective randomized study compared to a standard approach. *J. Arthroplasty* 22 8-13.

Kurtz S, Ong K, Lau E, Mowat F, Halpern M 2007 Projections of primary and revision hip and knee arthroplasty in the United States from 2005 to 2030. *J. Bone Joint Surg.* 89A 780-5.

Laskin RS 2003 An oxidized Zr ceramic surfaced femoral component for total knee arthroplasty. *Clin. Orthop. Rel. Res.* 416 191-6.

Laskin RS 2005 Minimally invasive total knee arthroplasty: the results justify its use *Clin. Orthop. Rel. Res.* 440 54-9.

Lau YCA, Khan WS. Literature Review in Robotic Arm-Assisted Orthopaedic Knee Arthroplasty. pp 139-46. In *Advances in Medicine and Biology*, Volume 54, Editor Berhardt LV, 2012, Nova Science Publishers, New York.

Lee JK, Maruthainar K, Wardle N, Haddad F, Blunn GW 2009 Increased force simulator wear testing of a zirconium oxide total knee arthroplasty *Knee* 16 269-74.

Malik A, Dorr LD 2007 The science of minimally invasive total hip arthroplasty. *Clin. Orthop. Rel. Res.* 463 74-84.

Manning DW, Chiang PP, Martell JM, Galante JO, Harris WH 2005 In vivo comparative wear study of traditional and highly crosslinked polyethylene in total hip arthroplasty. *J. Arthroplasty* 20 880-6.

Mason JB, Fehring TK, Estok R, Banel D, Fahrbach K 2007 Meta-analysis of alignment outcomes in computer-assisted total knee arthroplasty surgery. *J. Arthroplasty* 22 1097-106.

Matziolis G, Krocker D, Weiss U, Tohtz S, Perka C 2007 A prospective, randomized study of computer-assisted and conventional total knee arthroplasty. Three dimensional evaluation of implant alignment and rotation. *J. Bone Joint Surg.* 89A 236-43.

Mehin R, Burnett RS, Brasher PMA 2010 Does the new generation of high-flex knee prostheses improve the post-operative range of movement? A META analysis. *J. Bone Joint Surg.* 92 1429-34.

Minocha A, Khan WS (2014). Knee osteoarthritis: review of treatment options. *GM: Midlife & Beyond.* 44(9): 88-91.

Mullaji A, Kanna R, Marawar S, Kohli A, Sharma A 2007 Comparison of limb and component alignment using computer-assisted navigation versus image intensifier guided conventional total knee arthroplasty: a prospective, randomized, single surgeon study of 467 knees. *J. Arthroplasty* 22 953-9.

Noble PC, Conditt MA, Cook KF, Mathis KB 2006 The John Insall Award: Patient expectations affect satisfaction with total knee arthroplasty. *Clin. Orthop. Relat. Res.* 452 35-43.

National Joint Registry for England and Wales: Summary Report the 7th Annual Report 2010 http://www. njrcentre.org.uk (date last accessed 20 October 2010).

Oral E, Malhi AS, Wannomae KK, Muratoglu OK 2008 Highly cross-linked ultrahigh molecular weight polyethylene with improved fatigue resistance for total joint arthroplasty: recipient of the 2006 Hap Paul *Award J. Arthroplasty* 23 1037-44.

Ries MD, Bellare A, Livingston BJ, Cohen RE, Spector M 1996 Early delamination of a Hylamer-M tibial insert. *J. Arthroplasty* 11 974-6.

Ritter MA, Faris PM, Keating EM et al. 1994 Postoperative alignment of total knee replacement. Its effect on survival. *Clin. Orthop. Rel. Res.* 299 153.

Ritter MA, Berend ME, Meding JB, Keating EM, Faris PM, Crites BM 2001 Long-term follow up of anatomic graduated components posterior cruciate-retaining total knee replacement. *Clin. Orthop. Relat. Res.* 388 51-7.

Seon JK, Song EK 2006 Navigation-assisted less invasive total knee arthroplasty compared with conventional total knee arthroplasty: a randomized prospective trial. *J. Arthroplasty* 21777-82.

Sharkey PF, Hozack WJ, Rothman RH, et al. 2002 Insall Award paper. Why are total knee arthroplasties failing today? *Clin. Orthop. Rel. Res.* 404 7.

Shetty AA, Tindall A, Ting P and Heatley FW 2003 The evolution of total knee arthroplasty. Part III: surface replacement. *Curr. Orthop.* 17 478-81.

Sohail MZ, Aresti N, Hanna SA, Malik AA, Khan WS (2015). The Peri-operative Management of the Rheumatoid Patient Undergoing Total Knee Arthroplasty: A Review of Literature. *Curr. Rheumatol. Rev.* (in press).

Swedish Knee Arthroplasty Register 2010. Department of Orthopedics, Lund University Hospital http://www.knee.nko.se/english/online/uploadedFiles/113_SVK2009 ENGL1.0. pdf (date last accessed 20 October 2010).

Stulberg SD, Loan P, Sarin V 2002 Computer-assisted navigation in total knee replacement: results of an initial experience in thirty-five patients. *J. Bone Joint Surg.* 84A (Suppl 2) 90.

Tsukamoto R, Chen S, Asano T, Ogino M, Shoji H, Nakamura T, Clarke IC 2006 Improved wear performance with crosslinked UHMWPE and zirconia implants in knee simulation. *Acta. Orthop.* 77 505-11.

Tsukamoto R, Williams PA, Shoji H et al. 2008 Wear of sequentially enhanced 9-Mrad polyethylene in 10 million cycle knee simulation study. *J. Biomed. Mater. Res. B Appl. Biomater.* 86 199-24.

Varela-Egocheaga JR, Suarez-Suarez MA, Fernandez-Villa M, Gonzalez-Sastre V, Varela-Gomez JR, Rodrıguez-Merchan CD 2010 Minimally Invasive Subvastus Approach Improving the Results of Total Knee Arthroplasty: A Prospective, Randomized Trial. *Clin. Orthop. Rel.* Res 468 1200-8.

Wannomae KK, Christensen SD, Micheli BR, Rowell SL, Schroeder DW, Muratoglu OK 2010 Delamination and adhesive wear behavior of alpha-tocopherol-stabilized irradiated ultrahigh-molecular-weight polyethylene. *J. Arthroplasty* 25 635-43.

Weeden SH, Schmidt R 2007 A randomized, prospective study of primary total knee components designed for increased flexion. *J. Arthroplasty* 22 349-52.

Wong JM, Khan WS, Saksena J (2013). The Role of Navigation in Total Knee Replacement Surgery. *J. Periop. Pract*. 23(9): 202-7.

Wulker N, Lambermont JP, Sacchetti L, Lazaro JG, Nardi J 2010 A Prospective Randomized Study of Minimally Invasive Total Knee Arthroplasty Compared with Conventional Surgery. *J. Bone Joint Surg*. 92A 1584-90.

In: Perioperative Practice in Trauma and Orthopaedic Surgery ISBN: 978-1-63483-325-7
Editor: Wasim S. Khan

Chapter 24

THE ROLE OF NAVIGATION IN TOTAL KNEE REPLACEMENT SURGERY

James Min-Leong Wong, Wasim S. Khan [*]
and Joyti Saksena

Department of Trauma and Orthopaedics, Chase Farm Hospital, Royal Free Hospitals NHS Trust, Enfield, Middlesex, UK

ABSTRACT

Since the introduction of modern implants in the 1970's, Total Knee Replacement surgery has been a great clinical and commercial success. Implants and techniques have continued to evolve, driven by the desire for improved function and longevity. However, inaccurate insertion of these implants may cause them to loosen and fail. Computer navigation has been introduced as a modification to existing surgical techniques to improve the accuracy with which the bones are cut prior to inserting the knee replacement implants. Research continues to see if this potentially costly and time consuming technique can contribute to improved longevity of knee replacements.

Keywords: Total knee replacement, navigation, implants, accuracy, longevity, computer

INTRODUCTION

This chapter deals with the role of navigation in Total Knee Arthroplasty, or Replacement (TKR) surgery (Wong et al. 2012). Over the past 20 years TKR surgery has enjoyed great clinical and commercial success. Modern implants have been shown to have excellent long term results (Berger 2001, Rodriguez 2001, Laskin 2001) with a high level of patient satisfaction (Ethgen 2004, Noble 2006, Bourne 2010). The most recent published National

---

[*] Corresponding Author: Mr Wasim S Khan, Clinical Lecturer, University College London Institute of Orthopaedic and Musculoskeletal Sciences, Royal National Orthopaedic Hospital, Stanmore, Middlesex, HA7 4LP, UK, Telephone number: +44 (0) 7791 025554, E-mail address: wasimkhan@doctors.org.uk.

Joint Registry figures show almost 80,000 TKR's were performed in the UK alone in 2009/10 (NJR 2010). This figure is expected to rise, with some estimates projecting a 673% increase from 2005 levels by the year 2030 (Kurtz 2007).

Although better implant designs, materials and patient education has improved the longevity of implants, some knee replacements, due to a combination of surgical, patient and implant factors, do fail. The most common cause for a TKR requiring revision is infection, followed by aseptic loosening and wear (Hossain 2010). Although some of these causative factors for failure are out of the surgeon's control, malpositioning of implants, which can lead to aseptic loosening and early failure (Lotke 1977, Tew 1985, Ritter 1994), is. The final position of the tibial and femoral components of a knee replacement are strongly influenced by the cuts the surgeon makes in these bones, resecting the arthritic articular surfaces and preparing them to accept the knee prosthesis. The accuracy of these cuts will affect the ultimate alignment and stability of the prosthetic joint, in addition to soft tissue and ligament balancing.

Computer assisted surgery, or navigation, has been developed to improve the accuracy of these cuts. An increasing number of navigation options are now commercially available, usually designed by implant manufacturers to be used solely with a specific knee implant system. Despite ongoing advances, the use of these systems has thus far been limited as they are cumbersome and time consuming to use, as well as costly.

The vast majority of TKR implants in use today are versions of the "condylar" knee replacements developed in the 1970's. The introduction of this design resulted in not only a marked improvement in results and longevity, but also reproducibility. Jigs and guides were introduced to enable the surgeon to reliably determine the orientation and alignment of the tibia and femur, and use this to guide his subsequent bony cuts. Most knee systems utilise a combination of intramedullary and extramedullary instrumentation, together with extensive visual referencing, to guide appropriate resection of bone.

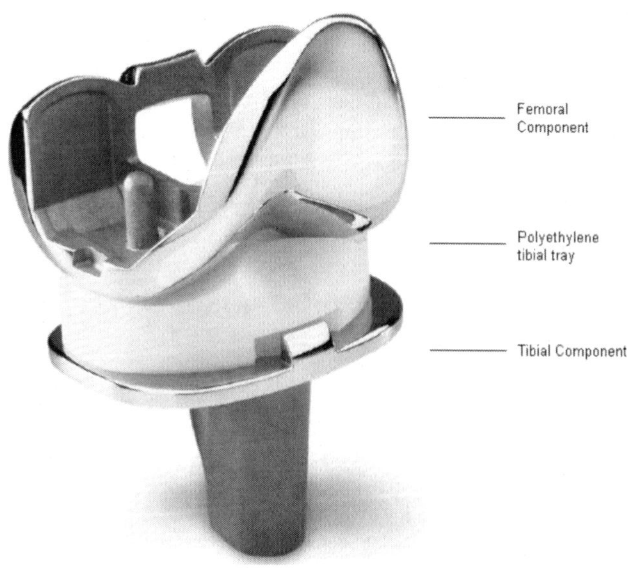

Figure 1. A modern knee replacement prosthesis (Picture reproduced courtesy of Zimmer Inc., Warsaw, Indiana USA).

Condylar knee replacements incorporate an anatomically shaped femoral component, with an anterior flange to articulate with the patella. The cobalt chrome femoral component articulates with a polyethylene tibial insert, which is usually attached to a titanium tibial component (Fig 1). Inserting these implants involves resection of the bone ends to create parallel and equal spaces in flexion and extension, and then balancing the soft tissues to convey stability.

These implants are usually cemented in place using acrylic polymethylmethacrylate cement, but can be coated in materials which enable an uncemented, biological fixation.

The majority of surgeons are guided in cutting the femur with the aid of intramedullary guide. A rod is inserted up the femoral canal, thus defining its anatomical axis. A cutting jig is then applied to this rod, enabling the distal femur to be cut in at the desired angle relative to the anatomical axis of the femur.

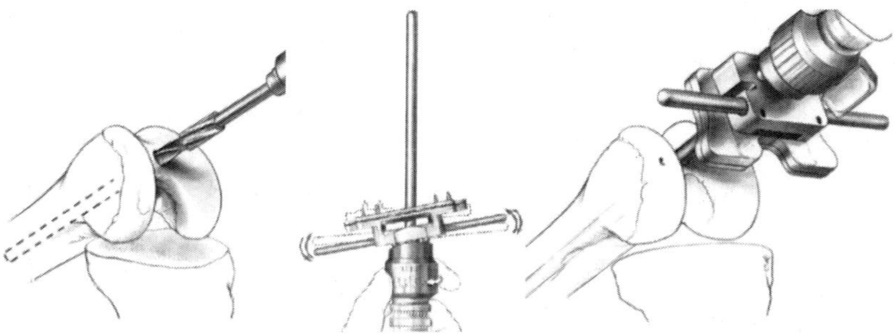

Figure 2. Intramedullary femoral instrumentation. A drill is passed up the intramedullary femoral canal, approximating the anatomical axis. Cutting the distal femur is guided by a rod passed up the drill hole and a cutting jig set to resect bone. This is usually set at 5-7 degrees from the estimated anatomical axis (Images courtesy of Zimmer Inc. Warsaw, Indiana).

Cutting guides are then applied to allow further bone cuts to be made to accommodate the anatomically shaped femoral component, with the majority of surgeon's using a guide which enables them to place these cuts in 3 degrees of external rotation relative to the posterior femoral condyles.

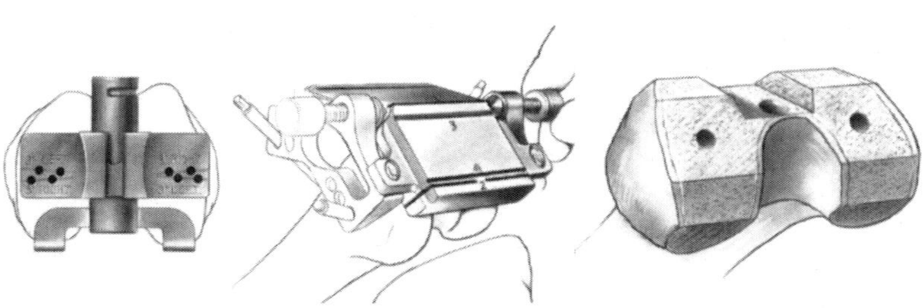

Figure 3. Further femoral instrumentation determines the size and rotation of the femoral component and then guide further bone cuts (Images courtesy of Zimmer Inc. Warsaw, Indiana).

When cutting the tibial component, many surgeons use extramedullary instrumentation, placing an alignment guide parallel to the tibia, and cutting the tibia in a plane perpendicular to this.

Once these cuts have been made to the surgeon's satisfaction, the gap between the cut femoral and tibial surfaces is checked to ensure a symmetrical gap in flexion and extension. If the gap is found to be asymmetrical, it is corrected by a combination of soft tissue releases or further bony cuts. Only after the soft tissues have been appropriately balanced are the implants inserted and secured in place.

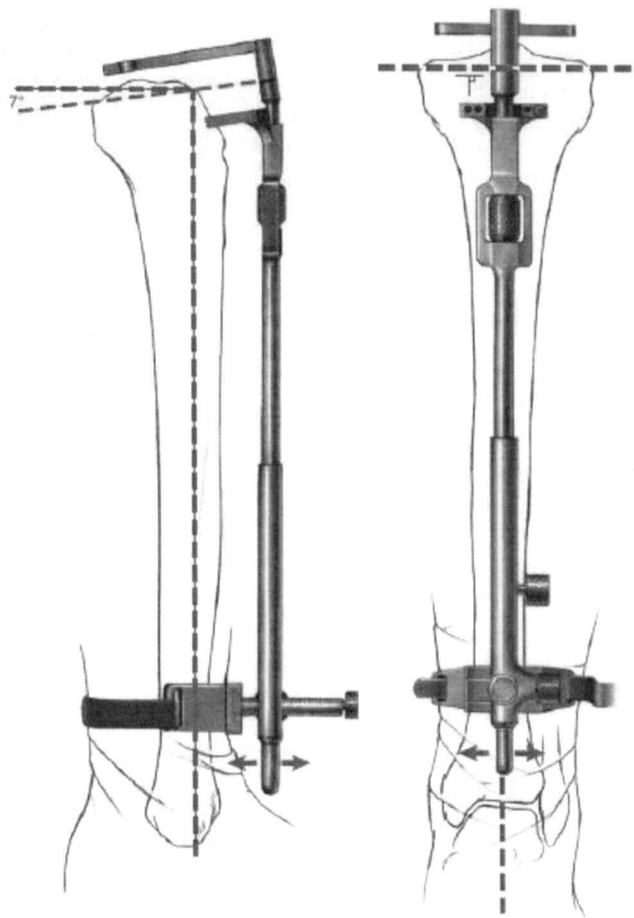

Figure 4. Extramedullary tibial instrumentation. This guide is placed on the anterior surface of the tibia. The mechanical axis is estimated by placing this guide over anatomical landmarks and a cutting jig is then applied to guide bone cuts perpendicular to this (Images courtesy of Zimmer Inc. Warsaw, Indiana).

The need for Navigation

The conventional instrumentation described above is largely similar amongst manufacturers and has not changed significantly over the past 20 years. Even in experienced hands, using conventional instrumentation to guide bone resection can still result in component malposition. It is estimated that up to 10% of total knee replacements have significant (> 3 degrees) errors in mechanical alignment (Stulberg 2002). Mechanical axis malalignment has been proven to adversely affect implant function and survival (Jeffery 1991, Ritter 1994, Wasielewski 1994), particularly if the erroneous bony cuts result in a significant varus deformity (Jeffery).

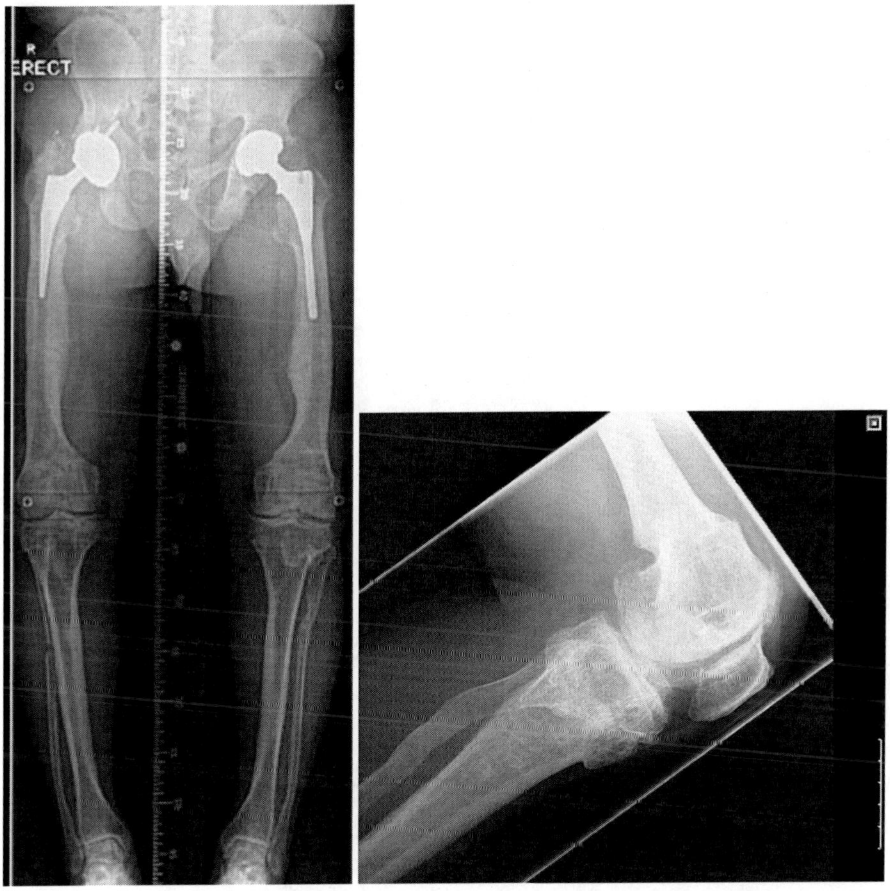

Figure 5. Preoperative long leg and lateral x-rays of a patient previously affected by rickets and previous bilateral total hip replacements. The bowed femurs and hip replacements make femoral intramedullary instrumentation difficult.

Furthermore, the use of conventional instrumentation to accurately resect bone can be technically very difficult in the presence of abnormal patient anatomy, poor exposure and preoperative bone loss. There are occasions when using intramedullary instrumentation is not possible at all. For example patients with previous trauma and residual bony deformity, or with pre-existing metal implants such as a total hip replacement, which may prevent the use of an intramedullary guide.

At a time when TKR's are now being performed in ever younger and more demanding patients, there is a need to improve the accuracy of existing surgical techniques, in the hope this will maximise the longevity and function of these implants. Computer assisted, or navigated, surgery is a technique previously well known in neurosurgery to guide precise surgery. It has now been adapted to aid the accurate implantation of total knee replacements.

Navigation systems

Various types of navigated surgical systems are now available. Most are produced by manufacturers of total knee replacement implant systems and are generally recommended to be used with specific TKR implants. All these systems develop a three dimensional model of the patient's knee and maps the position of the surgeon's instruments in relation to this model. This can then be used to guide the surgeon to make accurate bony cuts.

Image-guided navigated systems utilise data obtained preoperatively or intraoperatively to build a three dimensional model of the knee which is then used to guide bony cuts. Most of these systems utilise preoperative imaging, usually in the form of CT scans, but some also use intraoperative fluoroscopy to map anatomical landmarks.

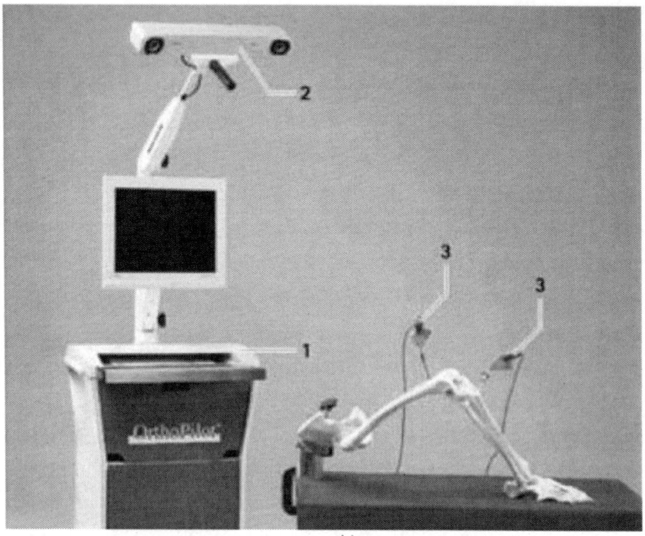

A)

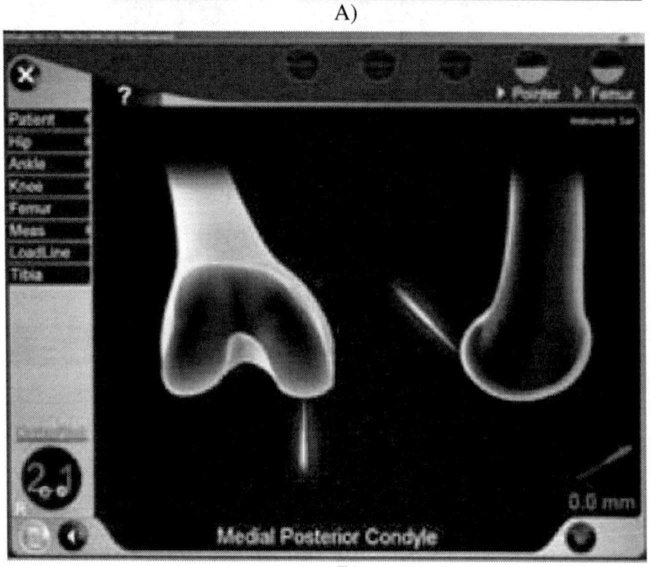

B)

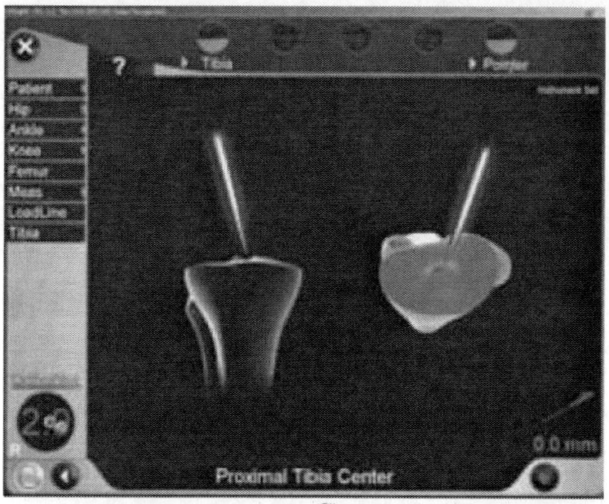

C)

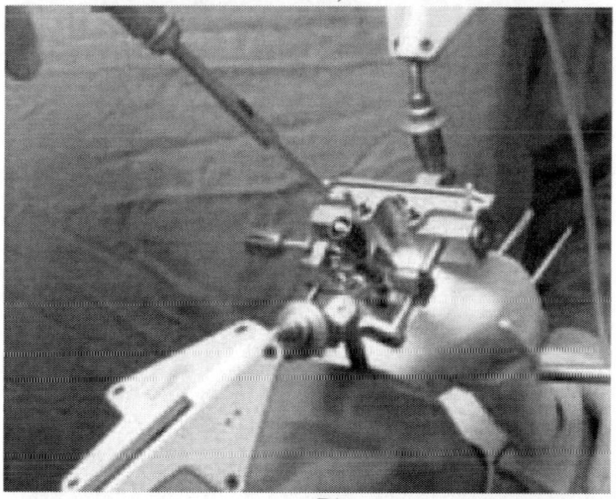

D)

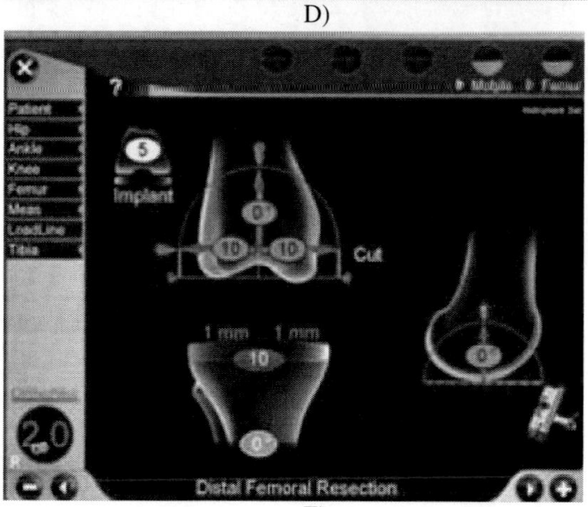

E)

Figure 6. A. An example of an imageless navigation system. Reflective markers are drilled into the femur and tibia (3), and their location is detected by an infrared (2) camera attached to a computer (1). B,C. A stylus with another reflective marker attached is then used to register multiple anatomical landmarks to enable the computer to develop a three-dimensional model of the knee D. Cutting guides with a further reflective marker attached are then placed on the knee. E. The monitor display is used to guide the positioning, angulation and rotation of the cutting guide to ensure that the bone is accurately cut (Images courtesy of B Braun Inc., Tuttlengen, Germany).

Once the computer has developed a three dimensional model of the patient's lower limb, bone cuts can then be accurately planned. Navigation systems can then use this information intraoperatively. The position of the patient's knee is registered into the navigation system, which then correlates this with the three dimensional model. The most common means of doing this is the use of reflective markers which are drilled into the femur and tibia, and a further marker which can be placed on surgical instruments and cutting jigs. Infrared cameras which are coupled to an emitter and the navigation computer can track the movements of the markers drilled into bone and marked surgical instruments relative to each other. The computer can thus guide the surgeon to ensure that the cutting jigs are deployed in exactly the correct position.

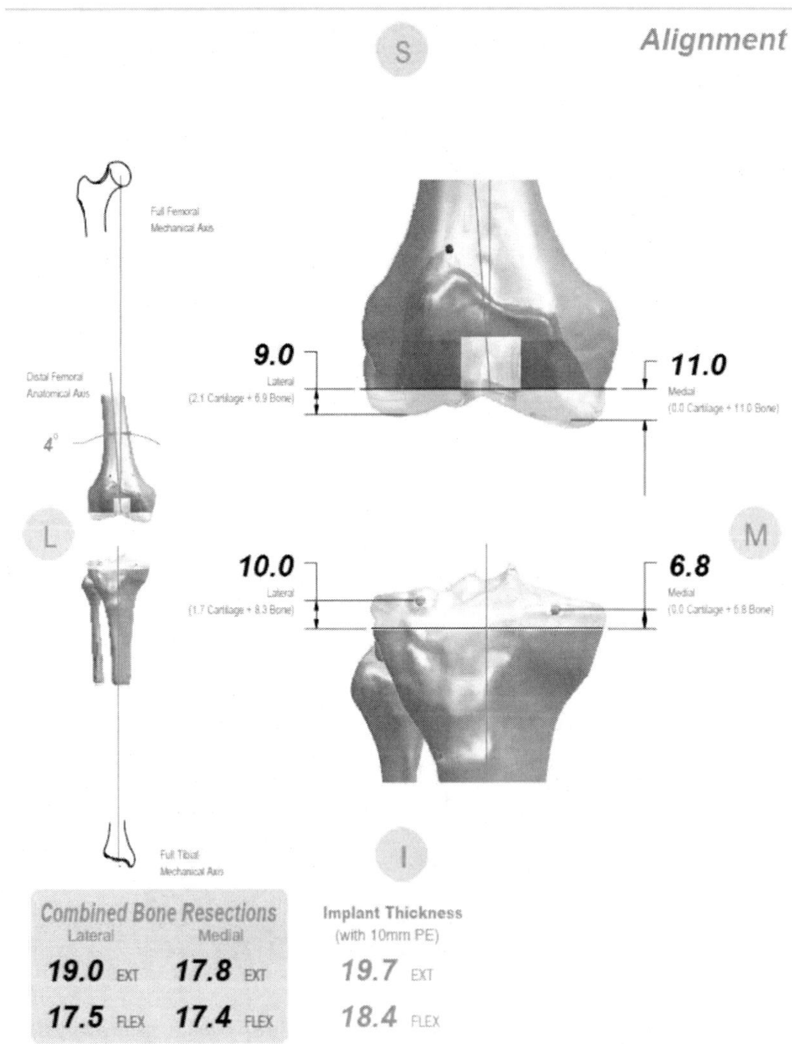

Figure 8. A three-dimensional model of the knee has been produced based on a patient's CT scan, allowing the desired cuts to be planned by the surgeon prior to surgery (Image courtesy of Depuy Orthopaedics Inc., Warsaw, Indiana).

A variation of this approach is an imageless navigation system. This is also called morphing surface navigation and utilizes a large database of knee CT scans. Once the markers have been drilled into the femur and tibia, a marked stylus is used to register multiple anatomical landmarks (Figure 6). The computer system then uses the information on its database to build or morph a three dimensional model of the patient's knee which fits the registered anatomical landmarks.

It should be recognised that all of these systems increase the operative time required to perform a knee replacement (Weng 2009). Furthermore, in the current health economy the cost of installing and maintaining these systems may prove prohibitive, with one author estimating the cost of purchasing the computer system and software approaches $150,000, with a further $20,000 a year spent on maintenance. These factors have limited the use of navigated systems, particularly at a time when the need for increased efficiencies and cost reduction in operating theatres is being stressed.

Customised Patient Instrumentation

The next evolution of navigated knee surgery is the manufacture of instrumentation or cutting guides to specifically fit an individual patient. These systems involve building a model of the knee based on preoperative CT or MRI scans and taking images of the hip and ankle to determine mechanical alignment. The ideal cuts are planned by the surgeon based on this model (Figure 7) and then custom designed cutting blocks are manufactured using three-dimensional printing techniques to fit that individual patient's knee and produce the planned cuts. Some of these systems produce patient specific cutting guides that fit directly onto a patient without the need for any conventional instrumentation, others guide the placement of pins into the bone, and conventional cutting blocks are then passed over these pins (Figure 8).

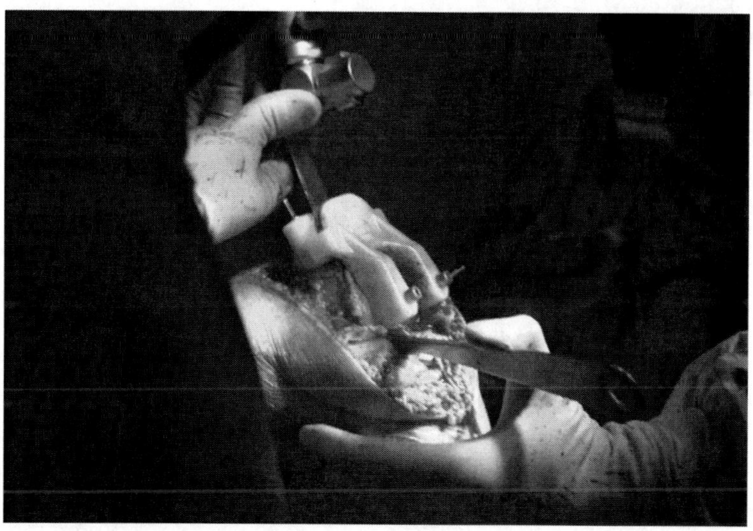

Figure 9. Customised patient specific instruments are manufactured to fit over the patient's bone and guide a saw blade to accurately.

This strategy has the advantage of being a faster procedure, with reduced tourniquet times when compared with conventional knee replacement surgery (Hafez 2006). There is no need to drill markers into the tibia and femur, as the time consuming anatomical landmark registration is no longer necessary and, unlike conventional knee replacements, no intra- or extra-medullary guides are required. All patients will however, need to undergo a preoperative CT or MRI, and this, combined with the need to manufacture cutting guides for each procedure, does mean that there is a lead time for each surgery and an added cost.

RESULTS

Multiple prospective randomised controlled trials have now been performed comparing various navigated systems with conventional total knee replacements. Many have shown significant improvements in coronal alignment (Mullaji 2007, Dutton 2008), with better restoration of the mechanical axis of the limb on post operative radiographs. CT scans have also been used to assess postoperative implant position showing improved accuracy in the coronal (Mizu-uchi 2008, Hernandez-Vacquero 2010) and sagittal planes (Chauhan 2004, Matziolis 2007).

Two of these trials also showed significantly improved rotational alignment of implanted prostheses (Chauhan 2004, Mizu-uchi 2008). Other trials, however, have showed no difference in alignment and rotation (Kim 2007, Lutzner 2008), although one of these did show a reduction in large deviations of mechanical axis in the navigated group. It should be noted that errors in alignment have not been completely eradicated by navigation, and errors in inserting and cementing implants in place has been shown to cause malpositioning despite perfect bony cuts (Catani 2008)

Studies have also investigated the potential improved accuracy of navigation in the presence of significant deformity.

When used in the presence of significant femoral bowing in a Taiwanese population, navigated TKR's were found to be significantly better at reproducing a normal mechanical axis than conventional TKR (Huang 2011). A further study also showed improved leg alignment when performing navigated TKR's in the presence of large frontal plane deformities (Hernandez-Vacquero 2010).

With an increasing number of trials available, two META-analyses have now been published, with mixed results. Whilst one has shown significantly improved alignment and rotational orientation when compared to conventional TKR (Mason 2007), another showed no overall difference in alignment, but a decrease in critical deviations from the mechanical axis in excess of 3 degrees (Bauwens 2007).

Whether these improvements in accuracy will translate to improved function and implant survival, however, remains to be seen. A functional analysis of patients at two years post surgery has shown no difference in clinical outcome between navigated and conventional TKR's (Spencer 2007). As yet, no studies have been able to demonstrate a survival benefit for Navigated TKR's.

A further study has investigated whether the added cost of navigation (an estimated $1500 per operation) is justified (Novak 2007). The argument was made that the improved alignment will reduce the need for a potentially very costly early revision procedure, and this study concluded that navigated surgery was a cost-saving and cost-effective modification to conventional total knee replacement.

Conclusion

Whilst excellent results continue to be reported for the vast majority of total knee replacement implants, even the best implants can fail due to malpositioning. Using conventional instrumentation, significant errors in position can occur in up to 10% of patients. Navigated knee replacement systems have been devised to reduce the amount of error in implant positioning.

Despite advances in navigation technology, however, many surgeons still find these systems cumbersome and time-consuming to use. They are, of course, also expensive to acquire and may require additional CT or MRI scans. As a result, navigated knee replacement systems have not entered widespread use.

Customised patient instrumentation may achieve more widespread acceptance, although these systems are still in their infancy and long term results are yet to be published.

It should also be remembered that TKR is not just a procedure on bony abnormality, but also a procedure to correct soft tissue imbalances. Despite many studies showing improved alignment none have as yet shown a functional improvement or improved implant survival.

As navigation continues to improve, its role in future knee replacement will become clearer. Whether this role is its involvement in all total knee replacements, or limited to difficult patients with distorted anatomy, is dependent on future clinical results, improvements to navigated systems and of course the long term health economy.

References

Bauwens K, Matthes G, Wich M, Gebhard F, Hanson B, Ekkernkamp A, Stengel D. Navigated total knee replacement. A meta-analysis. *Journal of Bone and Joint Surgery [Am]*. 2007; 89:261-9.

Berger RA, Rosenberg AG, Barden RM, Sheinkop MB, Jacobs JJ, Galante JO. Long-term followup of the Miller-Galante total knee replacement. *Clin Orthop Relat Res*. 2001;388:58–67.

Bourne RB, Chesworth BM, Davis, AM, Mahed NN, Charon KDJ. Patient Satisfaction after Total Knee Arthroplasty. *Clinical Orthopaedics & Related Research*. 2010; 468:57–63.

Catani F, Biasca N, Ensini A, Leardini A, Bianchi L, Digennaro V, Giannini S. Alignment deviation between bone resection and final implant positioning in computer-navigated total knee arthroplasty. *Journal of Bone and Joint Surgery [Am]*. 2008;90:765-71.

Chauhan SK, Scott RG, Breidahl W, Beaver RJ. Computer-assisted knee arthroplasty versus a conventional jig-based technique: a randomised, prospective trial. *J Bone Joint Surg Br*. 2004;86: 372–377.

Dutton AQ, Yeo S-J, Yang K-Y, Lo N-N, Chia K-U, Chong H-C. Computer-Assisted Minimally Invasive Total Knee Arthroplasty Compared with Standard Total Knee

Arthroplasty A Prospective, Randomized Study. *Journal of Bone and Joint Surgery [Am]*. 2008;90:2-9.

Ethgen O, Bruyère O, Richy F, Dardennes C, Reginster JY. Health-related quality of life in total hip and total knee arthroplasty. A qualitative and systematic review of the literature. *J Bone Joint Surg Am*. 2004;86:963-74.

Hafez MA, Chelule KL, Seedhom BB and Sherman KP. Computer-assisted Total Knee Arthroplasty Using Patient-specific Templating. *Clinical Orthopaedics and Related Research* 2006; 444: 184–192.

Hernandez-Vaquero MD, Suarez-Vazquez A, Sandoval-Garcia M, Noriega-Fernandez A. Computer Assistance Increases Precision of Component Placement in Total Knee Arthroplasty with Articular Deformity. *Clin Orthop Relat Res* (2010) 468:1237–1241.

Hossain F, Patel S, Haddad FS. Midterm Assessment of Causes and Results of Revision Total Knee Arthroplasty. *Clin Orthop Relat Res*. 2010 468:1221–1228.

Huang TW, Hsu WH, Peng KT, Hsu RWW Total knee replacement in patients with significant femoral bowing in the coronal plane. *J Bone Joint Surg [Br]* 2011;93B:345-50.

Jeffery RS, Morris RW, Denham RA. Coronal alignment after Total Knee Replacement. JBJS [Br] 1991 73B: 709-14

Kim YH, Kim JS, Yoon SH. Alignment and orientation of the components in total knee replacement with and without navigation support *J Bone Joint Surg [Br]* 2007;89-B:471-6.

Kurtz S, Ong K, Lau E, Mowat F, Halpern M. Projections of primary and revision hip and knee arthroplasty in the United States from 2005 to 2030. *Journal of Bone and Joint Surgery [Am]*. 2007;89:780-5.

Laskin RS. The Genesis total knee prosthesis: a 10-year followup study. *Clin Orthop Relat Res*. 2001;388:95–102.

Lotke PA, Ecker ML. Influence of positioning of prosthesis in total knee replacement.J Bone Joint Surg Am. 1977;59:77-

Lützner J, Krummenauer F, Wolf C, Günther P, Kirschner S. Computer-assisted and conventional total knee replacement. *J Bone Joint Surg [Br]* 2008;90-B:1039-44.

Mason JB, Fehring TK, Estok R, Banel D, Fahrbach K. Meta-analysis of alignment outcomes in computer-assisted total knee arthroplasty surgery. *J Arthroplasty*.2007;22:1097-106.

Matziolis G, Krocker D, Weiss U, Tohtz S, Perka C. A prospective, randomized study of computer-assisted and conventional total knee arthroplasty. Three dimensional evaluation of implant alignment and rotation. *Journal of Bone and Joint Surgery [Am]*.2007;89:236-43.

Mizu-uchi H., S. Matsuda, H. Miura, K. Okazaki, Y. Akasaki, Y. Iwamoto. The evaluation of post-operative alignment in total knee replacement using a CT-based navigation system. *J Bone Joint Surg [Br]* 2008;90-B:1025-31

Mullaji A, Kanna R, Marawar S, Kohli A, Sharma A. Comparison of limb and component alignment using computer-assisted navigation versus image intensifier guided conventional total knee arthroplasty: a prospective, randomized, single surgeon study of 467 knees. *J Arthroplasty*. 2007;22:953-9.

National Joint Registry for England and Wales: Summary Report the 7th Annual Report. 2010. http://www. njrcentre.org.uk (date last accessed 20 October 2010).

Noble PC, Conditt MA, Cook KF, Mathis KB. The John Insall Award: Patient expectations affect satisfaction with total knee arthroplasty. *Clinical Orthopaedics & Related Research.* 2006; 452:35-43.

Novak Erik J., Marc D. Silverstein and Kevin J. Bozic The Cost-Effectiveness of Computer-Assisted Navigation in Total Knee Arthroplasty. *J Bone Joint Surg Am.* 2007;89:2389-2397 156.

Ritter MA, Faris PM, Keating EM et al. Postoperative alignment of total knee replacement. Its effect on survival. *Clinical Orthopaedics & Related Research.*1994;299:153.

Ritter MA, Faris PM, Keating EM et al. Postoperative alignment of total knee replacement. Its effect on survival. *Clinical Orthopaedics & Related Research.*1994;299:153.

Rodriguez JA, Bhende H, Ranawat CS. Total condylar knee replacement: a 20-year followup study. *Clin Orthop Relat Res.* 2001; 388:10–17.

Spencer JM, Chauhan SK, Sloan K, Taylor A, Beaver RJ Computer navigation *versus* conventional total knee replacement. *J Bone Joint Surg [Br]* 2007;89-B:477-80.

Stulberg SD, Loan P, Sarin V (2002) Computer-assisted navigation in total knee replacement: results of an initial experience in thirty-five patients. *J Bone Joint Surg Am* 84-A(Suppl 2):90–98.

Tew M, Waugh W. Tibiofemoral alignment and the results of knee replacement. *J Bone Joint Surg Br.* 1985;67:551-6.

Wasielewski RC, Galante JO, Leighty R, et al. Wearpatterns on retrieved polyethylene inserts and their relationship to technical considerations during total knee arthroplasty. *Clin Orthop Relat Res* 1994;299:31.

Weng YJ, Hsu RW, Hsu WH. Comparison of computer-assisted navigation and conventional instrumentation for bilateral total knee arthroplasty. *J Arthroplasty.* 2009;24(5):668-673.

Wong JM, Khan WS, Saksena J (2013). The Role of Navigation in Total Knee Replacement Surgery. *J Periop Pract.* 23(9): 202-7.

In: Perioperative Practice in Trauma and Orthopaedic Surgery ISBN: 978-1-63483-325-7
Editor: Wasim S. Khan

Chapter 25

RECENT DEVELOPMENTS IN TOTAL HIP REPLACEMENTS

Wasim Khan*, Sujay Dheerendra, Mohammed Saeed and Nicholas Goddard
Royal Free Hospital NHS Trust, London, UK

ABSTRACT

Total hip replacement is a commonly performed procedure with good results. The implants could be cemented or cementless, and there has been a resurgence of resurfacing procedures. It is important that special consideration is given to the choice of the material used at the bearing surfaces. There have been many developments in recent years that influence our choice of implant and have shaped our practice including minimal invasive surgery and computer-assisted surgery. This chapter aims to provide an overview of these developments.

Keywords: Total hip replacement, cement, resurfacing, bearing surface, minimal invasive surgery, computer-assisted surgery

This chapter discusses recent developments in total hip replacements including cementation, articulation, minimal-invasion and navigation (Dheerendra et al. 2010). Total hip replacement as a surgical treatment has developed over the last two centuries. Following unsuccessful attempts, that included interposition of materials such as ivory, gold foil, glass, stainless-steel, acrylic and ceramic between the joint bearing surfaces to relieve pain, in 1938 Philip Wiles at the Middlesex Hospital, London undertook the first prosthetic joint replacement (Wiles 1958). In 1948 Smith-Petersen used cups or moulds designed to cover the femoral head to interpose between the articulating surfaces, and this was deemed to produce

* Corresponding author: Mr W Khan, Department of Trauma & Orthopaedics, Royal Free Hospital, London, NW3 2QG, UK; E-mail: wasimkhan@doctors.org.uk; Telephone number: +44 (0) 7791 025554; Fax number: +44 (0) 1707 655059.

satisfactory results (Smith-Petersen 1948). The latter half of the last century witnessed pioneering development during an impressive era of development of total hip arthroplasty initially by George Kenneth Mckee from Norwich and later by Sir John Charnley at Wrightington. Charnley revolutionised hip replacement by developing a metal-on-polymer arthroplasty and using acrylic cement to fix components to living bone, which dominated the field as the Gold Standard for at least half a century (Charnley 1961). It is thanks to these pioneers that a total hip replacement is described as the greatest achievement in orthopaedic surgery in the twentieth century.

Total hip replacement is a viable option for nearly all patients with diseases of the hip that cause chronic discomfort and significant functional impairment. This chapter gives an insight into the various more recent developments in total hip replacement that determine the use of cement, choice of bearing surfaces, and include minimal invasive and computer-assisted surgery.

Cemented Total Hip Replacement

Sir John Charnley popularised the use of polymethyl methacrylate bone cement to obtain a better fixation of the femoral prosthesis (Charnley 1960). Cement acts as a grout rather than glue, and mechanical interlock rather than adhesion is essential for fixation. Cementing the femoral prostheses is the key step of a cemented hip replacement as it is technique dependant in which the surgeon creates the bone-cement-implant interface during the surgery. Although the constituents of cement have remained the same, cementation technique has evolved over the years.

In the earlier years, cement was finger packed into the femoral canal without pressurisation which led to inadequate cement mantle and early implant failure (Hashemi-Nejad et al. 1994). Currently third generation cementation technique is used and it entails the preparation of the femoral, insertion of a distal cement restrictor, cleaning with pulsed lavage of normal saline and drying the canal. The cement is mixed in a vacuum container and loaded into a cement gun that allows pressurised insertion into the femoral canal and is facilitated by a proximal pressuriser. Proximal and distal centralisers facilitate reproducible creation of a complete and uniform cement mantle around the prosthesis (Gozzard et al. 2003).

Improved cementing techniques have remarkably extended the durability of the cemented femoral implants and reduced the incidence of loosening. Aseptic loosening is mainly attributed to bone resorption activated by an *in vivo* macrophage response to particulate debris generated by wear debris. There are many cemented femoral prostheses available and one example is shown in Figure 1. Carrington et al., (2009) have reported 100% survival of the Exeter femoral stem at 17 year follow-up with revision for aseptic loosening being the end point. Wroblewski et al., (2009) have shown good results of the Charnley femoral stem at 30 to 40 year follow-up. Barrack et al., (1992) noted loosening of cemented cups in 44% of patients aged less than 50 years at 12 year follow-up. An alternate approach to the use of a cemented acetabular component with the cemented femoral component is to use a cementless acetabular component, called the hybrid total hip replacement as shown in Figure 2. These cementless acetabular cups were popularised after difficulties with the fixation of cemented polyethylene cups. Cementless acetabular cups are hemispherical in shape and can be completely porous coated to encourage bone ingrowth. They are primarily press fit components but could also have additional attachments with pegs, spikes, screws or threaded cups.

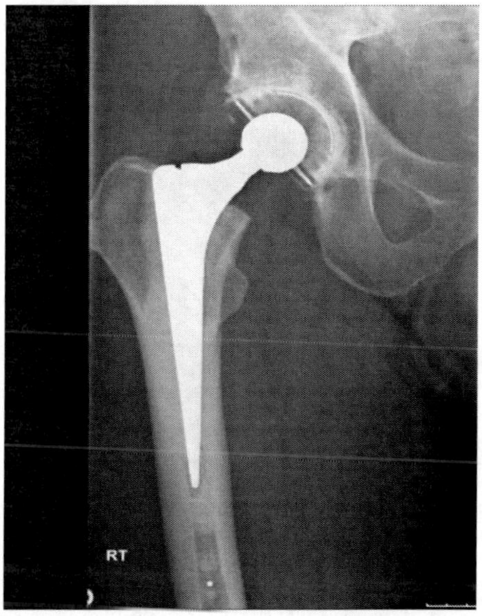

Figure 1. A cemented femoral and acetabular component. Note the radio-opaque cement mantle around the femoral and acetabular components, and the femoral cement restrictor beyond the tip of the femoral prosthesis.

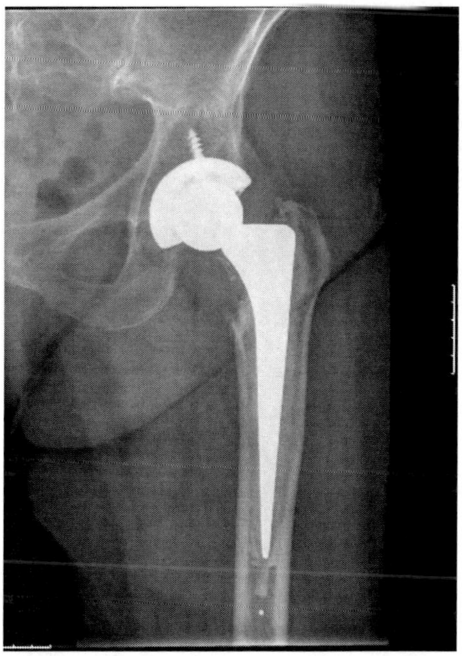

Figure 2. A hybrid hip replacement with a cemented femoral component and an uncemented acetabular component. Note the screw used for fixation of the acetabular component.

UNCEMENTED TOTAL HIP REPLACEMENT

For many years, acrylic cement was regarded as the only available means for a long-term secure fixation of components in hip replacement. First generation cementing techniques frequently resulted in bone destruction and resorption leading to early failure of the femoral prostheses. This was incorrectly attributed to a local inflammatory process triggered by the cement debris (Harris et al. 1976), and lead to an interest in cementless femoral prosthesis. Cementless components were designed in the 1980's and required biological fixation where bone integrates onto or into the implant to secure fixation. Cementless implants theoretically reduce the chances of infection and loosening of the component as there is one less interface that could potentially fail. Figure 3 shows an example of an uncemented total hip replacement.

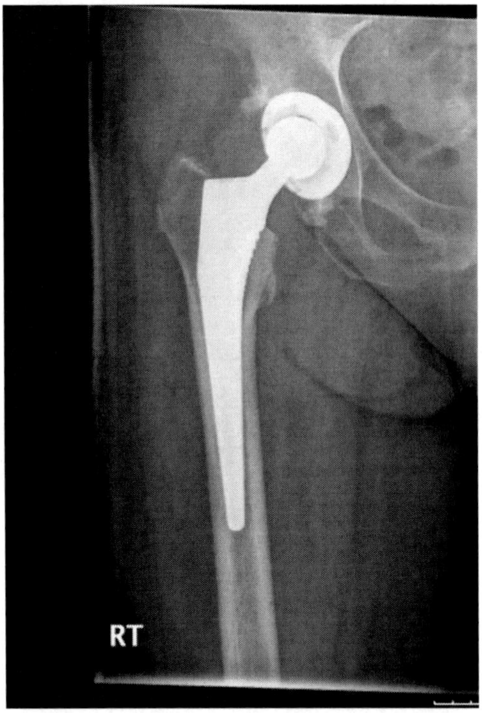

Figure 3. An uncemented femoral and acetabular component. The acetabular component is press-fitted without the use of screws or pegs.

In uncemented hip replacements, early revision rates however are almost two-fold greater for cementless hip replacement than those for cemented prostheses (Swedish Hip Registry). In a systematic literature review, cemented femoral components fared better than uncemented components in the short- and mid-term (Ni et al. 2005). In a meta-analysis comparing cemented and uncemented hip replacements, cemented fixation outperformed uncemented fixation in large subsets of study populations (Morshed et al. 2007). Recent literature however suggested that the performance of uncemented implants was improving. Parvizi et al., (2004) noted that the overall medium- to long-term outcome of cementless femoral prosthesis was excellent, with a low revision rate and high patient satisfaction.

A new generation of uncemented implants coated in hydroxyapatite became available in the mid-1980s, aiming to provide a 'biological interface' between metal and surrounding bone, and thus was distinct from plain porous fixation. Hydroxyapatite particles are biodegradable and do not produce any inflammatory reaction in the surrounding bone or debris resulting in osteolysis or third body wear. Comparison between hydroxyapatite and plain porous femoral components in the literature has demonstrated better results with hydroxyapatite in terms of the quantity and quality of bone remodelling, and the migration and subsidence of the stem (Epinette & Manley 2008). Epinette & Manley (2008) also demonstrated a 99% survival rate at 17-year follow-up using hydroxyapatite coated femoral stems.

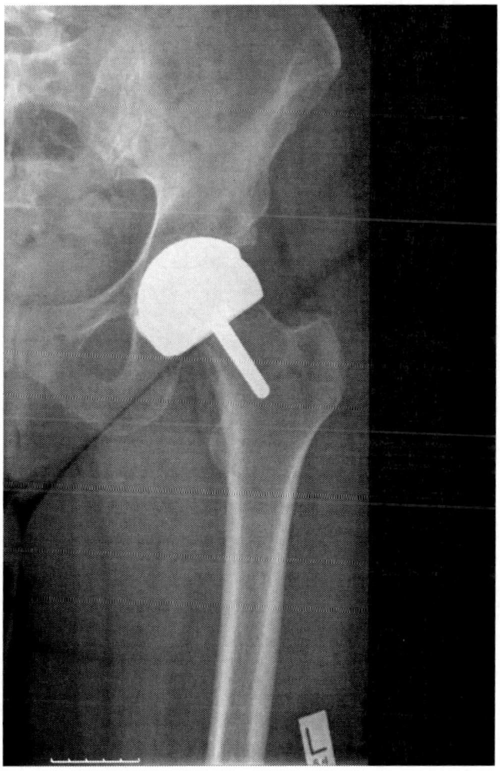

Figure 4. A hip resurfacing prosthesis. Compared with a traditional total hip replacement, resurfacing is a bone conserving procedure with more of the neck and part of the femoral head being preserved.

BEARING SURFACES

The initial belief that cement debris was the main cause of osteolysis in cemented hip replacement was found to be untrue as osteolysis was observed in uncemented hip replacements. Further histological studies revealed that osteolysis was related to the macrophage response to polyethylene debris (Archibeck et al. 2001). Willert et al., (1977) noted the role of wear particles generated by joint prostheses in the pathogenesis of osteolysis and aseptic loosening. The polyethylene wear debris cause synovitis, osteolysis, joint instability and loosening. Ceramic femoral heads have been associated with up to 50% lower *in vivo* polyethylene wear rates than metal heads (Heisel et al. 2004).

The wear resistance of polyethylene has been improved by cross-linking. Gamma irradiation of the polyethylene causes cross-linking which has greater resistance to wear (Saikko et al., 2002, D'Antonio et al. 2009). This however is associated with progressive decreases in other material properties, which theoretically increase the risk of component failure from very high and localized stresses. Total hip replacement with ceramic on ceramic or highly cross-linked ultra high molecular weight polyethylene (UHMWPE) bearing surfaces have all shown good mid-term results with regards to wear (Callaghan et al. 2008).

Metal-on-polyethylene total hip replacements are prone to wear with secondary osteolysis and aseptic loosening, especially in younger and active patients. Metal-on-metal bearings although initially favoured when introduced in the late 1980s, have now fallen out of favour due to the association with metalloses, pseudotumours, aseptic lymphocyte-dominated vasculitis-associated lesions (ALVAL), and raised serum cobalt and chromium levels.

Many hip replacement bearing surfaces are composed of cobalt-chromium alloys, and an increasing number of metal-on-metal prostheses are being revised. These bearings release metal wear debris that include chromium ions that are metabolised and redistributed in fluid and tissue compartments. Patients with metal-on-metal hips have higher levels of cobalt and chromium in their blood and urine than either patients with metal-on-polyethylene devices or control subjects. The potential biological effects of chromium are controversial and include DNA and chromosomal damage, reduction in CD8 lymphocyte levels and possible type IV hypersensitivity reactions or ALVAL (Afolaranmi et al., 2008, Khan et al. 2008). We raised concerns that the true incidence of these problems will become apparent over the coming years leading to the need for a significant number of revision procedures almost five years ago.

Ceramics including alumina have been used as a bearing surface in total hip replacements for over 35 years. Properties that make it particularly attractive as a bearing surface include its hardness, high compression strength, and excellent wettability (Lang et al. 2008). This results in improved fracture toughness as well as a low incidence of biologically significant particle generation and clinically significant osteolysis. Improvements in the processing of ceramic as well as advances in engineering have led to a decrease in the incidence of ceramic fracture and dislocation. These bearings have the lowest wear rates but these are sensitive to implant position and are the most expensive bearing option (Heisel et al. 2004). Other concerns related to ceramic on ceramic bearings are squeaking and chip fractures at the rim of acetabular liners due to implant malpositioning.

Minimally Invasive Surgery

As the emphasis of healthcare shifted to cost-effectiveness and patient choice, the last decade ushered in newer developments such as minimally invasive surgery (MIS). MIS can either be a single-incision or two-incision technique. The National Institute of Clinical Excellence (NICE) in the UK has approved the use of single-incision surgery using the same approaches as conventional surgery but with an incision less than 10 cm (NICE 2006). The benefits of two-incision technique are controversial and NICE concluded that there was insufficient evidence for it to be used without special arrangements (NICE 2005). Proponents of MIS claim improved patient satisfaction and cost reduction due to early discharge from hospital and return to work as a result of decreased intra-operative blood loss, reduced soft tissue trauma and post-operative pain. DiGioia et al., (2003) reported that patients had a significant improvement with respect to limp and ability to climb stairs at three months following MIS, and no difference to conventional hip replacement at one year follow-up.

MIS is complex and at any given moment not all the surgical field is visible (Howell et al. 2004). Considering the decreased visualisation of anatomical landmarks and greater difficulty in component positioning, computer navigation will aid technical performance and improve outcomes (Malik et al. 2007).

Computer-Assisted Surgery in Total Hip Replacement

Malpositioning of the acetabular component in total hip replacement may result in limited range of movement, joint dislocation and increased wear reducing survival of the prosthesis (Kennedy et al. 1998). Computer-assisted surgery is growing in popularity and aids precise placement of acetabular cups especially in MIS. Two forms of computer-assisted surgery exist for total hip replacements; one is an active system, which uses a robot to implant the cup, and the other is a passive system, whereby the surgeon navigates the instruments and components within a virtual picture intra-operatively. Kalteiss et al., (2006) reported that the operating time was increased by 17 minutes in CT-based navigation, and by eight minutes with imageless navigation, compared with conventional hip replacement. There was no significant difference in intra-operative blood loss.

Critics of computer-assisted surgery point to the costs associated with specialised equipment and increased operating time. In 2008 a meta-analysis of three randomised controlled prospective trials comparing computer-navigated against conventional total hip replacement showed that computer-assisted surgery significantly improved the placement of the acetabular cup within the desired alignment, but results on whether this translates to improved long-term outcomes are awaited (Gandhi et al. 2009). There is still a lack of substantial evidence supporting computer-assisted surgery and few surgeons are actually using navigation for total hip arthroplasty (Rubash & Paganano 2009).

National Joint Registry

A wide variety of implants are used in the thousands of total hip replacement surgeries carried out across England and Wales. The National Joint Registry of England and Wales was set up in 2002 by the Department of Health and Welsh Assembly Government to collect information on all hip and knee replacement operations and to monitor the performance of hip and knee joint implants. The Registry monitors the performance of various implants and the effectiveness of different types of surgery. It also collects data relating to patient demographics, surgical approach, cementation technique, intra-operative complications and deep vein thromboses prophylaxis. The aim is to result in improved clinical standards that benefit patients, clinicians and the orthopaedic industry. The Fifth Annual Report by the

Registry shows that the overall revision rate following primary hip replacement was 0.6% at one year and 1.2% at 3 years. It showed that the 3 year revision rates were lowest in patients with cemented prosthesis (0.7%) and highest after hip resurfacing, and metal-on-metal implants.

CONCLUSION

Total hip replacement has been shown to be a relatively safe and successful treatment method to alleviate pain and improve quality of life. Good results have been demonstrated with both cemented and uncemented hip replacements. There is a number of bearing surfaces available, as well as surgical techniques including computer-assisted surgery, and our practice is likely to continue to evolve with time. Patient's expectations from a hip replacement have changed with time and modern technology is continuously evolving to meet the challenges.

REFERENCES

Afolaranmi GA, Tettey J, Meek RM, Grant MH 2008 Release of chromium from orthopaedic arthroplasties *Open Orthopaedic Journal* 24 10-8.

Allen DJ, Beaulé PE 2008 Rationale for metal-on-metal total hip replacement *Journal of Surgical Orthopaedic Advances* 17 6-11.

Archibeck MJ, Jacobs JJ, Roebuck KA, Glant TT 2001 The basic science of periprosthetic osteolysis *Instructional Course Lectures* 50 185-195.

Australian Orthopaedic Association 2006 *National Joint Replacement Registry. Annual report* Adelaide, Australia.

Ball ST, Le Duff MJ, Amstutz HC 2007 Early results of conversion of a failed femoral component in hip resurfacing arthoplasty *Journal of Bone & Joint Surgery* 89A 735-741.

Barrack RL, Mulroy RD Jr, Harris WH 1992 Improved cementing techniques and femoral component loosening in young patients with hip arthroplasty. A 12-year radiographic review *Journal of Bone & Joint Surgery* 74B 385-389.

Beaulé PE, Dorey FJ, LeDuff M, Gruen T, Amstutz HC 2004 Risk factors affecting outcome of metal-on-metal surface arthroplasty of the hip *Clinical Orthopaedics & Related Research* 418 87-93.

Callaghan JJ, Cuckler JM, Huddleston JI, Galante JO 2008 Implant Wear Symposium 2007 Clinical Work Group. How have alternative bearings affected the prevention and treatment of osteolysis? *Journal of American Academy of Orthopaedic Surgeons* 16 S33-S38.

Carrington NC, Sierra RJ, Gie GA 2009 The Exeter Universal cemented femoral component at 15 to 17 years: an update on the first 325 hips *Journal of Bone & Joint Surgery* 91B 730-737.

Charnley J 1960 Anchorage of the femoral head prosthesis to the shaft of the femur *Journal of Bone & Joint Surgery* 42B 28-30.

Charnley J 1961 Arthroplasty of the hip: a new operation *Lancet 1* 1129-1132.

D'Antonio JA, Pagnano MW, Naughton M et al., 2009 Controversies regarding bearing surfaces in total hip replacement *Journal of Bone & Joint Surgery* 91A S5-S9.

Dheerendra S, Khan WS, Saeed MZ, Goddard NJ (2010). Recent Developments in Total Hip Replacements: Cementation, Articulation, Minimal-Invasion and Navigation. *J Perioper Pract.* 20(4): 133-8.

DiGioia AM 3rd, Plakseychuk AY, Levison TJ, Jaramaz B 2003 Mini-incision technique for total hip arthroplasty with navigation *Journal of Arthroplasty* 18 123-128.

Dumbleton JH, Manley MT 2005 Metal-on-Metal total hip replacement: what does the literature say? *Journal of Arthroplasty* 20 174-188.

Epinette JA, Manley MT 2008 Uncemented stems in hip replacement--hydroxyapatite or plain porous: does it matter? Based on a prospective study of HA Omnifit stems at 15-years minimum follow-up *Hip International* 18 69-74.

Gandhi R, Marchie A, Farrokhyar F, Mahomed N 2009 Computer navigation in total hip replacement: a meta-analysis *International Orthopaedics* 33 593-597.

Gozzard C, Gheduzzi S, Miles AW, Learmonth ID 2003 An in-vitro investigation of the CPS-Plus femoral stem: influence of the proximal centraliser on cement pressurisation during stem insertion *Acta Orthopaedica Scandinavia* 74 154-158.

Harris WH, Schiller AL, Scholler JM, Freiberg RA, Scott R 1976 Extensive localized bone resorption in the femur following total hip replacement *Journal of Bone & Joint Surgery* 58A 612-618.

Heisel C, Silva M, dela Rosa MA, Schmalzried TP 2004 Short-term in vivo wear of cross-linked *polyethylene Journal of Bone & Joint Surgery* 86A 748-751.

Hashemi-Nejad A, Birch NC, Goddard NJ 1994 Current attitudes to cementing techniques in British hip surgery *Annals of the Royal College of Surgeons of England* 76 396-400.

Howell JR, Garbuz DS, Duncan CP 2004 Minimally invasive hip replacement: rationale, applied anatomy, and instrumentation *Orthopaedic Clinics of North America* 35 107–118.

Kalteis T, Handel M, Bathis H et al., 2006 Imageless navigation for insertion of acetabular component in total hip arthroplasty: Is it accurate as CT based navigation *Journal of Bone & Joint Surgery* 88B 163-167.

Kennedy JG, Rogers WB, Soffe KE et al., 1998 Effect of acetabular component orientation on recurrent dislocation, pelvic osteolysis, polyethylene wear, and component migration *Journal of Arthroplasty* 13: 530-534.

Khan WS, Agarwal M, Malik AA et al., 2008 Chromium, cobalt and titanium metallosis involving a Nottingham shoulder replacement *Journal of Bone & Joint Surgery* 90B 502-505.

Lang JE, Whiddon DR, Smith EL, Salyapongse AK 2008 Use of ceramics in total hip replacement *Journal of Surgical Orthopaedic Advances* 17 51-57.

Lavigne M, Masse V, Girard J, Roy AG, Vendittoli PA 2008 Return to sport after hip resurfacing or total hip arthroplasty: a randomized study *Revue de Chirurgie Orthopédique et Réparatrice de L'appareil Moteur* 94 361-367.

Malik A, Dorr LD 2007 The science of minimally invasive total hip arthroplasty *Clinical Orthopaedics and Related Research* 463 74-84.

Marker DR, Seyler TM, Jinnah RH et al., 2007 Femoral neck fractures after metal-on-metal total hip resurfacing: a prospective cohort study *Journal of Arthroplasty* 22 66-71.

Mont MA, Seyler TM, Ragland PS et al., 2007 Gait analysis of patients with resurfacing hip arthroplasty compared with hip osteoarthritis and standard total hip arthroplasty *Journal of Arthroplasty* 22 100-108.

Morshed S, Bozic KJ, Ries MD, Malchau H, Colford JM Jr 2007 Comparison of cemented and uncemented fixation in total hip replacement: a meta-analysis *Acta Orthopaedica* 78 315-326.

Ni GX, Lu WW, Chiu KY, Fong DY 2005 Cemented or uncemented femoral component in primary total hip replacement? A review from a clinical and radiological perspective *Journal of Orthopaedic Surgery* 13 96-105.

National Institute for Health and Clinical Excellence 2005 *Minimally invasive two-incision surgery for total hip replacement: interventional procedure guidance* 112 London.

National Institute for Health and Clinical Excellence 2006 *Single mini-incision hip replacement: interventional procedure guidance* 152 London.

Parvizi J, Keisu KS, Hozack WJ, Sharkey PF, Rothman RH 2004 Primary total hip arthroplasty with an uncemented femoral component: a long-term study of the Taperloc stem *Journal of Arthroplasty* 19 151-156.

Rubash HE, Paganano MW 2009 Navigation in Total Hip Arthroplasty *Journal of Bone & Joint Surgery* 91A 17.

Saikko V, Calonius O, Keranen J 2002 Wear of conventional and cross-linked ultra high-molecular-weight polyethylene acetabular cups against polished and roughened CoCr femoral heads in a biaxial hip simulator *Journal of Biomedical Material Research* 63 848-853.

Smith-Petersen MN 1948 The classic: evolution of mould arthroplasty of the hip joint *Journal of Bone & Joint Surgery* 30B L59.

Swedish National Hip Registry: Citing References [online] Available from: http://www.jru.orthop.gu.se/documents.htm [Accessed August 2009].

Tennent TD, Goddard NJ 2000 Current attitudes to total hip replacement in the younger patient: results of a national survey *Annals of the Royal College of Surgeons of England* 82 33-38.

Treacy RB, McBryde CW, Pynsent PB 2005 Birmingham hip resurfacing arthroplasty: a minimum follow-up of five years *Journal of Bone & Joint Surgery* 87B 167-170.

Wiles P 1958 The surgery of the osteoarthritic hip *British Journal of Surgery* 45 488-497.

Willert HG 1977 Reactions of the articular capsule to wear products of artificial joint prostheses *Journal of Biomedical Material Research* 11 157-164.

Wroblewski BM, Siney PD, Fleming PA 2009 Charnley low-frictional torque arthroplasty: follow-up for 30 to 40 years *Journal of Bone & Joint Surgery* 91B 447-450.

In: Perioperative Practice in Trauma and Orthopaedic Surgery ISBN: 978-1-63483-325-7
Editor: Wasim S. Khan

Chapter 26

THE USE OF NON-STEROIDAL ANTI-INFLAMMATORY DRUGS IN TRAUMA AND ORTHOPAEDICS

W. Khan**, *M. Al-Rashid and D. R. Marsh
University College London Institute of Orthopaedics and Musculoskeletal Sciences, Royal National Orthopaedic Hospital, Stanmore, Middlesex, UK

ABSTRACT

Non-steroidal anti-inflammatory drugs are powerful and effective anti-inflammatory, analgesic and anti-pyretic drugs. They are routinely used in orthopaedic conditions and in the perioperative setting. They are however associated with potentially life-threatening side-effects and it is important to appreciate these before these drugs are given. There is evidence suggesting that these drugs adversely affect bone formation, and this has implications on their use in patients with fractures and other pathologies that involve bone remodelling.

Keywords: NSAIDs, side-effects, bone formation

In this chapter we look at Non-steroidal anti-inflammatory drugs (NSAIDs) and discuss how they word, as well as their side-effects (Khan et al. 2009). One of the most significant morbidity experienced by patients is the symptom of pain. This is relevant in acute and chronic injuries and disease, and also in the perioperative setting. Pain causes great suffering and disability, not only physical but also emotional and psychosocial. Pain can have a complex multi-factorial aetiology, and it is plausible to utilise different modalities of

* Corresponding Author: Mr WS Khan, Clinical Lecturer, University College London Institute of Orthopaedic and Musculoskeletal Research, Royal National Orthopaedic Hospital, Stanmore, Middlesex, HA7 4LP, UK; Telephone number: +44 (0) 77791 025554; Fax number: +44 (0) 1707 655059; E-mail address: wasimkhan@doctors.org.uk.

treatment in combination rather than to rely on one single modality to achieve complete efficacy.

NSAIDs are powerful and effective anti-inflammatory, analgesic and anti-pyretic drugs. They are commonly used in orthopaedic practice to manage acute soft tissue injuries as well as chronic degenerative conditions like osteoarthritis. The evidence for the effectiveness of NSAIDs is overwhelming with several studies comparing it against placebo in acute or chronic conditions (Towheed et al. 1997). In combination with opioids (e.g. morphine), it has been shown that NSAIDs reduce the amount of opioids needed. NSAIDs act as disease-modifying agents in rheumatoid arthritis, ankylosing spondylitis and acute gout. They are also used as a prophylaxis for heterotopic ossification (Balboni et al. 2006).

How NSAIDs work

NSAIDs inhibit both isoforms of the enzyme cyclo-oxygenase (COX). COX converts arachidonic acid to prostaglandins and leukotrienes. COX1 is primarily present in the stomach and kidneys, and blocking it can result in gastrointestinal and renal side-effects. COX2 is primarily associated with inflammation, and blocking it is the main clinical objective of NSAIDs. Inflammation is the hallmark of many musculoskeletal disease processes, and by blocking it NSAIDs acts as a potent analgesic.

NSAIDs reduce vasodilator prostaglandins resulting in anti-inflammatory action. Reducing prostaglandins also makes nerve endings transmitting pain less sensitive resulting in analgesic action. NSAIDs also reduce prostaglandin production associated with the pyrogen interleukin-1 resulting in anti-pyretic action.

Although studies have shown a correlation between concentration of NSAIDs and effect, they do not explain the observed differences in individual patient responses. It is thought that the pharmacokinetic (process by which a drug is absorbed, distributed, metabolised, and eliminated) differences among NSAIDs may account for these differences.

Different Types of NSAIDs

There are many groups of NSAIDs including propionic acid derivatives (e.g. ibuprofen), salicylic acid derivatives (e.g. aspirin), acetic acid derivatives (e.g., diclofenac), indole derivatives (e.g. indomethacin) and oxicam derivatives (e.g., piroxicam). Cochrane reviews on NSAIDs in hip and knee disease found that no conclusions could be drawn about which NSAID was best (Towheed et al. 1997). More recently there has been considerable interest in COX2 inhibitors (e.g. celecoxib) due to their selective action against COX2 and thus avoiding the gastrointestinal and renal side-effects associated with COX1 blockage (Ankarath et al. 2003).

NSAIDs can be given through the oral, parenteral and topical routes. The oral route is routinely used in clinical practice. The parenteral route is particularly suitable in the perioperative setting. The topical route possibly reduces gastrointestinal side-effects by maximising local delivery and minimising systemic toxicity (Evans et al. 1995).

SIDE-EFFECTS OF NSAIDS

NSAIDs are routinely used in the perioperative analgesic armoury due to an appreciation that it is better to utilise different modalities of treatment in combination rather than to rely on one single modality to achieve complete efficacy. All healthcare professionals involved in the perioperative care of patients must be aware of the potential side-effects of NSAIDs and this would allow them to have an appreciation of the risks and benefits.

1. Adverse Effects on Bone Formation

Bone healing is a complex process that involves several cell types and molecules in a number of complex pathways. The COX enzymes play an important role in fracture repair, and the activation and differentiation of progenitors cells (Xie et al. 2008). Prostaglandins are needed for the inflammatory responses, increase osteoclast activity that results in bone resorption, and increase osteoblast activity that results in new bone formation (Dumont et al., 2000, Zhang et al. 2002). NSAIDs, especially COX2 inhibitors, block the COX pathway inhibiting prostaglandin synthesis. This results in inhibition of bone formation. Inhibition of bone formation can be clinically useful in preventing heterotopic ossification, but is not desirable in fractures and in situations where bone remodelling is needed. These include surgeries where uncemented implants or bone grafts are used, and fusion procedures. In fractures, the inhibition of bone formation can result in delayed or non-union.

Animal studies on fracture healing show that NSAIDs impair bone healing (Huo et al., 1991, Altman et al., 1995, Murnaghan et al. 2006). Limited clinical data also suggests that COX2 inhibition by NSAIDs delays healing (Giannoudis et al., 2000, Goodman et al. 2004). The evidence regarding bone healing is sometimes however contradictory, with issues over type of drug, dose and duration (Bauer et al. 1996). Disagreement might be a function of type of NSAID; proprionic NSAIDs may prevent bone loss in some circumstances while acetic acid NSAIDs may not. Further clinical studies are needed to ascertain the effects of NSAIDs on bone formation definitively

2. Cardiovascular and Haematostatic Side-Effects

NSAIDs have also been associated with increased risk of cardiovascular complications, especially in patients with a history of cardiovascular disease or its risk factors. These complications include myocardial infarction, oedema, thrombosis, haemodynamic instability and death, and are dose and treatment duration dependent. Cardiovascular toxicity was reported following the release of COX2 inhibitors in the pharmaceutical market, and further studies showed this to be a feature of all NSAIDs. Rofecoxib was associated with significantly higher risk when compared with celecoxib and other NSAIDs, and was withdrawn from the market (Mukerjee et al., 2001, Dajani & Islam 2008).

Platelet COX produces thromboxane that causes platelet aggregation and aids coagulation. This mechanism is disrupted by NSAIDs as they inhibit platelet COX, and this can lead to perioperative bleeding. NSAIDs also enhance the effect of warfarin by displacing it from the carrier protein albumin and increasing the amount of free warfarin in the blood. NSAIDs could also affect the blood clotting by causing abnormalities in the liver (Day et al. 1996), and this is an important consideration in the perioperative patient.

3. Gastrointestinal Side-Effects

NSAIDs, particularly oral preparations, can cause gastric mucosa erosions that may lead to ulceration. These ulcers may perforate or bleed with a high incidence of mortality (Blower et al., 1997, Hawkey et al., 1997, MacDonald et al. 1997). These effects could be limited by using NSAIDs with gastroprotective agents (e.g. lansoprazole or misoprostol). The risk is dose-dependent and short duration of use reduces the risk of a serious adverse event. Epidemiological studies have demonstrated that ibuprofen is associated with the lowest risk and piroxicam with the highest. Intermittent therapy with NSAIDs is safe, and it remains to be shown whether COX2 inhibitors have a clinically significant benefit (Wolfe 2003).

4. Renal Side-Effects

Prostaglandins have a role in renal vasodilation and their inhibition by the NSAIDS reduces the renal blood flow and glomerular filtration rate. This can ultimately lead to acute and chronic interstitial nephritis, and renal failure (O' Callaghan 1994). The perioperative patient with hypotension and hypovolaemia is particularly vulnerable. Other risk factors include a history of renal impairment or cardiac failure, and patients taking other concurrent nephrotoxic drugs (e.g. gentamicin), angiotensin-converting enzyme inhibitors and diuretics. Although NSAIDs should not be withheld from patients with normal preoperative renal function, vigilance is required in all cases (Weir 2002).

5. Respiratory Side-Effects

NSAIDS are known to exacerbate asthma in some patients but, despite this well-known complication, cases of mortality in asthmatic patients given NSAIDs continue to be reported (Titchen et al. 2005). It should be remembered that NSAID-exacerbated asthma can occur in children as well as adults, and some studies describe an incidence of 30% in children with severe asthma. The asthmatic reaction is dose-dependent and can occur with sub-therapeutic doses. NSAIDs should be avoided when sensitivity is known or suspected in patients with severe asthma, and alternative modalities should be utilised (Palmer 2005). If the patient has a history of asthma, a trial dose should only be given in a setting where an acute exacerbation can be managed.

Clinical Considerations in Perioperative Practice

It is important to take a detailed medical history before commencing NSAIDs. If the patient is sedated or anaesthetised, this may not be possible and a review of the patient's medical records is essential. This should include a subjective and objective assessment of the pain. It should also include past medical history of cardiovascular problems, respiratory diseases, peptic ulcer disease, renal impairment, and recent fractures. A drug history should also be taken and a note made of any allergies. With the potential risks of NSAIDs on bone healing, it is important to identify other risk factors that may adversely affect bone healing e.g. smoking, diabetes mellitus and peripheral vascular disease. This will allow the practitioner to determine whether or not the patient is suitable for NSAIDs. It will also allow the practitioner to gauge the severity of the symptoms and to determine what has worked in the past.

Conclusion

NSAIDs are likely to continue to provide a very effective mode of treating pain in orthopaedic patients, and also in the perioperative setting. In view of the potential side-effects, it is important that a thorough clinical assessment is made before NSAIDs are used. The limited evidence available suggests that NSAIDs do adversely affect bone formation. In patients with pathologies that involve bone remodelling, and especially in the presence of other risk factors that adversely affect bone healing, NSAIDS should be avoided.

References

Altman RD, Latta LL, Keer R et al., 1995 Effect of nonsteroidal anti-inflammatory drugs on fracture healing: a laboratory study in rats *Journal of Orthopaedic Trauma* 9 392-400.

Ankarath S, Raman R, Giannoudis PV 2003 Non-steroidal anti-inflammatory drugs in orthopaedic practice: an update *Current Orthopaedics* 17 144-149.

Balboni TA, Gobezie R, Mamon HJ 2006 Heterotopic ossification: Pathophysiology, clinical features, and the role of radiotherapy for prophylaxis *International Journal of Radiation Oncology, Biology & Physics* 65 1289-1299.

Bauer DC, Orwoll ES, Fox KM et al., 1996 Aspirin and NSAID use in older women: effect on bone mineral density and fracture risk *Journal of Bone & Mineral Research* 11 29-35.

Blower AL, Brooks A, Fenn CG et al., 1997 Emergency admissions for upper gastrointestinal disease and their relation to NSAID use *Alimentary Pharmacology & Therapeutics* 11 283-291.

Dajani EZ, Islam K 2008 Cardiovascular and gastrointestinal toxicity of selective cyclo-oxygenase-2 inhibitors in man *Journal of Physiology & Pharmacology* 59 117-133.

Day JP, Lanas A, Rustagi P, Hirschowitz BI 1996 Reversible prolonged skin bleeding time in acute gastrointestinal bleeding presumed due to NSAIDs *Journal of Clinical Gastroenterology* 22 96-103.

Dumont AS, Verma S, Dumont RJ, Hurlbert RJ 2000 Nonsteroidal anti-inflammatory drugs and bone metabolism in spinal fusion surgery. A pharmacological quandary *Journal of Pharmacological & Toxicological Methods* 43 31-39.

Evans JM, McMahon AD, McGilchrist MM et al., 1995 Topical non-steroidal anti-inflammatory drugs and admission to hospital for upper gastrointestinal bleeding and perforation: a record linkage case-control study *British Medical Journal* 311 22-26.

Giannoudis PV, MacDonald DA, Matthews SJ et al., 2000 Nonunion of the femoral diaphysis. The influence of reaming and non-steroidal anti-inflammatory drugs *Journal of Bone & Joint Surgery* 82B 655-648.

Goodman SB, Ma T, Genovese M, Lane Smith R 2003 COX-2 selective inhibitors and bone International *Journal of Immunopathology & Pharmacology* 16 201-205.

Hawkey CJ, Cullen DJ, Greenwood DC, Wilson JV, Logan RF 1997 Prescribing of nonsteroidal anti-inflammatory drugs in general practice: determinants and consequences *Alimentary Pharmacology & Therapeutics* 11 293-298.

Huo MH, Troiano NW, Pelker RR, Gundberg CM, Friedlaender GE 1991 The influence of ibuprofen on fracture repair: biomechanical, histologic, and histomorphometric parameters in rats *Journal of Orthopaedic Research* 9 383-390.

Khan WS, Al-Rashid M, Marsh DR (2009). Non-Steroidal Anti-Inflammatory Drugs in Orthopaedic and Perioperative Practice. J Perioper Pract. 19(9): 287-90.

MacDonald TM, Morant SV, Robinson GC et al., 1997 Association of upper gastrointestinal toxicity of non-steroidal anti-inflammatory drugs with continued exposure: cohort study *British Medical Journal* 315 1333-1337.

Mukherjee D, Nissen SE, Topol EJ 2001 Risk of cardiovascular events associated with selective COX-2 inhibitors *Journal of the American Medical Association* 286 954-959.

Murnaghan M, Li G, Marsh DR 2006 Nonsteroidal anti-inflammatory drug-induced fracture nonunion: an inhibition of angiogenesis? *Journal of Bone & Joint Surgery* 88A 140-147.

O' Callaghan CA 1994 Acute renal failure associated with NSAIDS *British Medical Journal* 308 857-858.

Palmer GM 2005 A teenager with severe asthma exacerbation following ibuprofen *Anaesthetic Intensive Care* 33 261-265.

Titchen T, Cranswick N, Beggs S 2005 Adverse drug reactions to nonsteroidal anti-inflammatory drugs, COX-2 inhibitors and paracetamol in a paediatric hospital *British Journal of Clinical Pharmacology* 59 718-723.

Towheed T, Shea B, Wells G, Hochberg M 1997 Osteoarthritis: a systematic review of randomized controlled trials of analgesia and anti-inflammatory therapy in osteoarthritis of the hip *Cochrane Library* Issue 4.

Weir MR 2002 Renal effects of nonselective NSAIDs and coxibs *Cleveland Clinic Journal of Medicine* 69 53-58.

Wolfe MM 2003 Risk factors associated with the development of gastroduodenal ulcers due to the use of NSAIDs *International Journal of Clinical Practice* 135 32-37.

Xie C, Ming X, Wang Q et al., 2008 COX-2 from the injury milieu is critical for the initiation of periosteal progenitor cell mediated bone healing *Bone* 43 1075-1083.

Zhang X, Schwarz EM, Young DA et al., 2002 Cyclooxygenase-2 regulates mesenchymal cell differentiation into the osteoblast lineage and is critically involved in bone repair *Journal of Clinical Investigation* 109 1405-1415.

In: Perioperative Practice in Trauma and Orthopaedic Surgery ISBN: 978-1-63483-325-7
Editor: Wasim S. Khan

Chapter 27

STEM CELL APPLICATIONS AND TISSUE ENGINEERING APPROACHES IN SURGICAL PRACTICE

W. S. Khan*, A. A. Malik and T. E. Hardingham

UK Centre for Tissue Engineering and Wellcome Trust Centre for Cell Matrix Research, Faculty of Life Sciences, Michael Smith Building, University of Manchester, Manchester, UK

ABSTRACT

There has been an increasing interest in stem cell applications and tissue engineering approaches in surgical practice to deal with damaged or lost tissue. Although there have been developments in almost all surgical disciplines, the greatest advances are being made in orthopaedics, especially in bone repair. Significant hurdles however remain to be overcome before tissue engineering becomes more routinely used in surgical practice.

Tissue is frequently damaged or lost in injury and disease, and this review discusses the use of stem cells and tissue engineering in surgical practice (Khan et al. 2009). Current strategies to deal with the damaged or lost tissue include the use of tissue from the same patient e.g. bone grafting, the use of donated tissue e.g. heart transplant, and the use of prosthetic materials e.g. a total knee replacement. These are all associated with disadvantages and complications. The use of tissue from the same patient is associated with donor site morbidity and the replacement tissue does not tend to function optimally. The usc of donated tissue as with organ transplantation is limited by the dearth of donor availability and the complications associated with immunosuppression that is frequently required. The use of prosthetic materials is associated with wear and tear and a frequent need for revision surgery.

* Corresponding Author: Mr WS Khan, Clinical Lecturer, University College London Institute of Orthopaedic and Musculoskeletal Research, Royal National Orthopaedic Hospital, Stanmore, Middlesex, HA7 4LP, UK; Telephone number: +44 (0) 77791 025554; Fax number: +44 (0) 1707 655059; E-mail address: wasimkhan@doctors.org.uk.

Tissue engineering is an exciting strategy being explored to deal with damaged or lost tissue. It is the science of generating tissue using molecular and cellular techniques, combined with material engineering principles, to replace tissue. This could be in the form of cells with or without matrices. Unfortunately significant hurdles remain to be overcome in many areas before tissue engineering becomes more routinely used in clinical practice.

Cells used in tissue engineering could be autologous, allogeneic or xenogeneic. Autologous cells are derived from the same individual and avoid the issues of immunogenicity, rejection and disease transmission. Allogeneic cells are derived from another individual of the same species, and xenogeneic cells are derived from a different species. The use of allogeneic and xenogeneic cells raises concerns regarding immunogenicity, rejection, disease transmission and importantly ethical disquiet.

The cells for tissue engineering could be stem cells or cells further down the differentiation pathway. The use of embryonic stem cells is associated with religious, political and social concerns, but the use of adult stem cells is generally well accepted. Stem cells have been identified in a number of adult tissues, albeit in small numbers. In addition to bone marrow, mesenchymal stem cells (MSCs) have been identified in a number of tissues including adipose tissue and fat pad (Zuk et al., 2001, Wickham et al. 2003). Although most of the literature on MSCs concerns bone marrow derived cells, these cells show age related decline in cell proliferation and differentiation. We have shown that fat pad derived MSCs maintain their proliferation and osteogenic differentiation in later life (Khan et al., in press) and may present an interesting therapeutic option in an ageing population. The MSCs are generally isolated from the tissue and expanded in culture. These cells are characterised or defined using a set of cell surface markers; MSCs are generally positive for CD44, CD90 and CD105, and are negative for haematopoetic markers CD34 and CD45, and the neurogenic marker CD56. Figure 1 shows staining of MSCs *in vitro* using CD105. These cells can be differentiated down a particular differentiation pathway e.g. osteoblast or chondrocyte, using predefined culture conditions before being used for clinical applications.

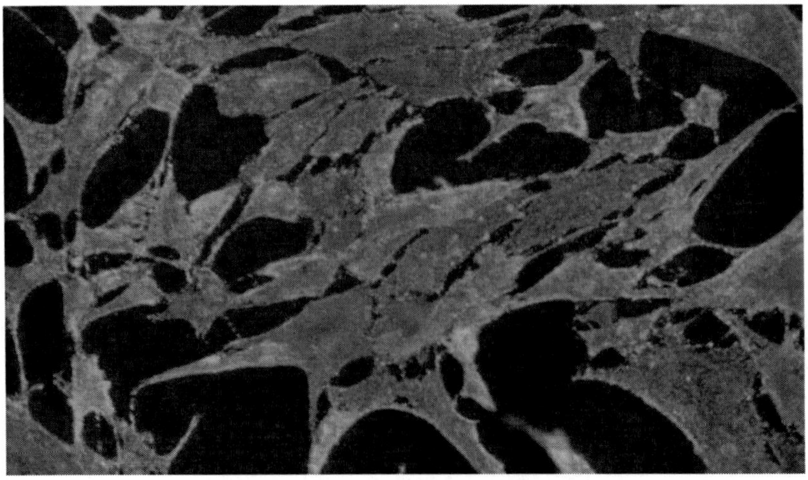

Figure 1. Cell surface epitope characterisation of mesenchymal stem cells using cell surface staining with a primary antibody that recognises CD105 and a fluorescent secondary antibody that shows up green. The nuclei are counterstained with a blue dye. The figure shows strong staining for CD105, a mesenchymal stem cell marker.

Cells are often used with scaffolds that provide a three-dimensional structural template. Scaffolds are natural (e.g. collagen and alginate) or synthetic (e.g. polyglycolic acid and polyacrylonitrile polyvinyl chloride) materials used for cell attachment and proliferation. The ideal scaffold is biocompatible and meets the biological needs of growing tissue. Tissue engineering approaches are being developed in almost all surgical fields and below are some examples of developments.

1. BONE TISSUE

Bone defects occur due to trauma, surgery or disease. Non-union is a significant problem complicating 5–10% of fractures (Axelrad et al. 2007). The approaches to deal with bone defects need to address three fundamental features for bone repair: osteoconduction, osteoinduction and osteogenesis. The management of bone defects is challenging, and the current 'gold standard' autologous cancellous bone grafting is limited by tissue availability and donor site morbidity. Allogenic bone grafting has the potential for disease transmission. The use of growth factors including BMPs has shown promising results (Geesink et al., 1999, Friedlaender et al. 2001) but their role is limited in the absence of an osteoconductive and osteogenic component.

A possible alternative is to use MSCs (Khan & Marsh 2010). Some clinical sites are deficient in MSCs and benefit from the additional application of bone marrow derived MSCs to the non-union site to reactivate fracture healing. The therapeutic options for using MSCs include the use of bone marrow, the use of selected but unexpanded bone marrow derived MSCs, or the use of expanded bone marrow derived MSCs.

The use of bone marrow in the clinical setting has been described with good results for the treatment of tibial non-union (Healey et al., 1990, Goel et al. 2005), but the results may not be directly attributed to bone marrow derived MSCs. The use of selected unexpanded bone marrow derived MSCs relies on the use of cell surface markers. The number of bone marrow derived MSCs in the bone marrow however is low and only 0.001-0.01% of the mononuclear cells in the bone marrow is a MSC (Muschler et al. 2001). So the supply of unexpanded cells is very limited.

The use of expanded cells allows the selection of bone marrow derived MSCs and the expansion of these cells to a number suitable for clinical applications. In an animal model, coral scaffold and expanded bone marrow derived MSCs performed better than autologous bone marrow injection or scaffolds alone (Petite et al. 2000). Further work has also showed better results with culture expanded cells (Kruyt et al. 2007). These expanded cells can also be used to augment bone integration into prostheses. Ohgushi et al., (2005) used bone marrow derived MSCs on ceramic ankle arthroplasty implants in three patients with good bone–implant integration and clinical results.

Animal studies have shown the satisfactory treatment of bony defects with bone marrow derived MSCs in an osteoconductive scaffold (Bruder et al., 1998, Kon et al. 2000). There are a number of clinical studies describing the use of MSCs to treat bone loss. The first report was from Vacanti et al., (2001) who reported successful tissue engineering of the distal thumb phalanx following an avulsion injury using periosteum derived MSCs embedded in a coral scaffold. Quarto et al., (2001) reported on the use of expanded bone marrow derived MSCs combined with porous hydroxyapatite (HA) scaffolds in three patients with 4–7 cm segmental defects. All patients had good graft integration and function. Morishita et al., (2006) reported on the use of bone marrow derived MSCs and HA scaffolds to fill three patient's bone cavity after tumour curettage with good results. Hibi et al., (2006) reported on the use of percutaneous bone marrow derived MSCs and platelet-rich plasma percutaneously injected to augment bone formation during distraction osteogenesis in an irradiated mandible.

2. Articular Cartilage

Articular cartilage is a particularly suitable tissue for tissue engineering applications as it is avascular, aneural and alymphatic. Articular cartilage shows a limited capacity for repair following injury. Cartilage injuries that extend down to the subchondral bone show some signs of repair due to the release of bone marrow derived MSCs from the subchondral bone, a principle used in the surgical procedure of microfracture. More recently there has been an interest in cell-based strategies for the repair of articular cartilage including autologous chondrocyte implantation (ACI) (Peterson et al. 2003), but the results are variable (Lee et al. 2000).

MSCs have been shown to differentiate into chondrocytes and represent an alternative cell source for therapeutic repair. Animal studies have successfully reported on the use of bone marrow derived MSCs embedded in a collagen gel to repair chondral defects (Wakitani et al. 1994). In a clinical trial, bone marrow derived MSCs injected into the medial femoral condylar cartilage defects at the time of high tibial osteotomy in twelve patients resulted in clinical improvement compared to the control group where no cells were used (Wakitani et al. 2002). Although the score for clinical improvement was not significantly different, the patients treated with bone marrow derived MSCs did have better arthroscopic and histological grading scores.

The optimal conditions for chondrogenic differentiation in MSCs derived from various sources are still being developed. We have shown that chondrogenesis in fat pad derived MSCs can be optimised by expanding cells in FGF-2 (Khan et al., 2008) and allowing them to differentiate under hypoxic culture conditions (Khan et al. 2007).

3. Tendons and Ligaments

In animal models tenocytes seeded onto polyglycolic acid scaffolds have been successfully used for the repair of 3-4 cm flexor tendons defects (Cao et al. 2002).

Using tenocytes for repair however is practically difficult and MSCs are a more easily accessible and relatively abundant possible alternative cell source. Animal studies involving bone marrow derived MSCs seeded onto 1 cm achilles tendon defects showed good cross-sectional collagen fibre formation (Young et al. 1998). Bone marrow derived MSCs seeded on a collagen carrier in patellar tendon defects showed higher maximum stresses and moduli when compared to natural healing in contralateral defects (Awad et al. 2003).

Clinical regeneration of tendons and ligaments remains a challenging problem, not least due to the need for an appropriate scaffold, and is one of the fields where there are significant collaborations between biologists and engineers.

4. Spinal Cord

Spinal cord injuries have a huge impact on patients and on society. Recovery from spinal cord injuries is difficult even though endogenous stem cells are present. It has been shown that bone marrow derived MSCs can successfully differentiate down the neuronal lineage *in vitro* (Sanchez-Ramos et al. 2000). In animal models of spinal cord injury, bone marrow derived MSC implantation resulted in the formation of neural and myelin-producing cells, axonal regeneration and functional recovery (Akiyama et al. 2002).

In clinical studies intra-lesional injections of bone marrow mononuclear cell fraction in five patients with acute spinal cord injury resulted in improvement in sensory and motor functions (Park et al. 2005). Similar results were also obtained in another study involving 20 patients who underwent intravenous injections, but only if the injections were given in the acute period following injury (Sykova et al. 2006).

There are however no randomised controlled trials and in the studies that have been performed, it is difficult to establish if the improvements in function were due to the injections or to spontaneous regeneration and recovery.

5. Nerve Tissue

The use of autografts results in variable regeneration and is associated with donor site morbidity. Current tissue engineering approaches are looking at nerve guidance conduits. Animal studies have shown Schwann cells expanded in culture to successfully be used with polylactic acid and polylactic-co-glycolic acid scaffolds (Hadlock et al. 1998) demonstrating the feasibility of *in vivo* regeneration through the conduit.

A nerve conduit that successfully delivers inosine, a purine analogue and axonal growth promoting substance, yielded neural regeneration with histological features suggesting superior motor function (Hadlock et al. 1999).

6. Small Intestine

Short bowel syndrome following small bowel resection procedures results in significant morbidity and mortality. Total parenteral nutrition has improved survival but prolonged intravenous hyperalimentation is associated with significant complications. Small intestine transplantation is still in its infancy and is associated with complications of immunosuppression. Tissue engineering approaches have included intestinal progenitor crypt cells seeded on sheets of polyglycolic acid wrapped around a silastic stent in animal models (Organ et al. 1993).

function at four months follow-up (Janssens et al. 2006). Longer-term follow-ups and studies are awaited.

9. Liver Tissue

The only realistic expectation of a cure in acute liver failure lies with transplantation. The availability of donor livers is limited compared with requirements. As there is no reliable liver support device available, one tissue engineering approach is to create an extracorporeal liver support system that consists of a system of isolated hepatocytes, often porcine and with a short functional life-span, in a synthetic suspension through which plasma is driven (Stockmann & Ijzermanns 2002). This approach is limited by donor availability and is also associated with significant costs and the risk of zoonoses transmission.

Another approach is the *in vivo* transplantation of hepatocytes. In a clinical case, the intraportal injection of allogeneic human hepatocytes under immunosuppression therapy cover allowed the regeneration of the native liver and recovery from hepatic failure (Fisher et al. 2000).

10. Breast Tissue

There is an increasing trend towards breast sparing and reconstruction surgery for malignancy. These are associated with donor site morbidity such as abdominal wall weakness and herniation after transabdominal myocutaneous flaps, or shoulder weakness and scarring after latissimus dorsi myocutaneous flaps.

Work is being done on trying to optimise the differentiation of MSCs into adipocytes and has improved our understanding of differentiation pathways. Insulin and Insulin-like growth factor-1 are being delivered using synthetic microspheres in animal models to enhance adipogenic differentiation and are producing good short-term results (Shenaq & Yuksel 2002), but longer-term studies are needed.

11. Urinary Bladder

The urinary bladder serves an important function and is difficult to replace. Surgical management options include the creation of a reservoir using the bowel but this involves injury and complications to the gastrointestinal tract and systemic metabolic abnormalities (McDougal 1992, Gilbert et al. 2005). More recently Atala et al., (2006) have reported of the use of autologous urothelial and smooth muscle cells seeded onto collagen and polyglycolic acid composite matrices and used for augmentation cystoplasty in clinical trials in seven patients. They noted improved bladder function with no reported complications over a mean follow-up of four years.

In the future, tissue engineering strategies will probably look at the use of MSCs rather than using urothelial cells; urothelial cells may be limited in availability or unsuitable for use due to the nature of the pathology. There have been reports of using MSCs for bladder tissue

Healey JH, Zimmerman PA, McDonnell JM et al., 1990 Percutaneous bone marrow grafting of delayed union and non-union in cancer patients *Clinical Orthopaedics* 256 280–285.

Hibi H, Yamada Y, Kagami H et al., 2006 Distraction osteogenesis assisted by tissue engineering in an irradiated mandible: a case report *International Journal of Oral and Maxillofacial Implants* 21 141–147.

Hori Y, Nakamura T, Matsumoto K, Kurakowa Y, Satomi S, Shimizu Y 2001 Tissue engineering of the small intestine by acellular collagen sponge scaffolding *International Journal of Artificial Organs* 24 50-54.

Janssens S, Dubois C, Bogaert J et al., 2006 Autologous bone marrow-derived stem-cell transfer in patients with ST-segment elevation myocardial infarction: double-blind, randomised controlled trial *Lancet* 367 113–121.

Kamihata H, Matsubara H, Nishiue T et al., 2001 Implantation of bone marrow mononuclear cells into ischaemic myocardium enhances collateral perfusion and regional function via side supply of angioblasts, angiogenic ligands, and cytokines *Circulation* 104 1046–1052.

Kanematsu A, Yamamoto S, Iwai-Kanai E et al., 2005 Induction of smooth muscle cell-like phenotype in marrow-derived cells among regenerating urinary bladder smooth muscle cells *American Journal of Pathology* 166 565–573.

Khan WS, Adesida AB, Hardingham TE 2007 Hypoxic conditions increase hypoxia-inducible transcription factor 2alpha and enhance chondrogenesis in stem cells from the infrapatellar fat pad of osteoarthritis patients *Arthritis Research and Therapy* 9 R55.

Khan WS, Tew SR, Adesida AB, Hardingham TE 2008 Human infrapatellar fat pad-derived stem cells express the pericyte marker 3G5 and show enhanced chondrogenesis after expansion in fibroblast growth factor-2 *Arthritis Research and Therapy* 10 R74.

Khan WS, Malik AA, Hardingham TE (2009). Stem Cell Applications and Tissue Engineering Approaches in Surgical Practice. J Perioper Pract. 19(4): 130-5.

Khan WS, Adesida AB, Tew SR, Hardingham TE The epitope characterisation and osteogenic differentiation potential of fat pad derived stem cells is maintained with ageing in later life *Injury* (in press).

Kon E, Muraglia A, Corsi A et al., 2000 Autologous bone marrow stromal cells loaded onto porous hydroxyapatite ceramic accelerate bone repair in critical-size defects of sheep long bones *Journal of Biomedical Materials Research* 49 328–337.

Kruyt MC, Dhert WJ, Oner FC et al., 2007 Analysis of ectopic and orthotopic bone formation in cell-based tissue-engineered constructs in goats *Biomaterials* 28 1798–1805.

Lee CR, Grodzinsky AJ, Hsu HP, Martin SD, Spector M 2000 Effects of harvest and selected cartilage repair procedures on the physical and biochemical properties of articular cartilage in the canine knee *Journal of Orthopaedic Research* 18 790-799.

Leri A, Kajstura J, Anversa P, Frishman WH 2008 Myocardial regeneration and Stem cell repair *Current Problems in Cardiology* 33 91-153.

Makino S, Fukuda K, Miyoshi S et al., 1999 Cardiomyocytes can be generated from marrow stromal cells in vitro *Journal of Clinical Investigation* 103 697–705.

Mazzucotelli JP, Moczar M, Zede L, Bambang LS, Loisance D 1994 Human vascular endothelial cells on expanded PTFE pre-coated with an engineered protein adhesion factor *International Journal of Artificial Organs* 17 112-117.

McDougal WS 1992 Metabolic complications of urinary intestinal diversion *Journal of Urology* 147 1199–1208.

McKenzie IA, Biernaskie J, Toma JG et al., 2006 Skin-derived precursors generate myelinating Schwann cells for the injured and dysmyelinated nervous system *Journal of Neuroscience* 26 6651–6660.

Messina E, De Angelis L, Frati G et al., 2004 Isolation and expansion of adult cardiac stem cells from human and murine heart *Circulation Research* 95 911–921.

Morishita T, Honoki K, Ohgushi H et al., 2006 Tissue engineering approach to the treatment of bone tumors: three cases of cultured bone grafts derived from patients' mesenchymal stem cells *Artificial Organs* 30 115–118.

Muschler GF, Nitto H, Boehm CA, Easley KA 2001 Age and gender related changes in the cellularity of human bone marrow and the prevelance of osteoblastic progenitors *Journal of Orthopaedic Research* 19 117-125.

Niklason LE, Gao J, Abbott WM et al., 1999 Functional arteries grown *in vitro Science* 284 489-493.

Ohgushi H, Kotobuki N, Funaoka H et al., 2005 Tissue engineered ceramic artificial joint– *ex vivo* osteogenic differentiation of patient mesenchymal cells on total ankle joints for treatment of osteoarthritis *Biomaterials* 26 4654–4661.

Organ GM, Mooney DJ, Hansen LK, Schloo B, Vacanti JP 1993 Enterocyte transplantation using cell-polymer devices to create intestinal epithelial-lined tubes *Transplant Procedures* 25 998-1001.

OrlicD, Kajstura J, Chimenti S et al., 2001 Bone marrow cells regenerate infarcted myocardium *Nature* 410 701–705.

Park HC, Shim YS, Ha Y et al., 2005 Treatment of complete spinal cord injury patients by autologous bone marrow cell transplantation and administration of granulocyte-macrophage colony stimulating factor *Tissue Engineering* 11 913–922.

Peterson L, Minas T, Brittberg M et al., 2003 Treatment of osteochondritis dissecans of the knee with autologous chondrocyte transplantation: results at 2–10 years *Journal of Bone and Joint Surgery* 85-A 17–24.

Petite H, Viateau V, Bensaid W et al., 2000 Tissue-engineered bone regeneration *Nature Biotechnology* 18 959–963.

Quarto R, Mastrogiacomo M, Cancedda R et al., 2001 Repair of large bone defects with the use of autologous bonemarrowstromal cells *New England Journal of Medicine* 344 385–386.

Roeder R, Wolfe J, Lianakis N, Hinson T, Geddes LA, Obermiller J 1999 Compliance, elastic modulus and burst pressure of small intestine submucosa (SIS), small diameter vascular grafts *Journal of Biomedical Materials Research* 47 65-70.

Sanchez-Ramos J, Song S, Cardozo-Pelaez F et al., 2000 Adult bone marrow stromal cells differentiate into neural cells *in vitro Experimental Neurology* 164 247–256.

Shenaq SM, Yuksel E 2002 New research in breast reconstruction *Clinics in Plastic Surgery* 29 111-125.

Stockmann HBAC, Ijzermanns JNM 2002 Prospects for the temporary treatment of acute liver failure *European Journal of Gastroenterology and Hepatology* 14 195-203.

Sykov´a E, Homola A, Mazanec R et al., 2006 Autologous bone marrow transplantation in patients with subacute and chronic spinal cord injury *Cell Transplant* 15 675–687.

Vacanti CA 2006 History of tissue engineering and a glimpse into its future *Tissue Engineering* 12 1137–1142.

Wakitani S, Goto T, Pineda SJ et al., 1994 Mesenchymal cell-based repair of large, full-thickness defects of articular cartilage *Journal of Bone and Joint Surgery* 76-A 579–592.

Wakitani S, Imoto K, Yamamoto T et al., 2002 Human autologous culture expanded bone marrow mesenchymal cell transplantation for repair of cartilage defects in osteoarthritic knees *Osteoarthritis and Cartilage* 10 199–206.

Wickham MQ, Erickson GR, Gimble JM, Vail TP, Guilak F 2003 Multipotent stromal cells derived from the infrapatellar fat pad of the knee *Clinical Orthopaedics* 412 196-212.

Wollert KC, Meyer GP, Lotz J et al., 2004 Intracoronary autologous bone-marrow cell transfer after myocardial infarction: the BOOST randomised controlled clinical trial *Lancet* 364 141–148.

Young RG, Butler DL, Weber W et al., 1998 Use of mesenchymal stem cells in a collagen matrix for Achilles tendon repair *Journal of Orthopaedic Research* 16 406–413.

Zuk PA, Zhu M, Mizino H et al., 2001 Multilineage cells from human adipose tissue: implications for cell-based therapies *Tissue Engineering* 7 211-228.

INDEX

A

B

C

D

E

F

G

H

I

N

O

P

Q

R

S

T